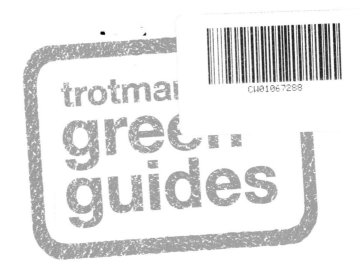

Healthcare Courses 2008

e definitive guide to degree courses for 2008 entry

Trotman's Green Guides: Healthcare Courses 2008

This third edition published in 2007 by Trotman Education
an imprint of Crimson Publishing
Westminster House, Kew Road, Richmond, Surrey TW9 2ND
www.crimsonpublishing.co.uk

Previously published by Trotman and Company Ltd in 2005, 2006

Author of front matter and introductory sections Beryl Dixon
Advertising Kerry Lyon, Senior Sales Executive (to contact the ad team, call 020 8334 1781)

Cover design by Pink Frog
Additional page design by James Rudge

Course information
Course information is supplied by TIS from its database of further and higher education courses. The TIS database holds details of over 120,000 courses at more than 1000 colleges and universities. The courses contained in this book are provided to TIS by higher education institutions in the UK and are recognised and accredited as award bearing qualifications. If you would like to update course information appearing in *Trotman's Green Guides*, please contact TIS on 01242 542680 or email data.collection@trotmanis.co.uk

The information in this book was correct to the best of the publisher's belief at the time of going to press. However, readers are advised to check details of courses they are interested in directly with the institution as course availability and entry requirements are subject to change.

British Library Cataloguing in Publication Data
A catalogue record for this book is available from the British Library

ISBN 978 1 90604 123 6

Typeset by RefineCatch Limited, Bungay, Suffolk
Printed and bound in Great Britain by Cambridge University Press, Cambridge

Contents

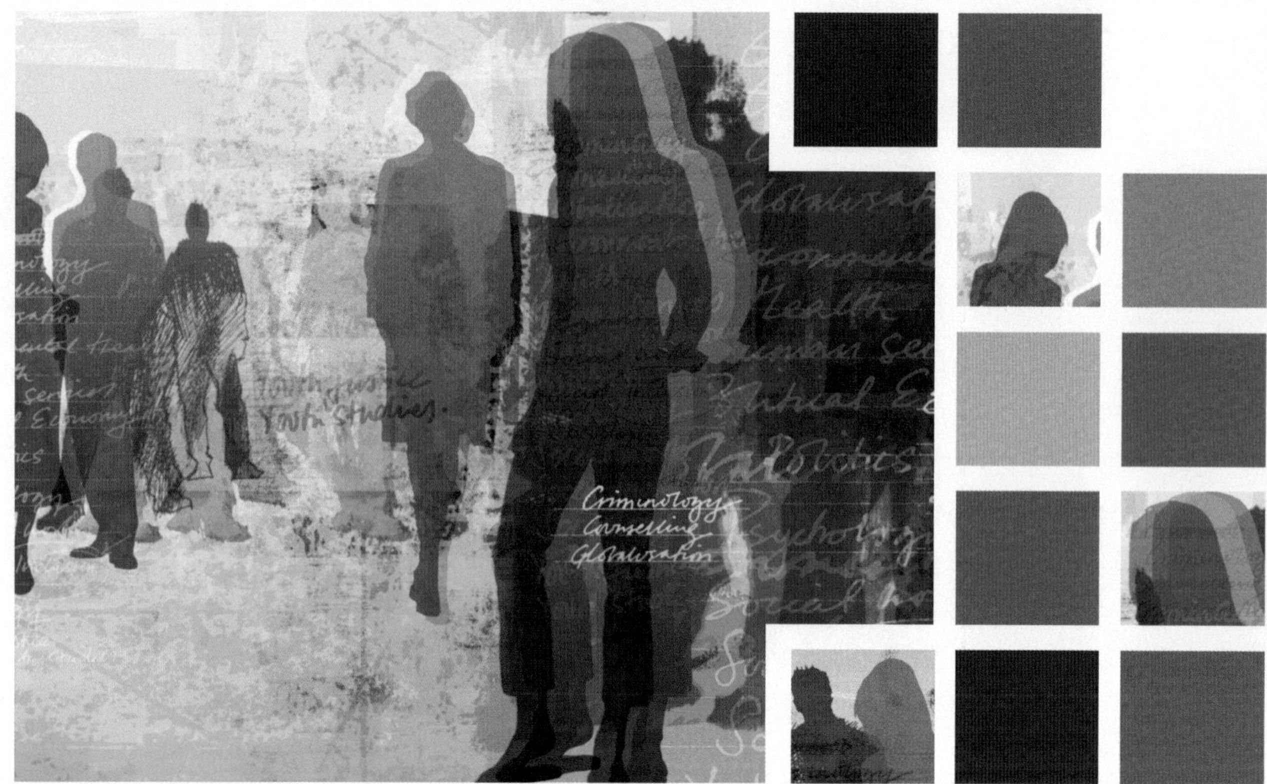

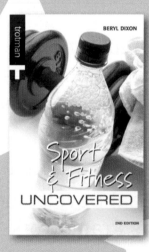

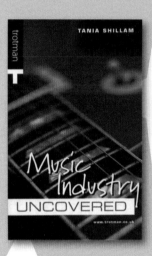

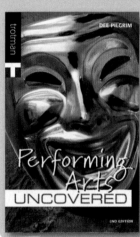

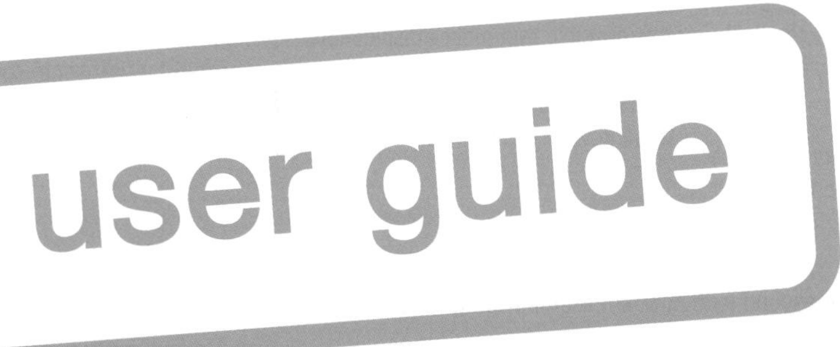

ɘlcome to **Trotman's Green Guides** series. This section will outline how ɘ guide is organised, so that you can find your way quickly to the ɔrmation you need.

otman's Green Guides are divided into three main sections:

- **Introduction** – provides a broad overview of healthcare, including the different courses available, advice and information on getting a place and a look at the employment prospects for healthcare graduates.
- **Course Listings** – green pages containing comprehensive listings of healthcare courses offered by universities and colleges throughout the UK, divided into 14 chapters, each of which has its own detailed introduction, followed by a list of courses in that subject area. For more information on the course listings, see the section below.
- **Institution Address Listings** – contact details of all the institutions featured in this guide.

ow to use the Course Listings section

ɜ course listings are divided into 14 chapters, each covering a different ject area:

atomy and Physiology
medical Sciences
mplementary Medicine
ntistry
tetics and Nutrition
alth Studies
dical Technology
dicine
rsing and Midwifery
ometry and Audiology
rmacology and Pharmacy
chology
rapies
erinary Science

h chapter has its own detailed introduction, which includes information on subject area as well as a case study of someone who is either studying subject now or who has their degree and is working in the industry.

nin each chapter, courses are arranged alphabetically by their title. ler each course title you will find an alphabetical list of institutions ring that course. The sample course entry explains how to read the a contained within each institution entry.

mple course entry

Physiotherapy

rse title. Any qualifying or additional information about the course ws in brackets – for example information about whether a nursing rse is for registered nurses or for pre-registration applicants.

Bristol, University of the West of England B80

Institution name, followed by its UCAS code. You will need the institution's UCAS code when you make your application. Square brackets around institution names signify the awarding body. Franchised courses (provided at one institution but applied for through another) are marked with the symbol ▲.

BSc (Hons): 3 years full-time – B160

Type of qualification, followed by duration and mode of study, followed by UCAS course code. For this course, the qualification offered is a Bachelor of Science degree, lasting three years. For a list of abbreviations used in this section, see page xiv. You will need the UCAS course code when you make your application. Courses offered on a specific campus or by a validated college can be distinguished by their UCAS course code: in addition to the standard four-digit format (eg A123), the code also contains an extra letter at the end (eg A123 B). For more information on this, see the **Before you apply** section on page xx.

Tariff: 280-340 IB: 32-34

List of entry requirements for this course. This list can include:

- **Tariff:** UCAS tariff points requirement. For more information on the UCAS tariff and how it corresponds with different qualifications and grades, see page xii.
- **A2:** GCE A level grade requirement. Lower case letters indicate AS level grades
- **BTEC:** BTEC grade requirement. Note that BTEC grades are expressed as Pass (P), Merit (M) or Distinction (D).
- **SQA:** Scottish Highers grade requirement. Where only two grades appear these refer to Advanced Highers rather than Highers.
- **ILC:** Irish Leaving Certificate grade or points requirement. For example, B2-B2 indicates two B2 grades. For more information on how ILC grades convert into ILC points, see page xiii.
- **IB:** IB points requirement. Where institutions have specified points, they have always been included separately.
- **FD/HND:** Indicates that a Foundation degree or Higher National Diploma is necessary to access the course. (Usually this only applies to top-up courses.)
- **HE credits:** Crdits awarded for HE level courses (eg Fd, HND etc)
- **RN/RM/HP:** Indicates that applicants must already have Registered Nurse (RN), Registered Midwife (RM) or Health Professional (HP) status.
- **UKCAT/MSAT/GAMSAT:** Indicates that applicants must take the UK Clinical Admissions Test (UKCAT), the Medical Schools Admissions Test (MSAT) or the Graduate Medical Schools Admissions Test (GAMSAT).

The entry requirements may also indicate that candidates are likely to be required to attend interview.

For the course shown here, a tariff points range is given, rather than qualifications being listed out individually. Students taking qualifications that form part of the UCAS tariff, such as A levels, Scottish Highers, BTEC National

Diplomas or Irish Leaving Certificates, must gain between 280 and 340 UCAS tariff points; IB students must gain 32–34 points. Where a range of points or grades is shown, you should investigate whether other factors will be taken into consideration. For example, nursing or physiotherapy courses may prefer applicants who have some relevant work experience.

Entry requirements included have been simplified, so tariff points or grades for the main qualifications are given, but no information has been included as to specific subjects required or minimum grades for those subjects. Yo are advised to check that your qualifications are suitable before you apply It is possible that other qualifications not mentioned in this guide, for example Access to HE courses, are also accepted for entry onto some courses; again you are advised to check with the relevant institution befo making your application.

UCAS tariff

You can use this table to calculate how the UCAS tariff totals correspond with different examination grades.

GCE/VCE Qualifications				BTEC Nationals[1]			OCR Nationals[2]			Points	Irish Leaving Cert		Scottish Qualifications				Advanced Placement Programme[3]	
GCE AS/ AS VCE	GCE AS Double Award	GCE A level/ AVCE	GCE/ AVCE Double Award	Award	Certificate	Diploma	Certificate	Diploma	Extended Diploma		Higher	Ordinary	Advanced Higher	Higher	Int 2	Standard Grade	Group A	Group B
						DDD			D1	360								
						DDM			D2/M1	320								
						DMM			M2	280								
			AA		DD	MMM		D	M3	240								
			AB							220								
			BB		DM	MMP		M1	P1	200								
			BC							180								
			CC		MM	MPP		M2/P1	P2	160								
			CD							140								
	AA	A	DD	D	MP	PPP	D	P2	P3	120			A				5	
	AB									110								
	BB	B	DE							100			B					
	BC									90	A1						4	
	CC	C	EE	M	PP		M	P3		80			C					
										77	A2							
										72			D	A				
										71	B1							
	CD									70								
										64	B2							
A	DD	D								60				B			3	
										58	B3							
										52	C1							
B	DE									50								5
										48				C				
										45	C2							
										42				D	A			
C	EE	E		P			P			40								
										39	C3	A1						
										38						Band 1		
										35					B			4
										33	D1							
D										30								
										28					C	Band 2		
										26	D2	A2						
E										20	D3	B1						3
										14		B2						
										7		B3						

[1] The points shown are for the newly specified BTEC National Award, Certificate and Diploma introduced into centres from September 2002
[2] Further information on OCR grades and Tariff points can be found on the UCAS website
[3] The points shown for the Advanced Placement Programme come into effect for entry to higher education in 2008 onwards. Details of the subjects covered by each group can be found on the UCAS website

BTEC Nationals in Early Years			CACHE Diploma in Child Care & Education		Points	Diploma in Foundation Studies (Art and Design)	Diploma in Fashion Retail[4]	iPRO[5]		AAT NVQ Level 3 in Accounting[6]
Theory		Practical	Theory	Practical				Certificate	Diploma	
Certificate	Diploma									
	DDD				320					
					285	D				
	DDM				280					
	DMM		AA		240					
					225	M				
	MMM				220					
DD			BB		200					
					165	P				
DM	MMP		CC		160		D			P
MM	MPP	D	DD	A	120		M			
				B	100				Pass	
MP	PPP	M	EE	C	80		P	Pass		
				D	60					
PP		P		E	40					

[4] The points for ABC's Diploma in Fashion Retail come into effect for entry to higher education in 2008 onwards
[5] The points for OCR's iPRO Certificate and Diploma come into effect for entry to higher education in 2008 onwards
[6] Points for the AAT Level 3 NVQ in Accounting come into effect for entry to higher education in 2009 onwards

British Horse Society[7]			Points	Music Examinations[8]						Speech & Drama Examinations[9]			
Stage 3 Horse Knowledge & Care	Stage 3 Riding	Preliminary Teacher's Certificate		Practical			Theory			Grade 6	Grade 7	Grade 8	PCertLAM[10]
				Grade 6	Grade 7	Grade 8	Grade 6	Grade 7	Grade 8				
			90										D
			80										M
			75			D							
			70			M							
			65									D	
			60		D							M	P
			55		M	P					D		
			50								M		
			45	D								P	
			40	M	P					D			
Pass	Pass	Pass	35							M	P		
			30						D				
			25	P					M				
			20					D	P	P			
			15				D	M					
			10				M	P					
			5				P						

[7] The points for the British Horse Society (BHS) Awards come into effect for entry to higher education in 2008 onwards
[8] Points shown are for ABRSM, Guildhall, LCMM, Rockschool and Trinity College London advanced level music examinations
[9] Points shown are for LAMDA, LCMM and Trinity Guildhall advanced level speech and drama examinations accredited by the National Qualifications Framework and come into effect for entry to higher education in 2008 onwards. A full list of the subjects covered can be found on the UCAS website.
[10] Points for the LAMDA Level 3 Certificate in Speech and Drama: Performance Studies (PCertLAM) come into effect for entry to higher education in 2009 onwards

International Baccalaureate[11]	Points
Diploma	
45	768
44	744
43	722
42	698
41	675
40	652
39	628
38	605
37	582
36	559
35	535
34	512
33	489
32	466
31	442
30	419
29	396
28	373
27	350
26	326
25	303
24	280

The points for the International Baccalaureate (IB) come into effect for entry to higher education in **2008** onwards and are awarded to candidates who achieve the IB Diploma

Free standing Maths[12]	IFS		COPE[15]	Advanced Extension Awards[16]	Points	Core Skills	Key Skills	Welsh Baccalaureate Core[17]
	CeFS[13]	DipFS[14]						
					120			Pass
			Pass		70			
	A	A			60			
	B	B			50			
	C	C		D	40			
	D	D			30		Level 4	
A	E	E		M	20	Higher	Level 3	
B					17			
C					13			
D					10	Int 2	Level 2	
E					7			

Covers free-standing Mathematics qualifications – Additional Maths, Using and Applying Statistics, Working with Algebraic and Graphical Techniques, Modelling with Calculus
Points shown are for the revised Institute of Financial Services Certificate in Financial Studies (CeFS) taught from September 2003
Points shown are for the Institute of Financial Services Diploma in Financial Studies (DipFS) and come into effect for entry to higher education in **2008**
Points are awarded for the Certificate of Personal Effectiveness (COPE) awarded by ASDAN and CCEA
Points for Advanced Extension Awards are over and above those gained from the A level grade
Points for the Core are awarded only when a candidate achieves the Welsh Baccalaureate Advanced Diploma

:e that in September 2005, VCEs in art and design, business, ICT, ence, engineering, health and social care, leisure and recreation, media mmunication and production), performing arts and travel and tourism re replaced by GCE A levels in applied art and design, applied business, lied ICT, applied science, engineering, health and social care, leisure dies, media: communication and production, performing arts and travel tourism. For more information see www.qca.org.uk.

our qualification is not listed in the table you can check on institutions' osites or in their prospectuses. If you need further help don't hesitate to tact the admissions department at an individual institution. (You can find addresses of the universities and colleges whose courses appear in this de in the **Institution Address Listings** section near the back of the book.)

sh Leaving Certificate points

Irish Leaving Certificate (ILC) is included in the UCAS tariff table shown the previous page. However, points can also be calculated for ILC results g an alternative method administered by the Central Applications Office O) in the Republic of Ireland. This calculation method is shown in the e below, and is unconnected with the UCAS tariff.

eaving Cert Grade	Higher Paper	Lower Paper
A1	100	60
A2	90	50
B1	85	45
B2	80	40
B3	75	35
C1	70	30
C2	65	25
C3	60	20
D1	55	15
D2	50	10
D3	45	5

Notes

- The six best results, in recognised subjects, in one Leaving Certificate Examination will be counted for points computation.
- One sitting only of the Leaving Certificate Examination will be counted for points purposes.
- In the case of certain subjects, eg home economics (general), Alternative Ordinary Level mathematics, Foundation Level mathematics or Foundation Level Irish, some higher education institutions may not award the points indicated on the points grid. If in any doubt, check with the Admissions Office of the appropriate institution.
- Some institutions also award bonus points for certain subjects. Check with the Admissions Office of the appropriate institution to find out.
- LCVP (Leaving Certificate Vocational Programme) points awarded: Distinction – 70, Merit – 50, Pass – 30
- For further information, see www.cao.ie

Qualification abbreviations

Access	Access to Higher Education (HE) Certificate (A qualification you can take as a mature student ie 21 or over in England, Northern Ireland and Wales; 20 or over in Scotland.)
BA	Bachelor of Arts
BCh	Bachelor of Surgery
BChD	Bachelor of Dental Surgery
BDS	Bachelor of Dental Surgery
BEng	Bachelor of Engineering
BHSc	Bachelor of Health Science
BM	Bachelor of Medicine
BM	Bachelor of Midwifery
BM BS	Bacheio of Midaiferg
BMedSc	Bachelor of Medical Science
BMedSci	Bachelor of Medical Science
BMid	Bachelor of Midwifery
BN	Bachelor of Nursing
BNurs	Bachelor of Nursing
BOptom	Bachelor of Optometry
BOst	Bachelor of Osteopathy
BOstMed	Bachelor of Osteopathic Medicine
BSc	Bachelor of Science
BTEC	BTEC National Certificate or Diploma
BTechnol	Bachelor of Technology
BVetMed	Bachelor of Veterinary Medicine
BVMS/BVM&S	Bachelor of Veterinary Medicine and Surgery
BVSc	Bachelor of Veterinary Science
DipHE	Diploma of Higher Education
DipSW	Diploma in Social Work
EFL	English as a Foreign Language
EN	Enrolled Nurse
Fd	Foundation Degree
FdA	Foundation Degree in Arts
FdEng	Foundation Degree in Engineering
FdSc	Foundation Degree in Science
GCE	General Certificate of Education Advanced Level
HND	Higher National Diploma
Hons	Honours
HP	Health Practitioner
IB	International Baccalaureate
MA	Master of Arts
MB	Bachelor of Medicine
MB BCh	Bachelor of Medicine/Bachelor of Surgery
MB BCh BAO	Bachelor of Medicine/Bachelor of Surgery/Bachelor of Obstetrics
MB BChir	Bachelor of Medicine/Bachelor of Surgery
MB BS	Bachelor of Medicine/Bachelor of Surgery
MB ChB	Bachelor of Medicine/Bachelor of Surgery
MBioSci	Master of Biological Science
MChem	Master of Chemistry
MChiro	Master of Chiropractic
MEng	Master of Engineering
MN	Master of Nursing
MNutr	Master of Nutrition
MPharm	Master of Pharmacy
MPharmSci	Master of Pharmaceutical Science
MSci	Master of Science
RM	Registered Midwife
RN	Registered Nurse
SQA	Scottish Qualifications Authority Highers
SWAP	Scottish Wider Access Programme
VetMB	Bachelor of Veterinary Medicine

; HPC

essional body/bodies approving the course. For a list of abbreviations in this section, see below.

ofessional body abbreviations

BDO	Association of British Dispensing Opticians	**IET**	Institution of Engineering and Technology
MLS	Academy of Medical Laboratory Science	**IFST**	Institute of Food Science and Technology
ACU	British Acupuncture Council	**IMC**	Institute of Measurement and Control
AOT	British Association of Occupational Therapists	**IMECHE**	Institution of Mechanical Engineers
APO	British Association of Prosthetists and Orthotists	**IOB**	Institute of Biology
ASES	British Association of Sport and Exercise Sciences	**IOM3**	Institute of Materials, Minerals and Mining
C	Bar Council	**IOSH**	Institution of Occupational Safety and Health
CO	British College of Optometrists	**LS**	Law Society
DA	British Dietetic Association	**NCA**	North Central Association of Colleges and Schools
PS	British Psychological Society	**NES**	NHS Education for Scotland
EH	Chartered Institute of Environmental Health	**NIMH**	National Institute of Medical Herbalists
OT	College of Occupational Therapists	**NMC**	Nursing and Midwifery Council
SP	Chartered Society of Physiotherapy	**PSNI**	Pharmaceutical Society of Northern Ireland
C	Engineering Council	**QAA**	Quality Assurance Agency
CCE	European Council on Chiropractic Education	**RCSLT**	Royal College of Speech and Language Therapists
S	Ergonomics Society	**RCVS**	Royal College of Veterinary Surgeons
DC	General Dental Council	**REHIS**	Royal Environmental Health Institute of Scotland
MC	General Medical Council	**RPSGB**	Royal Pharmaceutical Society of Great Britain
OC	General Optical Council	**RSC**	Royal Society of Chemistry
OSC	General Osteopathic Council	**SCP**	Society of Chiropodists and Podiatrists
PC	Health Professions Council	**SOR**	Society of Radiographers
PW	Health Professions Wales	**WFOT**	World Federation of Occupational Therapists
MS	Institute of Biomedical Science		

es

hroughout this Guide, the word 'institution' is used to mean 'university r college'.

he information in this book was correct to the best of the publisher's elief at the time of going to press. However, readers are advised to check details of courses they are interested in directly with the institution as course availability and entry requirements are subject to change. For further information on how the course data in this book is compiled, see page ii.

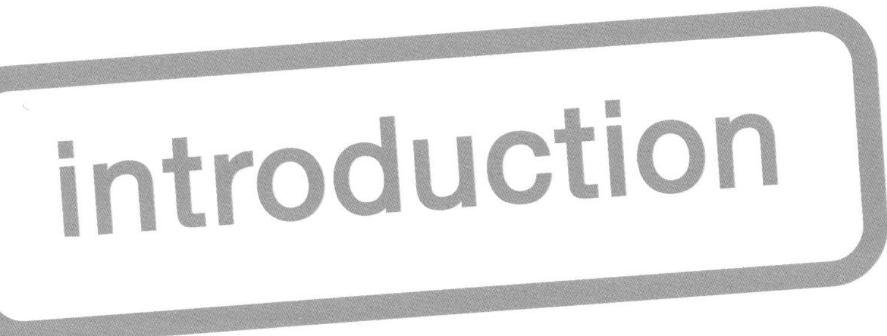

e world of healthcare revolves around highly professional and well-alified teams of doctors, nurses, therapists, lab-based staff and other erts providing diagnosis, treatment and aftercare to assist patients vards recovery. The theme of team work appears time and again.

re has never been a more interesting time to think about a career in lthcare. Change is in the air and things we take for granted now may l be different by the time you start your career. From a careers point of w, we are beginning to see significant change to the roles that each fession is playing in the healthcare process:

- More and more patients are being **treated in their own homes** wherever possible rather than being admitted to hospital. And more checkups, routine tests and minor procedures are carried out in doctors' surgeries.
- n **nursing**, while diagnosis and establishing a strategy for treating the more seriously ill patients is obviously still the preserve of the doctor, top grade nurses are now being trained to relieve some of the pressure by taking an increasingly prominent role.
- There is a new job of **nurse consultant**. Nurses now carry out many tasks previously done by doctors. For example intravenous chemotherapy was invariably administered by doctors, but is now routinely administered by specially trained nurses.
- **Ambulance paramedics** are being trained to higher levels so that they can deliver increasingly sophisticated urgent treatment before the patient even arrives in hospital.
- **Complementary medical professions** such as osteopathy and chiropractic, once considered to be on the fringes of medical provision, are now becoming increasingly accepted as mainstream medicine.

purpose of this book is to provide you with a broad introduction to the iness of gaining qualifications leading to careers within healthcare. The k also provides information on entry to Veterinary Science courses.

range of courses on offer is vast – whether you have already decided m for a specific career or whether you are simply interested in the ects for their own sake. What is more, while some courses (such as licine and Veterinary Science) demand the highest entry grades, others less demanding.

e readers might already have an idea about what some of the courses lve – particularly those studying for an A level in health and social care hose who have already built up a lot of relevant work experience. But e subjects, like radiography or pharmacology, might be completely to you. This guide will cater for readers coming from different starting ts, including those with 'non-relevant' A levels who might want to take a conversion course or a course with a foundation year. (For more information on how to navigate to the information you need, see the **User Guide** section on page xi.)

This introductory section will guide you through course/institution selection, application procedures, course structures and future career prospects for graduates in the healthcare sector.

Courses

Foundation years

A foundation-year course is a full-time, one-year course designed specifically for people who don't have the necessary qualifications for entry to a degree course. It gives you the 'foundation' to progress alongside students who come in with their science qualifications the following year. You study up to A level equivalent in the necessary subject or subjects and probably also improve your IT skills. Your exact programme is designed in consultation with a tutor, taking into account the degree course you hope to follow. A foundation year can be offered either as a stand-alone course or as an integral part of a degree course.

Foundation-year courses are offered in a wide range of the subject areas in this book – even in medicine. The standard medical degree is five years for those who apply with top grade science A levels. Some medical schools offer an initial foundation year to help high-grade non-science applicants acquire the science background to progress to the standard five-year course – but this should not be seen as a way in for people who have taken science A levels but not achieved the required grades for the five year course.

DipHE courses

DipHEs are normally two-year, full-time courses that have lower entry requirements than degree courses. They provide extra flexibility in surmounting the entry hurdles for mature students who may not possess the normal minimum requirements. DipHE courses are intended to be of a standard equivalent to the first two years of a degree programme and to provide an acceptable qualification in their own right. They are the standard qualification awarded to nurses who do not choose the degree route for example. They can also lead on to a programme of further study (honours or unclassified degree courses; BEd(Hons) etc).

Foundation degrees

These courses are designed in consultation with employers. They train people in specialist skills for careers in areas like business, engineering,

Take a look at yourself quiz

Answer 'yes' or 'no' to the questions below, then take a look at the Notes on the quiz section to find out why each question matters.

A. Subjects

- Do you like all the science subjects?
- Are you more inclined to biology ?
- Are you more inclined to chemistry?
- Are you more inclined to physics?
- Have you chosen not to study science subjects at all so far? Would you like, if possible, to pick them up later?

B. Your study skills

- Are you able to build on your lessons by using your research skills to find out more in your own time?
- Do you enjoy discovering theory from practical experiments?
- Are you comfortable with the practicals in which animals are dissected?
- Are you confident using IT to further your studies?
- Are you organised enough to be able to hand work in on time, most of the time?

C. Other abilities

- Do you enjoy helping people of all ages who are ill or need support?
- Do you enjoy working as part of a team?
- Can you explain scientific ideas clearly to your friends who don't do science subjects?
- Do you find that your friends are quite happy to discuss problems with you?
- Do you get on with people reasonably well, but find that what really interests you is the intricacies of the science you are studying, rather than the intricacies of people's relationships or problems?

D. Your personal qualities

- Can you keep calm under pressure?
- Can you work irregular hours if you have to?
- Have you had (or could you arrange) work experience or voluntary work in a medical or practical caring situation?
- Is your own health consistent with work in the healthcare field?

Notes on the quiz

A. Subjects

If you like all the science subjects then you are on course for any of the subject areas listed in this guide. Biology (or related subjects like nutrition) and chemistry feature strongly in most of the degree courses appearing in this book. Mathematics, especially in subjects like genetics or psychology, can be significant, as can physics for radiography or medical electronics. Science in general obviously features in all the courses in this book, but if you have not chosen to take science subjects, don't worry – the system offers ways round this:

- Some institutions, while especially welcoming applicants with science subjects, are not unhappy to take those without them – especially for some of the courses listed in the sections on complementary medicine, dietetics and nutrition, health studies and nursing. Normally these courses introduce scientific topics at a level that does not require advanced knowledge.
- Look out for the courses offering a preliminary extra year for non-scientists aimed at getting them up to speed so that they can work at the same pace as their fellow students in subsequent years. This extra year is usually referred to as a foundation year – see page xv for more information.

B. Your study skills

If you answered 'yes' to most of these, you are on the right lines. In between lectures, students often work in small groups doing their own research supervised by tutors. Most courses in the healthcare sector combine theory with practical experimental work in labs. You cannot afford to be squeamish where lab work is concerned. If you are used to computers, the internet and databases, you already have skills that appeal to admissions tutors. You need to be well-organised and able to work on your own to follow up the lectures and prepare work for your tutorials.

C. Other abilities

As far as working with people is concerned, there are two types of course listed in this directory. First there are courses like medicine, dentistry, the therapies and complementary medicine. These lead directly to careers where you will be on the front line working face-to-face with patients, many of whom may be nervous or distressed as a result of the condition that you are treating. They will need to have their treatment and progress explained to them in a calm and reassuring manner. (Many vets will tell you that it is not always the animal which is the problem but the owner!) All these courses need people who can contribute fully to the efforts of the team of experts working with patients. Second, there are courses (for example, many of those listed in sections four and five) that lead more to research work, often behind the scenes in hospital laboratories or in industry. In these jobs, communication skills are important – but are likely to be used more with professional colleagues than directly with patients.

D. Your personal qualities

It goes without saying that patients need to see someone who they feel is in control of their situation. Professionals in healthcare need to remain on top of all the working situations they find themselves dealing with during spells of duty which can be long and taxing. You may not be able to find work experience directly treating patients, but admissions tutors are looking for people who have worked or volunteered as assistants to nurses or carers in hospitals or care homes. With regard to your own health, there are some conditions which could restrict the range of work open to you – for example, some types of allergy or hepatitis B. Check carefully with admissions tutors and be open with them when you are applying if you think you may have a problem of this kind.

– but there are over 100 different courses. All Foundation degrees ؟ a practical slant, and aim to develop your:

- /ork skills, relevant to a particular careers area
- ey skills, for example communication and problem solving
- ieneral skills, such as reasoning and professionalism.

could study full-time, or by part-time or distance learning routes if you de to enter employment.

ıdation degrees take two years if studied on a full-time basis; longer if -time.

/ tend to place greater emphasis on work-based learning than esponding degree courses, and some institutions have established ng partnerships with companies in the industry to develop interesting <-based Foundation degree programmes. They are a qualification in own right and people with Foundation degrees can use the letters ;c', 'FdEng' or 'FdA' after their names, depending on whether their se is primarily science, engineering or arts-based. When you have ed a Foundation degree you'll be able to choose between entering loyment and continuing training there, or converting the qualification an Honours degree through further study – usually by transfer into second or third year of a related degree course. These degrees are ing popular with mature applicants who have been working for a e in the healthcare sector and wish to improve their formal ifications.

can find detailed information on www.foundationdegree.org.uk

nours degrees

time degrees take from three to six years. The healthcare field in icular features some of the longer ones such as Medicine, Veterinary nce and Dentistry. The usual three-year science course in Healthcare lead to the award of a BSc (Bachelor of Science). On the arts side, the ivalent is the BA (Bachelor of Arts) – some subjects, like Psychology, offered in both arts and science versions. Some of the longer Medical Veterinary courses lead to different qualifications, such as BMedSci :helor of Medical Science), MB BCh (Bachelor of Medicine/Bachelor of jery), BVetMed (Bachelor of Veterinary Medicine) or BVMS (Bachelor of rinary Medicine and Surgery).

w to choose a course

not easy! There are so many to choose from. You are about to invest eral years of your life and several thousand pounds of your money on a ıer education course: how do you maximise your chances of getting a rn on your investment?

two main things that are most likely to influence you are the content ıe course and its appropriateness to your future career plans. It's very ortant to know that courses vary from place to place. Even ones with ıtical names can be very different, and even the slightest variation in rse title can be significant. For example 'Sports Science and Music' is y to contain an equal amount of study in each subject, whereas 'Sports ence with Music' will be weighted towards Sports Science.

ık about the following questions:

- s it a professional qualification that you are after? If so, does the course neet the requirements of the relevant professional bodies? Where elevant, does it give the quickest possible route to NHS registration? Single-subject courses are often the best starting point to find this kind of course.)
- How employable are its graduates?
- Does the institution or department have a particular specialism?
- Has the department won any awards? Have its students?

Other more general points to take into consideration are:

- **Course structure:** do you want to specialise or take a more general course?
- **Assessment:** is it heavily exam-based or does it use continuous assessment – or a combination of the two?
- **Entry requirements:** are you doing the right subjects? Can you get the required grades?
- **Finance:** what help does the institution offer with fees? Are there bursaries and/or scholarships on offer?

Kate Elgood is a current student. She has the following advice.

'The course should come first. But it is important to find the right environment. Where you live can make all the difference to how happy your three or more years are. If you are a real city person you are likely to be miserable on a small campus for instance. I wouldn't go as far as some people I know who chose their university first and then decided what to study there!'

How to choose a university or college

There are all sorts of reasons for selecting a particular institution at which to study. You might have very little choice because only a limited number offer exactly the course you want. But if you have a wide choice, you could think about the following points:

- **Distance from home:** do you want to live at home and attend a local institution, or get as far away from home as possible?
- **Size:** will you be happiest in a small or a large institution?
- **Location:** do you prefer urban areas or the countryside?
- **Set-up:** would you prefer to be on a campus (with all the buildings on one site) or in the middle of a big city, or both?
- **Finances:** how much will it cost to live there?
- **Accommodation:** is there enough of it? Does it suit your preferences – eg self catering or with meals provided?
- **Disability:** if you have any form of disability, it is important to visit institutions to see the facilities for yourself and discuss the support you might need.

The list of points you'll be able to come up with could go on forever! What's important is to choose what is right for you. Luckily there are sources of information to help your decision. Read on ...

Information sources

- Institutions' websites: these are a good source of information on everything from intricate course details to local amenities.
- Higher education fairs.
- Visits and open days: attend these if you can. You will be able to talk to tutors, ask any questions you have, meet current students, see the facilities and get a 'feel' for the place.

How to apply

Nearly all applications for Foundation degrees and Honours degrees are handled initially by the Universities and Colleges Admissions Service (UCAS). You can apply for up to five courses, but applicants for medicine, veterinary science and dentistry courses are only allowed to apply for four while applicants for nursing courses may choose a maximum of five degrees and/or diplomas. Your application will be forwarded by the UCAS office in Cheltenham to all the institutions you have named. Their decisions on your application come to you through UCAS (but you may also receive a personal letter directly from the institution). The staff at UCAS act as agents: they do not make decisions, but they can help you with queries during the application process. There is an application fee of £15 (or £5 if you apply for only one course).

All applications for entry to courses at universities and colleges in the UK are made through **Apply** – UCAS' online system.

Before you apply

You need to double-check all details (particularly entry requirements) with the universities or colleges because things change and may have done so since this guide was prepared.

One thing to be aware of is that some institutions are divided into several large campus sites, and some courses may be offered on one campus only, or on a campus site many miles away from the main one. Make sure you have checked this out and know which campus delivers the course you are applying for.

Some colleges offer degree courses that are accredited by other universities. These are sometimes referred to as validated courses. In this guide, validated courses are listed under the college that provides the course rather than the institution that awards the qualification. When you apply to UCAS you need to apply to the institution that awards the qualification rather than the college at which the course is offered. It is therefore important that you check that the providing institution is the same as the awarding institution.

Courses offered on a specific campus or by a validated college can be distinguished by their UCAS course code: in addition to the standard four-digit format (eg A123), the code also contains an extra letter at the end (eg A123 B).

Consult all the information for applicants that is available from UCAS (www.ucas.com). Look at the institutions' own prospectuses and websites or contact them directly (you will find their contact details in the **Institution Address Listings** section of this book).

Timing

It's normal to make your UCAS application well before you want to start your course. The usual period for making applications is from 1 September to 15 January in the academic year before your course is due to start (ie 1 September 2007 to 15 January 2008 for courses due to start in September/October 2008). It is advisable to submit your application by the 15 January deadline – although universities *may* consider your application if it is late. And there are a few exceptions:

- If you want to apply to Oxford or Cambridge you must have submitted your application by 15 October of the academic year before you plan to start.
- If you want to apply for courses in Veterinary Science, Dentistry or Medicine at any institution you must have submitted your application by 15 October of the academic year before you plan to start.
- If you want to take a gap year and begin your course in autumn 2009 then you should still make your application, but state that you are applying for deferred entry in the relevant section.

Once you have received all your offers, you are expected to decide between them and keep one as your firm acceptance and a second as an insurance offer – in case you don't get the grades asked for. Because most applicants don't have their exam results at this stage, admissions tutors have to make offers conditional on their getting particular exam results.

Offers

You might be asked for a specific combination of grades in a certain qualification (eg BBC at A level) or for a number of UCAS tariff points (eg 280 points). For more information on the UCAS tariff, see page xii and for entry requirements to specific courses see the Course Listings in the subject chapters.

Remember that, even if you expect to comfortably achieve the minimum entry requirements given for a certain course, this does not guarantee that you will be offered a place. Institutions can ask for different entry grades/tariff totals according their popularity and also according to demand for the course.

How to get a place

In a perfect world everyone would be accepted on to their ideal course at their ideal institution. Unfortunately, entry to some courses is very competitive and you need to make your application stand out in order to give yourself an advantage. How can you do this?

First of all, you need to get an idea of what grades you are expecting to achieve. Talk to your teachers as they will be preparing your predicted grades to enter on your UCAS application. Having a good idea of these will help you target your application to suitable courses.

Once you've decided where to apply, try to think of things from the admissions tutors' point of view. Admissions tutors don't all follow the same pattern but in general they will want to know about your:

- Choice of subjects
- Qualifications
- Motivation to study for a healthcare qualification
- Reasons for applying for a particular institution and course
- Skills and personal qualities
- Work experience background (this is particularly important for healthcare courses).

They will get their evidence from:

- Your UCAS application – particularly the personal statement section
- Possibly an interview.

So how do you make yourself stand out? Start with your UCAS application. It sounds obvious, but it's crucial to send in a UCAS application with no errors or spelling mistakes – and it's amazing how many applicants fail to do this. Taking care over an application implies that you will be a conscientious student – and that is a quality admissions tutors are looking for.

The key area to spend time on is the personal statement. This is where you write all you can about why you want to do the course, your motivation and interests. It is your chance to impress. Guidance on how to do this is available from many sources: your teachers should be able to offer some suggestions and there are also books providing information and advice. One in particular to consult is *How to Complete Your UCAS Application* (Trotman, 2007). It can be worth paying attention to your email address too. One admissions tutor says that she was most definitely put off an applicant whose address was 'silent murderer'!!

At the beginning of this section you were advised to try to think of things from the admissions tutors' point of view. In the paragraphs below, three tutors offer their views on admissions.

Geraldine Giannopoulos, Admissions Officer for the Royal (Dick) School of Veterinary Studies at the University of Edinburgh

'We have around 1200 applicants per year and can only interview up to 250. We use the UCAS documentation to help us decide who to call for interview. We look first for evidence from academic results and school references that an applicant has, or is likely to achieve, the grades we are looking for.

'The personal statement then gives us crucial evidence about the applicant's awareness of veterinary science and level of motivation. We look for clear accounts of the length and type of relevant work experience the applicant has had, evidence of motivation and of extra-curricular activities.

'Most veterinary schools prefer the applicant to have had relevant work experience, which will have provided them with some prior practical knowledge. Examples of this kind of relevant experience include working:

- with a veterinary surgeon
- on livestock farms (such as dairying and lambing farms)
- on other types of farm
- at animal establishments such as zoos, kennels, catteries, stables
- at Veterinary Investigation (or 'VI') centres.

ou should also visit an abattoir.'

ue Locke, Senior Undergraduate Admissions Administrator at eninsula Medical School

ll applications are screened against a set of academic and non-academic iteria. Candidates whose applications are successful at this stage will be ked to attend an interview, which is a further part of the selection ocess. The interview is designed to determine whether applicants have e personal qualities to become a doctor. Examples of attributes assessed ring the course of the interview are:

- Communication skills
- Reflection
- Empathy
- Teamwork
- Insight into illness.

n the day of your interview you will attend an introductory talk about the terview selection process before being asked to complete a written estionnaire, which aims to investigate your commitment and motivation study medicine. You are then given three alternative scenarios to nsider, each of which centres upon a contemporary ethical issue related medicine, one of which you select as the basis for your interview.

ne Peninsula Medical School interview is structured and formal to ensure at every student is asked the same questions and receives the same ompts. It takes approximately 20 minutes. It is not a test of your medical owledge but aims to explore your attitudes, outlook and way of thinking. u will also be required to take part in a group problem-solving exercise.'

ckie Haigh is the admissions tutor for the BSC Hons programme Midwifery Studies at the University of Bradford.

e have a lot of applications — around 300 for 38 places so we have to a very close scrutiny of UCAS forms before we can decide which ndidates we can interview. We rule out anyone who does not seem likely meet our entry criteria. For standard entry applicants these are 280 AS points, including 200 points in two A2 subjects. We prefer one of se subjects to be a science. We also accept applications from ndidates who have completed an appropriate health specific Access or ndation course in the last five years.

e then look very carefully at the personal statements and references on UCAS form, looking for evidence of motivation, insight into the fession and the reasons they give to justify their choice. We like to see orts to read about midwifery issues, to talk to midwives and if possible, undertake activities like work experience placements that have helped increase their understanding of what is involved. We also look to see if y have done any relevant extra-curricular activities like volunteering caring work. Last, we look for transferable skills; communication, mwork, ability to develop their own learning — and to use IT.

me applicants are rejected at this stage.

then invite the remaining ones to an open day where they get the ortunity to look round, talk to staff and current students, to find out how course is structured and to decide whether they really want to come e. They are also invited to a final selection day where we divide them small groups and give them an enigma or scenario to analyse and cuss. Our curriculum is delivered through problem-based learning and up-work — so these activities help them to decide whether the roach is the right one for them. The group interaction is assessed by ervers, made up of staff, clinical practitioners and service users. At the of the day we all discuss the candidates and make our offers.

'We gave up one to one interviews some time ago because we found that although they confirmed our findings from the group interviews they did not add anything.'

What happens if you don't get any offers in the first round?

From mid-March to mid-June, UCAS will give you the chance to make one more application through a system known as **Extra**. If you have no offers, UCAS will automatically contact you and explain what to do.

What happens if you have no offers after this stage – or if you don't manage to get the grades asked for?

Then there is another safety net! UCAS operates Clearing during the summer when institutions advertise their empty places with the grades required and students apply for them. Vacancies are published on the UCAS website (www.ucas.com/clearing). By arrangement with UCAS the *Independent* and the *Independent on Sunday* also publish its official lists. Other national newspapers produce their own listings at this time.

How would you learn?

You would learn through a combination of lectures, practicals, tutorials and problem-solving classes. There will often be a major final year project. Higher education institutions tend refer to 'learning' in preference to 'being taught' because there is always some emphasis on self-directed study.

Lectures ...

... are given to large groups of students – sometimes as many as 200 in a large lecture hall. This is when you might find yourself with students from other courses who are studying some topics in common with you. The setting will be fairly formal. A member of staff gives a presentation (talk plus visual aids like PowerPoint or slides) and students make notes. There is usually an opportunity to ask questions at the end. Often, the lecturer hands out a summary of the lecture and a reading list.

Practicals ...

... can include laboratory work, exercises done on computer and individual and group projects. They are often based on a previous lecture. You might do some practicals on your own, or often with two or three other students. It is quite common practice for one section of the students to report back to the rest of the group – either a small tutorial group or the whole year group.

Tutorials or supervisions ...

... are discussion-based. A group of students meets regularly with a member of staff and works together. The topic of discussion might again be based on a lecture or on a practical. Group numbers vary at different institutions – they could be anything from two to over 15.

Problem-solving classes ...

... are rather like tutorials and are held mainly in science and technological subjects. Students will previously have been given a worksheet and meet to discuss their answers.

Case studies and patient contact

The trend in medicine, nursing and training for the therapies is to introduce patient contact into the practicals and problem-solving classes at an increasingly early stage, often as soon as the first few weeks of the course. The reason for this is to put the patient at the centre of professional training, and to give students as much opportunity as possible to develop and improve their communication skills. Students usually work in small groups and may be presented with a patient on whom to base a case study. They might be told something about the patient's health and they might then, under supervision, take the patient's case history, establish and discuss the symptoms and discuss treatment strategies. This leads on to discussion and exploration of the theoretical issues underlying that patient's condition.

Fees and funding

Nobody can pretend that doing a higher education course doesn't cost money. The thing is to look on it as an investment for the future. You will have to pay up to £3070 in tuition fees, depending on which university or college you choose since institutions are allowed to set their own fees up to this maximum figure.

Full-time home and EU undergraduate students will not have to pay any fees before starting their course *or* whilst studying. Instead, both new and existing students will be able to defer paying tuition fees by taking out a student loan for fees. Taking the fee deferment loan means that **you will not have to pay any up-front tuition fees** unless you wish to (see below for more details).

However, there are differences to the tuition fees you will be charged depending on where you live in the United Kingdom. We have what are rapidly becoming different systems in each country. For example:

- In **England, Northern Ireland and Wales**, the vast majority of institutions are charging the maximum of £3070 per year in tuition fees (although at some institutions there is a reduction for sandwich courses or years abroad, and some institutions are reducing fees for Foundation degree students). Students are eligible for a loan to cover tuition fees – for more information, see the **Financial support** section, overleaf.
- In **Scotland**, if you are a Scottish resident attending a Scottish institution, you will not have to pay any tuition fees.

The situation is further complicated by the fact that the level of fees students pay depends on the country in which they live. So, for example, if you are a Scottish student studying at an institution in England, you will have to pay the same fee as your English counterparts. Make sure you check out the situation thoroughly if you are planning to study in a different country to the one in which you live.

You'll have read horror stories of students graduating with large debts. Yes, they do have debts to pay off – and yes, they can be large. Graduates of some of the longer courses in the healthcare area like Medicine and Veterinary Science are particularly affected, and because these courses tend to be intense and challenging, little or no time is left for part-time work to ease the financial burden. But set against this is the fact that qualifications in these areas lead to well-paid, secure jobs and graduates will therefore be in a better position to pay off the debts they have built up.

A 2006 study by the NatWest Bank estimated that the average student in England and Wales now leaves higher education owing £13,252 (after a three year course). And this was for students paying fees at a much lower rate before the 2006 increase. But that's an average. Not every student leaves with the same level of debt. Some manage their money better than others. Some, of course, have more to start with. There are some useful books and websites that can give you more in-depth information and advise you on how to manage your money while at university or college. Try:

- www.interstudent.co.uk which is good for tips and advice from current higher education students and also has links to official sites
- *Students' Money Matters* (Trotman, 2007).

So tuition fees will be one expense. What else will you have to budget for? Books, equipment, visits or field trips and, unless you live at home, food and accommodation. The last two, plus expenditure on going out and general social life, are the biggest – and also the most variable. Do you intend to party every night or stay in by the TV eating toast?

Financial support

All students are entitled to borrow money from the **Student Loans Company** (www.slc.co.uk). You can take out two loans. The first is to help with your maintenance costs. (The maximum a student can borrow each year is currently £6315 but that's for students living in London. If you are studying outside London and living away from home, it's £4735. If you are living at home with your parents, husband, wife or partner it's £3495.) Loans available to Scottish students are smaller since they do not pay tuition fees. New figures will be announced for the year 2008/9.

The second loan is a fee deferment loan. If you are a full-time home or EU undergraduate student you will not have to pay any tuition fees during the course unless you choose to do so. Instead, you can defer paying tuition fees by taking out a student loan for fees. The Student Loans Company w pay the fees on your behalf, and the value of the fee will be added to you overall student loan.

Both loans are means-tested – in other words, the amount you can borrow will depend on family income. You will not have to start repaying either loan until after you have left higher education and are earning more than £15,000 a year. Repayments will be made in monthly instalments.

There are other sources of help. For example, students on low incomes can also apply for various kinds of support – and you might be able to claim more than you think. If your family income is £17,910 or less you a likely to be eligible for a full maintenance grant from the government (currently worth £2765 a year). Partial grants are available for those with family income of between £17,911 and £38,330. In addition every stude who receives the full £2765 maintenance grant may receive a further £3 from their university or college. Institutions may offer further bursaries – cash or kind (eg computers, travel vouchers or grants to purchase course materials).

Since support systems are different in England, Northern Ireland, Scotlan and Wales you will need to read the student support booklets relevant to different parts of the UK. You can get these from schools, colleges, local authority offices – or download them from the official websites given at end of this section.

Institutions also offer **bursary schemes** ranging from £300 to over £30 per annum. There is a great deal of variation between institutions on hov these are awarded: some are means-tested; some are not. To find out more, contact the institutions directly or visit the Office for Fair Access website (www.offa.org.uk). More general information on financial suppor offered by professional, commercial and other organisations is available *University Scholarships, Bursaries and Awards* (Trotman, 2007).

In addition, certain courses specific to the healthcare field attract **NHS bursaries**. An NHS bursary comprises an allowance to cover day-to-day living costs, such as accommodation, and allowances where payable for other expenses, such as extra weeks' attendance and abnormal placeme costs. Your tuition fees will also be paid.

NHS bursaries are available for full- or part-time pre-registration courses in:

- Audiology (professionally recognised courses)
- Chiropody (podiatry)
- Dental hygiene
- Dental therapy
- Dentistry
- Dietetics
- Medicine
- Midwifery (degree and diploma courses)
- Nursing
- Operating Department Practitioner
- Occupational therapy
- Orthoptics
- Physiotherapy
- Prosthetics and Orthotics

Radiography

Speech and language therapy.

ey are not available for pharmacy or complementary medicine. There are o types of NHS bursary. The first is non-means-tested and provides a t-rate income maintenance grant with a contribution required from you your parents. This is available for nursing and midwifery diploma urses. The second is a means-tested bursary, available for all courses ted above except nursing and midwifery diplomas. Your income and that your parents or spouse will be taken into account and the amount of aintenance grant will be reduced in proportion to that income, net of owable deductions. You can find out more at www.nhscareers.nhs.uk d www.nhsstudentgrants.co.uk

e amount of the non-means tested bursary, as this guide was being itten, was £7443 in London and £6372 elsewhere. Means-tested rsary rates were £3215 in London, £2672 elsewhere and £2231 for idents living in the parental home. These are the rates for the academic ar 2006/7. The new rates for 2007/8 were due to be announced. Means-sted bursary holders may also apply for student loans.

nd for students with disabilities

u might be able to claim several different allowances (depending on ether you need specialist equipment or a non-medical helper). These owances, unlike grants, are not means-tested. Again – check the bsites.

dditional points for mature students

st higher education staff like having mature students on their courses. ey find them very motivated and hardworking. Older students, however, en have particular worries – for instance:

ill I cope with the course?

ture students have a very good record in this respect. But if it is some e since you did any regular study, many admissions tutors will ask you undertake some as a preparation – perhaps a relevant evening class.

ill I qualify for entry?

titutions often relax the entry requirements for mature students – but ere many courses in this Guide are concerned, a certain background of hnical knowledge is required. If you don't have the right subjects you ld take an Access course. These are specially designed to prepare dents for study on particular courses.

n I afford it?

will have to work out your budget carefully, especially if you have endants. You will be entitled to the same level of support as younger dents but in addition might qualify for a range of other grants and loans elp you with additional costs such as travel and childcare. You can find ailed information on the websites given in the **Fees and funding** tion above and in the **Useful information** section at the end of the **roduction**. Staff at Student Services centres at the institutions to which might apply are also very knowledgeable about what may be claimed.

me common questions and answers

uld I change to science if I haven't done the ht A levels?

could consider taking a foundation course if the qualifications you are ently studying for do not match the requirements of the course you are rested in. For example, some courses require you to have A level nces (or equivalent). If you are not taking science(s) at A level then you d take a one-year conversion course that would provide you with the necessary background in science and/or mathematics to embark on the degree course you want to take. Foundation courses can be offered either as stand-alone courses or as part of a degree course.

What are sandwich courses?

They add a year to your degree course but the year is spent gaining work experience with an employer. The work placements can be in the form of a **thick** or **thin** sandwich. With a thick sandwich, the third year is spent in a work placement. With a thin sandwich, students usually spend two six-month periods of work experience in different years of the course.

Can I take a gap year?

There are good reasons why, if you are thinking about taking a higher education course in healthcare, you should consider taking a gap year and perhaps doing some form of volunteering. The first decision to make is whether you go before or after your course.

Taking a gap year before your course

Here are some reasons why going before your healthcare course begins might be a good idea:

- You may feel that you need a rest from purely academic work after your exertions at school or college.
- You may be attracted by the exciting gap year mix of broadening your social horizons, allowing you the chance to help out in communities and countries whose traditions and culture are different from yours, travelling and meeting people.
- Admissions tutors for many of the healthcare courses are keen to see reference to relevant work experience on your UCAS personal statement. You may not have had the chance, to date, to have worked in the type of caring environment which would give you sufficient understanding of the pressures of healthcare work. A well-chosen gap year project could help your application.
- In general admissions staff often find that students are more mature and independent when they arrive if they have had some time out after A levels, although there is often no institution-wide policy. Individual admissions tutors may have their own views, so it's always best to try to find out. Institutions' websites are usually a good starting point.

The range of gap year opportunities is quite bewildering and there is something for everyone – from learning drama in New York to teaching English in South America; from becoming a scuba diving instructor to helping on environmental projects in the Galapagos islands. See the **Useful information** section at the end of this **Introduction** to give you an idea of where to start.

Taking a gap year after your course

If you are reading this directory seriously then there is obviously a high chance that you will eventually qualify as some form of healthcare professional. It therefore makes sense for you to consider whether taking time out *after* you have qualified would be better than a gap year before you go to university. Volunteer organisations have a serious need for trained and qualified healthcare people to work in developing countries. You would have infinitely more to offer your host community working as a professional.

Graeme Chisholm, Marketing Adviser for Health and Social Development at VSO

'VSO recruits a range of health professionals – from GPs to community nurses, speech and language therapists to physiotherapists. Volunteers are usually working with limited resources in very challenging environments and, as well as administering care, they are working in partnership with colleagues to facilitate the training and professional development of their local colleagues. They may also be working at a management and policy level helping to strengthen an organisation's abilities and capacity to deliver much-needed services. For this reason it is important that VSO recruits skilled and confident health professionals and we usually ask for at least two years' professional experience.'

When you have your degree

What are employers looking for?

They expect a good knowledge of your subject naturally. But there is more to it than that. They are also looking for what are known as soft or personable transferable skills, such as communication, initiative and the ability to work in a team.

Applicants to many of the courses listed in this guide are being selected for employment at the same time as they are being considered for places on courses. No-one is going to admit a student to a place at medical school or on a course leading to registration in one of the professions related to medicine without also being as sure as possible that they will be suited to the career. Many selection panels include practising members of a particular profession to give their viewpoint. Sally Abel, who is quoted as an admissions tutor on page xxi, helped to interview students for several years while she was working as a radiographer. She now invites a practising radiographer to help select students for her course. She stresses that two of the things they look for are strong communication skill and a positive interest in technology.

So, if you successfully complete a degree that leads to a specific medical profession you can be sure that you have what employers are looking for. But, if several newly qualified students are competing for the same jobs, there might just be some extra qualities some students have that help them to get the job. They might have more work experience for instance or – if time permits (and it does not always do so on medically-related courses whose terms may be longer) – may have had term-time jobs in which they had a lot of contact with people, like catering or sales work.

Later on, as your career develops you will find that you need a set of skills relevant to the direction your career is taking. For instance, the following is a job advertisement that appeared for an experienced occupational therapist:

'We are looking for creative and flexible staff, who can communicate with ethnically diverse, troubled young people, aged 14–35 with a first episode of psychosis.

'You will have a limited caseload and work intensively in the community with the young person and his/her family to promote recovery. You need to be confident in your skills, keen to learn new ways of working and take responsibility as a senior worker in helping to develop a new team. Special interest in adolescents, family work, substance misuse, as well as in psychosis would be beneficial.'

What sort of jobs do healthcare graduates do?

The healthcare sector includes a vast range of careers: from aromatherapy to physiotherapy; from surgery to speech and language therapy – and those are just the professions involved in patient contact. In addition, there is work in scientific research and development, and administrative work ranging from health promotion initiatives to pharmaceutical sales and business management. With such a wide range of disciplines included under the healthcare umbrella, it is difficult to make generalisations about what healthcare jobs actually involve. The list below shows a range of tasks someone working in the area might perform – but it is a very rough indication:

- Giving physical or psychological support or treatment to help improve (or save) the lives of members of the public
- Carrying out research into the development of new treatments or medication
- Applying the latest technology to the needs of individual patients
- Working in the community with people in schools, the workplace and residential care establishments to maintain positive attitudes to healthcare
- Keeping abreast of new treatment techniques relevant to your professional area

and

- Working with colleagues
- Managing staff
- Managing projects
- Managing budgets.

The NHS is the largest employer in the healthcare field, with employee over 70 different professions. Careers in healthcare within the NHS are secure and carry a pension scheme. But while the NHS remains the biggest employer in the country, you would not necessarily find yourse working in a hospital after you qualify for your chosen healthcare care For example, dentists, doctors, vets, therapists, and complementary medicine professionals such as chiropractors and osteopaths often wo for small, privately-run businesses or are self-employed. And many of lab-based qualifications in this guide (such as pharmacy, food science biochemistry) could lead to work for large research and manufacturing companies. Many healthcare professionals will also find that work in t community takes them to people's homes, schools, factories and residential care establishments.

Whatever your eventual healthcare subject, employment or further stu prospects look good in the long term. More specific information on eac subject area is provided at the beginning of each chapter.

Salaries

NHS staff are paid on a pay system, called Agenda for Change which is intended to reduce the range of separate pay deals by establishing an across the board arrangement whereby all employees have their salary assessed according to their skill and responsibility levels. The Agenda Change pay system relates to all staff in the NHS, excluding dentists, doctors and very senior managers.

Under Agenda for Change the pay system is divided into nine pay band There are several pay points within each band and each post is placed pay band using the NHS job evaluation scheme.

The bands given below are those in force from 1 April, 2006. At the tim writing this book the public sector unions had not accepted the pay increase of around 2.5%, which had been offered in April 2007.

1. £11,782–£12,853
2. £12,177–£15,107
3. £14,037–£16,799
4. £16,405–£19,730
5. £19,166–£24,803
6. £22,886–£31,004
7. £27,622–£36,416
8. £35,232–£42,278 (Range A)
   £41,038–£50,733 (Range B)
   £49,381–£60,880 (Range C)
   £59,189–£73,281 (Range D)
9. £69,899–£88,397

Some job levels within these bands:

Band 5

Newly qualified allied health professional (ambulance paramedic, art therapist, drama therapist, music therapist, chiropodist/podiatrist, dietitian, occupational therapist, orthoptist, orthotist, prosthetist, physiotherapist, radiographer, speech and language therapist), healthcare scientist, hospital pharmacist, midwife, nurse, operating department practitioner.

and 6

llied health profession specialist or team leader, biomedical science team ader, health visitor, nursing or midwifery specialist or team leader.

and 7

dvanced health professional, nurse, midwife, scientist or team manager, inical psychologist.

and 8

onsultant clinical scientist, consultant pharmacist (Range B–D), consultant urse or midwife, consultant or principal occupational therapist (Range -B), consultant or principal radiographer (A–C), consultant or principal beech and language therapist (A–D), dental laboratory manager (A–C), odern matron (A–C).

and 9

onsultant clinical psychologist/head of psychology services, consultant inical scientist/head of service (molecular genetics/cytogenetics), diatric consultant (surgery)/head of service.

get a feel for what employees working in different areas of the NHS rn, the best thing to do is to visit the NHS's jobs website, ww.jobs.nhs.uk. You will see that salaries increase significantly as you in more experience and take on more responsibility.

edical consultants and specialists, normally after at least ten years' NHS perience, may find employment in the private healthcare sector – often a part-time addition to their NHS contract. For other professionals such nurses and therapists, the NHS is the dominant employer and its salary ructure tends to set the benchmark for salaries in the private sector. any employers match or exceed the NHS although some pay less.

e chapter introductions provide more details about salaries – but bear in nd that the salary levels quoted are intended as a guide only and are bject to change.

seful information

eneral

- *University and College Entrance: The Official Guide* (UCAS)
- *UCAS Universities Scotland* (UCAS)
- *Degree Course Offers*, Brian Heap (Trotman, 2007)
- *The Ultimate University Ranking Guide*, Catherine Harris (Trotman, 2004)
- *How to Complete Your UCAS Application* (Trotman, 2007)
- *Making the Most of University,* Kate Van Haeften (Trotman, 2003)
- *The Student Book*, Klaus Boehm & Jenny Lees-Spalding (Trotman, 2007)
- *The Virgin Alternative Guide to British Universities,* Piers Dudgeon (Virgin Books, 2007)

Healthcare

- CRAC/Trotman Degree Course Guides Series: *Medical & Related Professions,* (Trotman, 2006)
- *Getting into Dental School,* James Burnett (Trotman, 2007)
- *Getting into Physiotherapy Courses,* James Burnett & Andrew Long (Trotman, 2006)
- *Medicine Uncovered,* Laurel Alexander (Trotman, 2003)
- *Nursing & Midwifery Uncovered,* Laurel Alexander (Trotman, 2006)
- www.nhscareers.nhs.uk (National Health Service careers website)
- www.skillsforhealth.org.uk (Skills for Health website – the sector skills council for all staff groups working in the NHS, independent and voluntary health organisations
- For specialist websites see the individual subject chapters

Gap year

- *A Year off. A Year Oh?* (Lifetime Careers, 2005)
- *Taking a Gap Year*, Susan Griffith (Vacation Work Publications)
- *The Gap-Year Guidebook* (John Catt Educational Ltd, available via Trotman)

Finance

- *Students' Money Matters*, Gwenda Thomas (Trotman, 2007)
- http://direct.gov.uk/EducationAndLearning/fs/en
- www.saas.gov.uk (Scotland)
- www.studentfinanceni.co.uk
- www.studentfinancewales.co.uk
- www.nhsstudentgrants.co.uk
- www.interstudent.co.uk/channel_money.php (good for tips and advice from current higher education students and also has links to official sites)

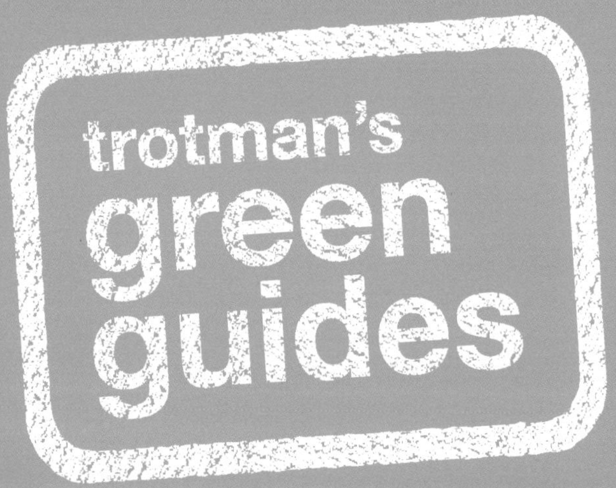

Green Pages: Course Listings

Anatomy and Physiology

Including:
Anatomy
Applied Physiology
Human Physiology
Pathology and Physiology

What would you study?

Whilst many of the higher education courses featured in this guide lead to a professional qualification, courses in this chapter are more likely to be chosen because you are simply interested in taking the subject. If you have a particular healthcare profession in mind, you should find the courses leading to it listed elsewhere. However, courses in this chapter have much in common with those in other chapters – especially biomedical sciences. The 'core' studies cover much of the same ground.

There is considerable overlap in the content of courses in this chapter. All of them help develop research skills, familiarity with statistical investigation techniques and other transferable skills which will be useful to a range of employers. Frequently they are offered in combination with each other and it is quite on the cards that you could transfer from one to the other as your studies progress. The paragraphs below give a broad overview of some of the different areas covered.

Anatomy

Anatomy is the study of the human structure. It looks at the bodies of humans and animals from the molecular level to the whole structure. Most courses will use dissection as one of the ways of learning – although other methods, using sophisticated electronic equipment, are now complementing dissection as a learning medium. These include computerised images, ultrasound and magnetic resonance imaging. Your own body and those of your student colleagues may also provide learning tools when studying living anatomy. Typical topics for study in an anatomy degree include:

- Anatomy
- Biochemistry
- Cell biology
- Genetics
- Immunology
- Neurobiology
- Zoology.

Students will acquire considerable expertise in research techniques by the end of the course and these in themselves will come in useful on a CV when looking at options after higher education.

Physiology

Physiology is a key part of medical sciences. It deals with how living organisms work and seeks to understand the processes which operate in structures from the level of cells to the whole body. Topics studied could include:

- Anatomy
- Biochemistry
- Study of a particular aspect or function of the body (for example nerve cells, respiratory systems or the reaction of the cell to drugs – so aspects of pharmacology could also feature as part of the course).

Pathology

Like anatomy and physiology, pathology is also biochemistry-based and encompasses topics such as:

- Bacteriology
- Cellular processes
- Molecular genetics
- Virology.

Study in these areas will lead to increased understanding of issues such as how cancer cells develop and the effect of chemo- and radiotherapy. But be warned: if you have been inspired by all those TV shows featuring pathologists cutting up corpses as part of a criminal investigation team, be aware that, in reality, the pathologists who carry out these tasks will have a full medical degree.

Getting in

The bottom line with these courses is that they have much in common with each other and therefore applicants need similar qualifications for entry to all of them. Each university decides on its own entry requirement You can see the range of UCAS points asked by each one by consulting t course listings on the following pages.

Linda Wilson, Admissions Tutor, BSc Human Physiology, University o Leeds

'When I get the applications I look first at GCSE grades and predicted A level grades. With the GCSE grades I am looking for evidence that the student has a good grounding in mathematics, English and science and is nice to see A and B grades in these subjects but I would not reject a student solely based on their performance at GCSE as some students are late developers when it comes to academic studies. However, if their predicted A level grades are much below our requirement (BBB, includin two sciences (one of which must be biology), or equivalent) they are rejected because realistically they are unlikely to improve that much. If they are marginally below, say BCC, next I'll still consider making an offe of BBB after reading the rest of the application in the hope that the stud may achieve these grades or be very near.

'I then read the personal statement, looking for evidence of strong commitment to the course. This would come out through reasons why students enjoy A level human biology or the human biology side of the general biology A level. I'm also looking for an indication that they would like to follow some kind of related career – in research perhaps, or in o of the professions related to medicine through postgraduate study. Som students apply for human physiology as an insurance choice for medici or dentistry and therefore their personal statement is geared towards th degrees. This does not matter as I can still extract the information I am looking for from it.

'Evidence of some work experience or strong interest in an out of schoo activity is important. I'm not thinking of the placements organised by schools and done in school time but something done on their own initiative. I want to know that the applicants do more than go to school sleep. So a description of a Saturday or holiday job, particularly if it is o that has been done for some time, is appropriate. So too is membership a sports team or club or society. They should not simply write a list but what they do and what they gain from it (like taking responsibility, deali with people or learning to manage time). I have a form in front of me at moment from a student who has written about a strong interest in musi On the face of it this is not relevant to the study of human physiology b to me playing in an orchestra shows commitment to something.

'I look at the reference of course – and this is where I might be influenc to lower the entry grades required if there is something describing any mitigating circumstances. I also look for something saying that the refe knows the applicant is committed to my subject and is recommended a good potential student.'

Graduate outlook

Around 20% of graduates in this area of courses continue with further study. They could go for further research, based on their subject, readi for a Master's degree (MSc) or a Doctorate (PhD). Those people will eventually be looking for work in research with companies in the healthcare field, such as pharmaceutical manufacturers, or for academ posts within higher education.

The remainder of those who stay in full-time postgraduate study go for further full-time courses leading to a professional qualification. Those w wish to try for qualification in one of the medical or veterinary professi ill find that their studies so far have much in common with the pre-inical parts of medicine, veterinary science or one of the therapies. They 'll therefore be able to compete for a place on one of the graduate fast-ack versions of the relevant degree.

e publication *What do graduates do?* provides statistics for Anatomy, ysiology and Pathology graduates. It shows that of 2630 students who sponded to a survey in 2005 (the latest year for which figures are ailable):

67.3% were in employment in the UK

16.2% were doing full-time further study.

4.5% were working and studying

5.8% were unemployed

six months after graduation.

(The figures do not total 100% because some graduates answered the survey stating that they were not available for work.)

The majority of those in employment were working as health professionals and associate health professionals (59.9%) while a further 2.9% were in scientific research and analysis. Around 3.5% were in commercial, industrial and public sector management. A number had used their degree as a level of qualification rather than as a specific vocational training and had entered careers as different as business, finance, marketing, sales, advertising, IT work and retailing.

What would you earn?

Some graduates going on to the employment market will go for similar careers to those discussed in the next chapter, **Biomedical Sciences**. Those who find lab work in industries such as pharmaceutical research and production may expect to earn starting salaries of around £22,000.

Case Study

Claire McKinley

Claire is a second-year student, studying for a BSc in Human Physiology at Leeds University.

'Physiology wasn't my original choice. I started a biology degree here but didn't like it. I soon realised that it was the human biology side that interested me most (as it had done for A level) and that I wanted to concentrate on that rather than do general biology also involving plants and animals. Luckily for me I was allowed to change during my first year.

'It was the right choice. I'm really interested in what I am doing now and it is a very good department to be in. All the staff are friendly and helpful and we are also assigned a personal tutor. We meet on a one to one basis once a term to discuss our progress; they give us their email details so that we can contact them at any time or arrange another meeting.

'We shared a common first semester with students doing anatomy, pharmacy and medicine. Many of the subjects were compulsory but we did have some choice of optional modules. Lectures were in large groups; some had more than 400 students. Teaching wasn't always as formal as this though. We also had practical classes – for the 75 of us doing physiology – but we worked at tables in small groups or sometimes in pairs. We also worked in groups of four on oral presentations. All this mixing was very good since we got to know each other.

'The practical topics in the first year were quite straightforward: microscope work, staining slides and fixing them, then studying them to explain what we saw or PCR (polymer chain reaction) analysis, through amplifying small amounts of DNA. We also learned how to measure blood pressure and do ECGs and hearing tests.

'In the second year we have tutorial groups of nine or ten on things like interpreting data to solve problems and discussing relevant topical issues, such as the impact of anorexia or obesity on the NHS. Usually one of us has to prepare a topic, for which we had been given two weeks to work on, present it and then take questions afterwards. In lectures we continue learning about the different body systems; nervous, cardiovascular, respiratory and renal for instance.

'There are a lot of optional modules and you can group them to form a specialism if you wish. I'm concentrating on the central nervous system and so have chosen ones like anatomy, pharmacology, chemotherapy (which is not just about cancer but includes anti-viral and anti-bacterial drugs). I'm also taking toxicology.

'I'm beginning to look now at the modules I shall choose for my third year. I also have to start thinking about a subject for my research project which can be either library or laboratory based, or could be a field work project involving a clinical survey.

'Ultimately I hope to go into a career in embryology and would like to do the NHS training which would allow me to do a Master's and then a PhD.'

Anatomical and Physiological Sciences

University of Dundee D65
BSc (Hons): 4 years full-time – B120
Tariff: 240 IB: 26

University of Dundee D65
BSc (Hons): 3 years full-time – B190
Tariff: 240 - 300 IB: 32

Anatomical Science

University of Bristol B78
BSc (Hons): 3 years full-time or 4 years sandwich – B110
A2: BBB SQA: BBBBB IB: 32 HND

Anatomical Sciences

University of Dundee D65
BSc (Hons): 4 years full-time – B110
Tariff: 240 IB: 26

University of Dundee D65
BSc (Hons): 3 years full-time – B111
Tariff: 300 IB: 32 HND

University of Manchester M20
BSc (Hons): 3 years full-time – B110
A2: BBB - AAB BTEC: DDM - DDD SQA: AABBB - AAAAB ILC: AAABB IB: 32 - 35 Interview

Anatomical Sciences (with industrial or professional experience)

University of Manchester M20
BSc (Hons): 4 years sandwich – B111
A2: BBB - AAB BTEC: DDM - DDD SQA: AABBB - AAAAB ILC: AAABB IB: 32 - 35 Interview

Anatomical Sciences with a Modern Language

University of Manchester M20
BSc (Hons): 4 years full-time with time abroad – B114
A2: BBB - AAB BTEC: DDM - DDD SQA: AABBB - AAAAB ILC: AAAABB IB: 32 - 35 Interview

Anatomy

University of Glasgow G28
BSc: 3 years full-time BSc (Hons): 4 years full-time – B110
A2: BCC SQA: BBBB ILC: BBBB IB: 28 HND

University of Glasgow G28
MSci (Hons): 5 years sandwich – B141
A2: BCC SQA: BBBB ILC: BBBB IB: 28 HND

Queen's University Belfast Q75
BSc (Hons): 3 years full-time – B110
A2: CCC - AB SQA: BBBC IB: 28

Anatomy and Human Biology

University of Liverpool L41
BSc (Hons): 3 years full-time – B110
A2: ABB - AAA BTEC: DDM - DDD SQA: AAAAA IB: 26

Anatomy and Physiology

University of Leeds L23
BSc (Hons): 3 years full-time or 4 years full-time including foundation year – B151
Tariff: 300 IB: 32

Applied Physiology and Pharmacology

Bristol, University of the West of England B80
BSc (Hons): 3 years full-time or 4 years sandwich or 5 years sandwich including foundation year – BB12
Tariff: 180 - 220 IB: 24 - 26

Biomedical Sciences (Anatomy)

Cardiff University C15
BSc (Hons): 4 years sandwich – B112
Tariff: 300 - 340 IB: 32

Cardiff University C15
BSc (Hons): 3 years full-time – B111
Tariff: 300 - 340 IB: 32

Biomedical Sciences (Physiology)

University of Aberdeen A20
BSc (Hons): 4 years full-time – B9B1
A2: BB SQA: ABBB ILC: ABBBB IB: 32

Cardiff University C15
BSc (Hons): 3 years full-time – B121
Tariff: 300 - 340 IB: 32

Cardiff University C15
BSc (Hons): 4 years sandwich – B122
Tariff: 300 - 340 IB: 32

Biomedical Sciences (Physiology/Pharmacology)

Leeds Metropolitan University L27
BSc (Hons): 3 years full-time or 5 years part-time – BB12
Tariff: 160 IB: 24

Biosciences (Medical Physiology)

University of Greenwich G70
BSc (Hons): 3 years full-time or 4 years sandwich or 5 years part-time – B100
Tariff: 180

Clinical Physiology

Castle College Nottingham [De Montfort University] C21
BSc (Hons): 4 years part-time
Tariff: 140

NESCOT [Open University] N49
FdSc: 2 years full-time or 3 years part-time – B121
A2: EE BTEC: PP - PPP

University of Portsmouth P80
BSc (Hons): 4 years part-time
Tariff: 140

University of Sunderland S84
BSc (Hons): 4 years part-time
A2: CC

University of Ulster U20
BSc (Hons): 4 years sandwich – B941 J
Tariff: 260 IB: 30

University of Wolverhampton W75
BSc (Hons): 3 - 4 years full-time or 4 years sandwich or 4 - 6 years part-time – B120
Tariff: 120 - 180 IB: 24

Clinical Physiology (Cardiology)

University of Essex E70
BSc (Hons): 4 years sandwich – BB18
Tariff: 240 - 260 IB: 26 - 27

University of Leeds L23
BSc (Hons): 4 years full-time – B101
A2: CCC SQA: CCCCC

Clinical Physiology with Cardiology

University of Wales, Swansea S93
BSc (Hons): 4 years full-time – B1B8
Tariff: 240

Clinical Physiology and Clinical Technology

Castle College Nottingham [De Montfort University] C21
BSc (Hons): 4 years part-time
Tariff: 140

Clinical Physiology with Clinical Technology

University of Wales, Swansea S93
BSc (Hons): 4 years full-time – B1F3
Tariff: 240

Clinical Physiology with Respiratory Physiology

University of Wales, Swansea S93
BSc (Hons): 4 years full-time – B121
Tariff: 240

Human and Medical Science

University of Westminster W50
BSc (Hons): 3 years full-time – B901
A2: CC

Human and Medical Science (with foundation)

University of Westminster W50
BSc (Hons): 4 years full-time including foundation year – B408
A2: EE

uman Musculoskeletal Science

niversity of Bristol B78
c (Hons): 3 years full-time – B111
: BBB BTEC: DDM SQA: BBBBB IB: 32

uman Physiology

niversity of Leeds L23
c (Hons): 3 years full-time or 4 years full-time with time
oad or 4 years sandwich – B120
: BBB SQA: BBBBB - AAAAA IB: 32

uman Physiology and Biomedical cience

niversity of Wolverhampton W75
(Hons)/BSc (Hons): 3 years full-time or 4 years
dwich – BC19
iff: 220 - 240

uman Physiology and Sport and xercise Science

iversity of Wolverhampton W75
(Hons)/BSc (Hons): 3 years full-time or 4 years sandwich
CC6
iff: 160 - 220

uman Sciences

g's College London (University of ndon) K60
(Hons): 3 years full-time or 4 years sandwich – B150
BBB SQA: ABBBB ILC: AABBBB IB: 32

iversity of Sussex S90
(Hons): 4 years full-time – BLV0
ABB - AAB IB: 34 - 36

ames Valley University T40
(Hons): 3 years full-time or 3 - 7 years part-time day –
1
f: 160

iversity College London, University of ndon U80
(Hons): 3 years full-time – BCL0
ABB - AAB BTEC: DDD SQA: AAB ILC: AAAAA IB: 36
view

uman Sciences and Law

iversity of Bolton B44
Hons)/BSc (Hons): 3 years full-time – CM91
: 220 IB: 20

man Sciences and Mathematics

versity of Bolton B44
(Hons): 3 years full-time – CG91
: 230 IB: 22

man Sciences and Philosophy

versity of Bolton B44
ons)/BSc (Hons): 3 years full-time – CV95
: 280 IB: 24

Human Sciences (pre-medical option) (top-up)

Thames Valley University T40
BSc (Hons): - 1 year full-time – B9C1
Tariff: 200 IB: 30

Human Sciences and Psychology

University of Bolton B44
BSc (Hons): 3 years full-time – CC98
Tariff: 240 IB: 24

Medical Physiology

University of Leicester L34
BSc (Hons): 3 years full-time or 4 years sandwich – B120
Tariff: 320 IB: 32 - 34

Pathology and Microbiology

University of Bristol B78
BSc (Hons): 3 years full-time or 4 years sandwich – BC15
A2: BBB BTEC: DDM SQA: BBBBB IB: 32

Physiological Science

University of Bristol B78
BSc (Hons): 3 years full-time – B120
A2: BBB BTEC: DMM - DDM SQA: AAABB IB: 32

Physiological Sciences

University of Dundee D65
BSc (Hons): 4 years full-time – B100
Tariff: 240 IB: 26

University of Dundee D65
BSc (Hons): 3 years full-time – B121
Tariff: 300 IB: 32 HND

Newcastle University N21
BSc (Hons): 3 years full-time – B100
A2: ABB ILC: ABBBB IB: 30 - 32

University of Oxford O33
BA (Hons): 3 years full-time – B100
A2: AAB - AAA SQA: AAAAB - AAAAA IB: 38

Physiology

University of Aberdeen A20
BSc (Hons): 4 years full-time – B120
A2: CDD SQA: BBBB ILC: BCCCC - BBCC IB: 26

University of Edinburgh E56
BSc (Hons): 4 years full-time – B120
A2: BBB SQA: BBBB IB: 30

University of Glasgow G28
BSc: 3 years full-time BSc (Hons): 4 years full-time –
B120
A2: BCC SQA: BBBB ILC: BBBB IB: 28 HND

University of Glasgow G28
MSci (Hons): 5 years sandwich – B121
A2: BCC SQA: BBBB ILC: BBBB IB: 28 HND

University of Hertfordshire H36
BSc/BSc (Hons): 3 years full-time or 4 years full-time including foundation year or 4 years sandwich or 5 years sandwich including foundation year – C1B1
Tariff: 200 IB: 24
IOB

King's College London (University of London) K60
BSc (Hons): 3 years full-time or 4 years sandwich – B120
A2: BBB SQA: ABBBB ILC: AABBB IB: 32

University of Liverpool L41
BSc (Hons): 3 years full-time – B120
A2: BBC - BBB IB: 26

University of Manchester M20
BSc (Hons): 3 years full-time – B120
A2: BBB - AAB BTEC: DDM - DDD SQA: AABBB - AAAAB
ILC: AAABB IB: 32 - 35 Interview

Queen's University Belfast Q75
BSc (Hons): 3 years full-time – B120
A2: BCC - AB SQA: BBBC IB: 28

University of St Andrews S36
BSc (Hons): 4 years full-time – B120
A2: BBB - ABC SQA: BBBBB - ABBB IB: 31

Physiology with Biochemistry (with 2+2 option)

University of Salford S03
BSc (Hons): 3 years full-time or 4 years sandwich or up to 6 years part-time – BC17
A2: CCD BTEC: DMM SQA: BBBCC ILC: 340 IB: 28

Physiology with Biochemistry (with previous studies in France)

University of Salford S03
BSc (Hons): 3 years full-time – BCC7
Tariff: 200 IB: 28

Physiology (with industrial or professional experience)

University of Manchester M20
BSc (Hons): 4 years sandwich – B121
A2: BBB - AAB BTEC: DDM - DDD SQA: AABBB - AAAAB
ILC: AAABB IB: 32 - 35 Interview

Physiology with a Modern Language

University of Manchester M20
BSc (Hons): 4 years full-time with time abroad – B122
A2: BBB - AAB BTEC: DDM - DDD SQA: AABBB - AAAAB
ILC: A2 A2 A2 B2 B2 - A1 A1 A1 B1 B1 IB: 32 - 35
Interview

Physiology and Pharmacology

King's College London (University of London) K60
BSc (Hons): 3 years full-time or 4 years sandwich – BB12
A2: BBB SQA: BBBBB ILC: AABBBB IB: 32

Nottingham Trent University N91
BSc/BSc (Hons): 3 years full-time or 4 years sandwich – BB12
Tariff: 160

University of Westminster W50
BSc (Hons): 3 years full-time – BB12
A2: CC

University of Westminster W50
BSc (Hons): 4 years full-time including foundation year – BBC2
A2: CC

University of Wolverhampton W75
BSc (Hons): 3 years full-time or 4 years sandwich or 5 - 6 years part-time – BB12
Tariff: 260 - 320 IB: 24

Physiology with Pharmacology

Manchester Metropolitan University M40
BSc (Hons): 4 years full-time including foundation year – B1BF
Tariff: 40 - 100

University of Sheffield S18
BSc (Hons): 3 years full-time – B1B2
A2: ABB SQA: AAAB ILC: AABBB IB: 33

University of Sheffield S18
MBioSci: 4 years full-time – B1BF
A2: ABB SQA: AAAB ILC: AABBB IB: 33

Physiology and Philosophy

University of Oxford O33
BA (Hons): 3 years full-time – BV15
A2: AAB - AAA SQA: AAAAB - AAAAA IB: 38

Physiology and Psychology

Cardiff University C15
BSc (Hons): 3 years full-time – BC18
Tariff: 320 IB: 33
BPS

University of Glasgow G28
BSc (Hons): 4 years full-time – BC18
A2: BCC SQA: BBBB ILC: BBBB IB: 28 HND

University of Oxford O33
BA (Hons): 3 years full-time – BC18
A2: AAB - AAA SQA: AAAAB - AAAAA IB: 38

Physiology with Sports Biomedicine

University of Dundee D65
BSc (Hons): 3 years full-time – B1CP
Tariff: 300 IB: 32 HND

University of Dundee D65
BSc (Hons): 4 years full-time – B1C6
Tariff: 240 IB: 26

Physiology with Sports Science

University of Glasgow G28
BSc: 3 years full-time BSc (Hons): 4 years full-time – B1C6
A2: BCC SQA: BBBB ILC: BBBB IB: 28 HND

University of Glasgow G28
MSci (Hons): 5 years sandwich – B1CP
A2: BCC SQA: BBBB ILC: BBBB IB: 28

Physiology, Sports Science and Nutrition

University of Glasgow G28
MSci (Hons): 5 years sandwich – BC96
A2: BCC SQA: BBBB ILC: BBBB IB: 28

University of Glasgow G28
BSc: 3 years full-time BSc (Hons): 4 years full-time – BC46
A2: BCC SQA: BBBB ILC: BBBB IB: 28 HND

Physiology with Studies in Pharmacology

Manchester Metropolitan University M40
BSc (Hons): 3 years full-time – B1B2
Tariff: 200 - 240 IB: 24

Physiology (with a year in Europe)

University of Hertfordshire H36
BSc (Hons): 4 years sandwich – B101
Tariff: 200

Physiology (with year in North America)

University of Hertfordshire H36
BSc (Hons): 4 years sandwich – B102
Tariff: 200

Physiology/Pharmacology

University of Central Lancashire C30
BSc (Hons): 3 years full-time – BB12
Tariff: 200

Biomedical Sciences

Including:
Biomedical Engineering
Biomedical Sciences
Immunology
Medical Biochemistry
Medical Genetics
Virology

What would you study?

This chapter has a great deal in common with the previous one (**Anatomy and Physiology**). Most of the courses are taught in conjunction with the university medical school or at least, where there is no medical school, in a life sciences department. You may enter courses with the intention at the start of taking one of the degrees in the department – but there will be scope for you to make choices as you progress which could take you to another department.

This is an advantage as biology tends to be taught in a fairly general way in schools. A department's initial task is to give its first year undergraduates a foundation on which they can build for the rest of the course. It follows that, with greater understanding of life science subjects, you will benefit from the flexibility which encourages you to think about your choices and develop them to suit your needs.

Like those in the previous chapter, the courses listed here give a fairly general life sciences grounding in subjects such as:

- Anatomy
- Genetics
- Microbiology
- Pathology
- Physiology.

This approach makes them attractive to mature students and many further education colleges have established Access courses designed to bring applicants up to the standards necessary to begin these degrees. There are also a number of Foundation degrees in this area. From these broad beginnings students will develop specialisms as they progress through the courses.

Biomedical Engineering

Biomedical engineering, however, stands out as being different. It is often a joint effort between institutions' engineering departments and their life sciences departments. There are a number of variations in title from one institution to another – for example: biomedical engineering, biomedical materials science, biomedical electronics, biomaterials and tissues engineering and so on. Courses in these areas cover subjects such as:

- Computer architecture
- Medical imaging
- Solid and fluid mechanics
- Study of artificial organs
- Systems and control.

All this goes alongside the more familiar biology-based topics such as cells and tissues and physiology. Courses in these areas lead to a range of specific career paths, covered in the Graduate outlook section, below.

Getting in

Each university decides on its own entry requirements. You can see the range of UCAS points asked by each one by consulting the course listings on the following pages.

For Biomedical Engineering, there is a preference for applicants offering physics and mathematics, which is not surprising bearing in mind some of the topics which this course could involve (see above).

However, many Foundation degree courses exercise a more flexible admissions procedure which enables them to take into account factors such as work experience in their entrance requirements and which cannot therefore be expressed as part of the UCAS tariff framework.

Graduate outlook

The outlook for graduates of courses in this chapter is similar to that of th anatomy and physiology graduates described in the previous chapter. If you have ever provided a sample of blood to a doctor, that sample will have been processed by a biomedical scientist. They provide analytical support to the front-line staff – identifying viruses, checking smears and monitoring the progress of treatment. They can also be found undertaking research at universities and working for the National Blood Authority, the Medical Research Council, various veterinary establishments, HM Forces and pharmaceutical manufacturers. Some of the specialist aspects of the work of a biomedical scientist are:

- Virology – testing for infections such as HIV, hepatitis, or herpes
- Immunology – analysing the body's response to infectious diseases, tissue grafts or organ transplants
- Clinical chemistry – analysing samples to check for signs of disease such as diabetes, or the presence of toxicological materials, or to assess how vital organs such as the liver and kidneys are functioning
- Medical microbiology – checking for disease-carrying micro-organism such as are present in conditions such as legionella, meningitis or foo poisoning
- Transfusion science – checking that blood samples from donors and patients are compatible
- Haematology – checking on abnormalities in blood samples which could occur in cases of anaemia or leukaemia
- Histopathology – processing and analysing tissue samples from operations
- Cytology – best known for its role in analysing cervical smears.

If you want to work for the NHS, you will need to qualify to the level approved by the Health Professions Council (HPC, www.hpc-uk.org). This usually means a practical first year on the job practising skills and gaining experience which you record in a log book and submit to the council for assessment.

Biomedical Engineering

The object for those wanting a career in this field is to qualify either as a chartered engineer or as a clinical scientist registered with the Health Professions Council (HPC), or both. The latter qualification enables you to work in the NHS. NHS biomedical engineers work in teams and have frequent contact with doctors, physiotherapists and occupational therapists, and with the actual patients. They assist patient rehabilitation by designing or customising equipment – for example by fitting a wheelchair with a control system within the capabilities of a particular client, or by creating systems to control devices at home when the patie returns. The chapter on **Therapies** covers prosthetics, which is a related area.

However, the NHS is not the only employer in this field. Graduates could apply for work with private companies who develop and supply medical equipment – from artificial hips and limbs to pacemakers – or for university research posts doing teaching, research or development work

What would you earn?

In general, salaries in private companies tend to be more than those in the NHS but many biomedical scientists get their job satisfaction from being nearer the patients and working with the medical teams in hospitals.

Salary scales for medical scientists working the NHS are on a scale from approximately £19,000 to £31,000. Promotion could bring salaries up to £36,400 and very senior posts are paid up to £88,000.

These examples are based on April 2006 salary scales. At the time of writing this book the public sector unions had not accepted the pay increase of around 2.5%, which had been offered in April 2007.

Case Study

Nicola Jones

Nicola is a third-year student studying for a BSc in Biomedical Science at the University of Chester.

'I came to higher education from an Access course at Llandrillo College. I had other things on my mind at 18 and, although I liked my A level sciences, I failed them. Llandrillo helped me back into science. I chose Biomedical Science as a degree because I was interested in working in the medical field as a lab scientist rather than on the front line with patients.

'Chester appealed as it was local and because of its size. It's a small, intimate and friendly college campus. The intake into my first year was about a dozen. The tutors know everyone personally. I found the first year relatively plain sailing as it built on my A level/Access course knowledge. I probably had slightly less scientific knowledge than the people who had come straight from A level, but the Access course gave me better skills in conducting independent research. I took physiology, chemistry, biology and a more practical module in biomedical science which, usefully, involved some work in hospital with the professionals. We had plenty of practical lab sessions. The year was assessed 50/50 exams and coursework. Typically each piece of coursework would be a 1500-word essay.

'Financially, I needed to find part-time work and managed two days a week at a supermarket, fitting the hours around my college commitments.

'The second year saw more challenging modules using specialised technology. Subjects included immunology and cellular pathology. The tutor added spice to one of our genetics modules by setting up a fictitious evidence file for a murder. We used various scientific techniques to look at the evidence, particularly Polymerase Chain Reaction – a process that amplifies DNA to allow analysis from a minute sample. Chester's second-year students all have a few weeks' work-based learning. I worked with North Wales Police on a project looking at reducing the time taken for accident victims to be transferred to hospital.

'I am now in my final year and the course is more difficult. We are studying topics like haematology and transfusion. In addition to the lectures and study modules, we have dissertations to write. Being a contact lens wearer, I chose to research the microbiological content of contact lens cases. I use the investigative techniques we have picked up on the course. I have to produce a 6000-word report – but I could sum it up in one sentence: "wash your hands before putting in your lenses"! My supermarket time is now down to one day per week.

'Most of my fellow students will go on to work in NHS hospital medical labs for a pre-registration year – essential for anyone wanting a hospital-based biomedical science career. However, I am getting married this year and will be living in the USA. My degree should help me find hospital work there.

'The most satisfying aspect of the course for me has been that it has restored my self-esteem and confidence, which had taken a battering after my A levels.'

Applied Biomedical Science

University of Lincoln L39

BSc (Hons): 3 years full-time or 4 years sandwich – C900 L
Tariff: 200 IB: 24

University of Portsmouth P80

BSc (Hons): 3 - 4 years part-time
A2: CC
HPC, IBMS

University of Wolverhampton W75

BSc (Hons): 3 years full-time or 4 years sandwich or 4 - 6 years part-time – C910
Tariff: 240 - 320
HPC, IBMS

Applied Biomedical Sciences

University of Brighton B72

BSc (Hons): 3 years full-time – B900
Tariff: 220 IB: 28

London Metropolitan University L68

BSc (Hons): 3 years full-time or 4 - 6 years part-time – C910
Tariff: 200 IB: 28

Northumbria University N77

BSc (Hons): 4 - 5 years part-time
A2: EE BTEC: PP - PPP

Biochemistry (Immunology)

University of Aberdeen A20

BSc (Hons): 4 years full-time – C7C9
A2: CDD SQA: BBBB ILC: BCCCC - BBCC IB: 26

Biochemistry (Immunology, with industrial placement)

University of Aberdeen A20

BSc (Hons): 5 years sandwich – C7CX
A2: CDD SQA: BBBB ILC: BCCCC - BBCC IB: 26

Biochemistry (Medical)

University of Surrey S85

BSc (Hons): 3 years full-time or 4 years sandwich – C721
Tariff: 260 - 300 IB: 30 - 32

Biological Sciences (Biomedical and Molecular)

Anglia Ruskin University A60

BSc (Hons): 3 years full-time – C900
Tariff: 200 IB: 24

Biological Sciences (Physiology with Pharmacology)

University of Leicester L34

BSc (Hons): 3 years full-time or 4 years full-time with time abroad or 4 years sandwich – B1B2
Tariff: 300 IB: 32 - 34

Biomaterial Science and Tissue Engineering

University of Sheffield S18

BEng (Hons): 3 years full-time – BJ89
A2: BBC SQA: ABBB ILC: ABBBB IB: 30 - 33

University of Sheffield S18

MEng: 4 years full-time – BJ8X
A2: BBB SQA: AAAB ILC: ABBBB IB: 33

Biomaterials and Tissue Engineering

Imperial College London I50

MEng (Hons): 4 years sandwich – BJ95
A2: ABB ILC: AABBB IB: 36
IoM3

Biomedical Engineering

University of Birmingham B32

MEng (Hons): 4 years full-time – HB19
Tariff: 320 IB: 32 - 36

Imperial College London I50

BEng (Hons): 3 years full-time – BH81
A2: AAB

Imperial College London I50

MEng (Hons): 4 years full-time – BH9C
A2: AAB

University of Sheffield S18

BEng (Hons): 3 years full-time MEng: 4 years full-time – BH81
A2: BBB SQA: AABB ILC: ABBBB IB: 32

University of Ulster U20

BSc (Hons): 4 years sandwich or 5 years full-time including foundation year – BH81 J
Tariff: 240 IB: 28
IET

Biomedical Engineering and Applied Physics

City University C60

BEng (Hons): 3 years full-time – BH66
A2: CCC SQA: BBBBB IB: 27

City University C60

BSc (Hons): 3 years full-time – BH6P
A2: CCC SQA: BBBBB IB: 27

Biomedical Engineering and Cybernetics

University of Reading R12

BSc (Hons): 3 years full-time – H655
Tariff: 280 IB: 30

Biomedical Informatics

St George's, University of London S49

BSc (Hons): 3 years full-time MSci: 4 years full-time – BG95
Tariff: 240

Biomedical Materials Science

University of Birmingham B32

BMedSc (Hons): 3 years full-time – BJ95
Tariff: 280 IB: 30

University of Manchester M20

BEng: 3 years full-time – J2BV
A2: ABC BTEC: DMM SQA: BBBBB ILC: ABBCC IB: 32

University of Manchester M20

MEng: 4 years sandwich – J2B8
A2: AAB BTEC: DDM SQA: AAABB ILC: AAABB IB: 35

University of Manchester M20

MEng: 4 years full-time – BJ82
A2: AAB BTEC: DDM SQA: AAABB ILC: AAABB IB: 35

University of Nottingham N84

BSc (Hons): 3 years full-time – BJ85
A2: BBB ILC: BBBBB IB: 32

Queen Mary, University of London Q50

BSc (Hons): 3 years full-time – J503
Tariff: 260 IB: 26 - 32

Biomedical Materials Science and Engineering

Queen Mary, University of London Q50

BEng (Hons): 3 years full-time – J501
Tariff: 280 IB: 26 - 32
IoM3

Biomedical and Molecular Sciences

University of Hull H72

BSc (Hons): 3 years full-time – C700
Tariff: 240 - 300

Biomedical Science

Anglia Ruskin University A60

BSc (Hons): 3 years full-time – B940
Tariff: 200 IB: 24
HPC, IBMS

University of Wales, Bangor B06

BSc (Hons): 4 years sandwich – C900
Tariff: 240 - 280 IB: 30

University of Bedfordshire B22

BSc (Hons): 3 years full-time – B940
Tariff: 160 - 200

University of Bedfordshire B22

BSc (Hons): 4 years full-time including foundation year – B903
Interview

University of Bedfordshire B22

FdSc: 2 years full-time – B902
Tariff: 160 - 200

University of Central Lancashire C30

BSc (Hons): 3 years full-time or 6 years part-time day – B940
Tariff: 200 IB: 24
IBMS

lasgow Caledonian University G42
Sc: 3 years full-time BSc (Hons): 4 years full-time –
940
2: CC SQA: BCCC - BBC
PC, IBMS

niversity of Hertfordshire H36
Sc (Hons): 3 years full-time or 4 years sandwich – B990
riff: 200
MS

niversity of Kent K24
Sc (Hons): 4 years sandwich – B942
: BCC IB: 28

niversity of Kent K24
c (Hons): 3 years full-time – B940
: BCC - BBC IB: 28

ng's College London (University of ondon) K60
c (Hons): 3 years full-time – BC99
: BBB SQA: BBBBB ILC: BBBBBB IB: 32

ngston University K84
c (Hons): 4 years full-time including foundation year –
48
iff: 40 Interview
C, IBMS

ngston University K84
c (Hons): 3 years full-time or 6 years part-time – B930
iff: 200 - 220
C, IBMS

ngston University K84
c (Hons): 4 years sandwich – B931
ff: 200 - 220

iversity of Lincoln L39
c (Hons): 3 years full-time or 4 years sandwich – B940 L
ff: 200 IB: 24
S

ndon Metropolitan University L68
c (Hons): 3 years full-time or 4 years sandwich or 4 - 6
s part-time day – B940
ff: 200 IB: 28
C, IOB, IBMS

anchester Metropolitan University M40
c (Hons): 4 years full-time including foundation year –
49
ff: 40 - 100
C, IBMS

anchester Metropolitan University M40
c (Hons): 3 years full-time or 4 years sandwich or 5 years
-time – B940
ff: 160 - 200 IB: 24
C, IBMS

pier University N07
: 3 years full-time or 4 years part-time BSc (Hons): 4
s full-time or 6 years part-time – B940
CC SQA: BBC HND
C, IBMS

SCOT [Open University] N49
(Hons): 3 years full-time or 4 years part-time – B940
EE BTEC: PP - PPP
, IBMS

ford Brookes University O66
(Hons): 3 years full-time – B900
BCC

University of Portsmouth P80
BSc (Hons): 4 years full-time including foundation year –
B948 C
Interview
HPC

University of Portsmouth P80
BSc (Hons): 3 years full-time – B940
Tariff: 200 - 280
HPC, IBMS

Queen's University Belfast Q75
BSc (Hons): 3 years full-time – B940
A2: BBC IB: 28

Robert Gordon University R36
BSc (Hons): 4 years full-time – B900
A2: CC SQA: BBC ILC: BBC

University of Salford S03
BSc (Hons): 3 years full-time or 4 - 6 years part-time –
B900
Tariff: 180

University of Sheffield S18
BSc (Hons): 3 years full-time – B900
A2: ABB SQA: AAAB ILC: AABBB IB: 33

University of Sheffield S18
MBioSci: 4 years full-time – B909
A2: ABB SQA: AAAB ILC: AABBB IB: 33

Staffordshire University S72
BSc (Hons): 3 years full-time – B900
Tariff: 240 IB: 32

Truro College [University of Plymouth]
FdSc: 2 years full-time or 3 years part-time – C700
Tariff: 60

University of Warwick W20
BSc (Hons): 3 years full-time – B900
A2: BBB

University of Westminster W50
BSc (Hons): 4 years sandwich – B900
A2: CC BTEC: MMM SQA: CCC ILC: CCCC
HPC, IBMS

University of Westminster W50
BSc (Hons): 4 years full-time including foundation year –
B948
A2: CC
HPC, IBMS

University of Westminster W50
BSc (Hons): 3 years full-time or 4 years sandwich or 4 years
part-time day-release – B940
A2: CC BTEC: MMM SQA: CCC ILC: CCCCC IB: 26
HPC, IBMS

University of Wolverhampton W75
BSc (Hons): 3 years full-time or 4 years sandwich or 4 - 6
years part-time day – B990
Tariff: 260 - 320 IB: 24
HPC, IBMS

Biomedical Science (Developmental Biology)

University of Aberdeen A20
BSc (Hons): 4 years full-time – B9C1
A2: BCC - ABB SQA: ABBB

Biomedical Science with Enterprise

University of Sheffield S18
BSc (Hons): 3 years full-time – B9N2
A2: ABB SQA: AAAB ILC: AABBB IB: 33

University of Sheffield S18
MBioSci: 4 years full-time – B9NF
A2: ABB SQA: AAAB ILC: AABBB IB: 33

Biomedical Science with Forensic Biology

Manchester Metropolitan University M40
BSc (Hons): 3 years full-time or 4 years sandwich or 5 years
part-time – C703
Tariff: 200 - 240 IB: 24

Manchester Metropolitan University M40
BSc (Hons): 4 years full-time including foundation year –
C704
Tariff: 40 - 100

Biomedical Science (Interdisciplinary)

Nottingham Trent University N91
BSc/BSc (Hons): 3 years full-time or 4 years sandwich –
B940
Tariff: 180
HPC, IBMS

Biomedical Science (with year in Europe)

University of Hertfordshire H36
BSc (Hons): 3 years full-time or 4 years sandwich or 5 years
part-time – B991
Tariff: 200

Biomedical Science (with year in North America)

University of Hertfordshire H36
BSc (Hons): 3 years full-time or 4 years sandwich or 5 years
part-time – B992
Tariff: 200

Biomedical Sciences

University of Abertay Dundee A30
BSc (Hons): 4 years full-time – B901
Tariff: 168 - 220
HPC, IBMS

University of Bradford B56
BSc (Hons): 3 years full-time or 4 years sandwich – B940
Tariff: 260 IB: 24
HPC, IBMS

University of Brighton B72
BSc (Hons): 3 years full-time or 4 years sandwich or 5 years
part-time – B940
A2: CCC - BCD BTEC: MM - MMM IB: 28
HPC, IBMS

Bristol, University of the West of England B80
BSc (Hons): 3 years full-time or 4 years sandwich or 5 years sandwich including foundation year or 5 years block-release – C980
Tariff: 180 - 220 IB: 24 - 26
HPC, IBMS

Bromley College of Further and Higher Education [University of Greenwich] ▲
BSc (Hons): 3 years full-time or 4 years part-time day and evening – B940 B
Tariff: 180

Brunel University B84
BSc (Hons): 3 years full-time – C900
Tariff: 280 IB: 30

Brunel University B84
BSc (Hons): 4 years sandwich – C901
Tariff: 280 IB: 30

Cardiff University C15
BSc: 4 years sandwich – BC9R
Tariff: 300 - 340 IB: 32

Cardiff University C15
BSc: 3 years full-time – BC97
Tariff: 300 - 340 IB: 32

University of Wales Institute, Cardiff C20
BSc (Hons): 3 years full-time or 4 years sandwich – B900
Tariff: 180
HPC, IBMS

University of Chester C55
BSc (Hons): 3 years full-time or part-time – B940
Tariff: 220 IB: 30
IBMS

Chichester College [University of Portsmouth] ▲
BSc (Hons) (Foundation): 1 year full-time – B948 C
Interview

Coventry University C85
BSc (Hons): 3 years full-time or 4 years sandwich – B940
A2: CC
HPC, IBMS

De Montfort University D26
BSc/BSc (Hons): 3 years full-time or 4 years sandwich – B940 Y
A2: CDD ILC: BBCCC IB: 26
HPC, IBMS

University of Dundee D65
BSc (Hons): 4 years full-time – B900
Tariff: 240 IB: 26

University of Dundee D65
BSc (Hons): 3 years full-time – B901
Tariff: 300 IB: 32 HND

University of Durham D86
BSc (Hons): 3 years full-time – B940 S
A2: ABB SQA: BBBBB ILC: BBBBBB IB: 28
HPC, IBMS

University of Durham D86
BSc (Hons): 4 years sandwich – B941 S
A2: ABB SQA: BBBBB ILC: BBBBBB IB: 28
HPC, IBMS

East Durham and Houghall Community College [University of Sunderland] ▲
BSc (Hons) (Foundation): 1 year full-time – B948 P
Tariff: 100

University of East London E28
BSc (Hons): 4 years full-time including foundation year or 5 years sandwich including foundation year – B948
Tariff: 60

University of East London E28
BSc (Hons): 3 years full-time or 4 years sandwich – B940
A2: CC BTEC: MMM SQA: CCCC

University of Essex E70
BSc (Hons): 3 years full-time – B990
Tariff: 240 - 280 IB: 26

University of Essex E70
BSc (Hons): 4 years sandwich – B991
Tariff: 240 - 280 IB: 26

University of Essex E70
BSc (Hons): 4 years full-time including foundation year – B992
Tariff: 120 IB: 24

University of Glasgow G28
MSci (Hons): 5 years sandwich – B941
A2: BCC SQA: BBBB ILC: BBBB HND

University of Glasgow G28
BSc: 3 years full-time BSc (Hons): 4 years full-time – B940
A2: BCC SQA: BBBB ILC: BBBB HND

University of Greenwich G70
BSc (Hons): 3 years full-time or 4 years sandwich or 4 years part-time – B940 M
Tariff: 180
IBMS

University of Hull H72
BSc (Hons): 3 years full-time – B941
Tariff: 240 - 300
HPC, IBMS

University of Hull H72
BSc (Hons): 4 years sandwich – B940
Tariff: 240 - 300
HPC, IBMS

University of Hull H72
BSc (Hons): 4 years full-time including foundation year – B942
Tariff: 240 - 300
HPC, IBMS

Imperial College London I50
MSci (Hons): 4 years full-time – B901
Tariff: 340

Imperial College London I50
BSc (Hons): 3 years full-time – B900
Tariff: 320

Keele University K12
BSc (Hons): 4 years full-time including foundation year – C933
Tariff: 240 - 260

Keele University K12
BSc (Hons): 3 years full-time or 4 years sandwich – C930
Tariff: 240 - 260 IB: 26 - 28
IBMS

Lancaster University L14
BSc (Hons): 3 - 4 years full-time – B990
Tariff: 280 - 300 IB: 32 - 33

Leeds Metropolitan University L27
BSc (Hons): 3 years full-time or 5 years part-time – B900
Tariff: 180 IB: 26

Liverpool John Moores University L51
BSc (Hons): 3 years full-time or 4 years sandwich or 5 - 8 years part-time – B940
Tariff: 180 - 240
HPC, IBMS

Liverpool John Moores University L51
BSc/BSc (Hons): 4 years full-time including foundation year – B948
Tariff: 100
HPC, IBMS

University of Manchester M20
BSc (Hons): 3 years full-time – B940
A2: BBB - AAB BTEC: DDM - DDD SQA: AABBB - AAAA
ILC: AAABB IB: 32 - 35 Interview

Middlesex University M80
BSc (Hons): 3 years full-time or 4 years sandwich – C700 E
Tariff: 260

Newcastle University N21
MSci (Hons): 4 years full-time – B900
A2: AAB ILC: AABBB IB: 32

Newcastle University N21
BSc (Hons): 3 years full-time – B940
A2: ABB ILC: ABBBB IB: 30 - 32

Northumbria University N77
BSc (Hons): 3 years full-time or 4 years sandwich – B94
Tariff: 240 IB: 28
HPC, IBMS

Northumbria University N77
BSc (Hons): 4 years part-time
A2: EE

University of Paisley P20
BSc: 3 years full-time BSc (Hons): 4 years full-time or 5 years sandwich – B940
A2: DD SQA: BBC HND
HPC, IBMS

Queen Mary, University of London Q50
BSc (Hons): 3 years full-time – B990
Tariff: 300 IB: 32

University of Reading R12
BSc (Hons): 3 years full-time – C741
Tariff: 300 IB: 32

Roehampton University R48
BSc (Hons): 3 years full-time or 4 - 7 years part-time – B940
Tariff: 160 - 200

Royal Holloway, University of London R72
BSc (Hons): 3 years full-time – C790
Tariff: 320 IB: 34

St George's, University of London S49
BSc (Hons): 4 years sandwich – B941
Tariff: 280

t George's, University of London S49
c (Hons): 3 years full-time – B940
iff: 280 IB
MS

heffield Hallam University S21
c (Hons): 4 years sandwich – B940
iff: 220
C, IBMS

niversity of Southampton S27
c (Hons): 3 years full-time – B940
: BCC BTEC: PPP SQA: BBCCC IB: 28

niversity of Southampton S27
ioSci: 4 years full-time – B941
: BCC BTEC: MMM SQA: ABBBB IB: 28

niversity of Strathclyde S78
c: 3 years full-time BSc (Hons): 4 years full-time –
92
: BBC SQA: BBB

iversity of Sunderland S84
c (Hons): 3 years full-time – B940
iff: 200
C, IBMS

ty of Sunderland College [University of
nderland] ▲
c (Hons) (Foundation): 1 year full-time – B948 K
iff: 100

iversity of Surrey S85
c (Hons): 3 years full-time or 4 years sandwich – B900
iff: 260 - 280 IB: 30 - 32

iversity of Surrey S85
c (Hons): 4 years full-time including foundation year or 5
s sandwich including foundation year – B901
BCC - BBC

iversity of Ulster U20
c (Hons): 4 years sandwich – B991 C
ff: 280 IB: 30
C, IBMS

iversity College London, University of
ndon U80
(Hons): 3 years full-time – B990
BBB - AAB BTEC: MMM SQA: BBB ILC: AABBB
32 - 36 Interview

omedical Sciences (Biochemistry)

unel University B84
(Hons): 3 years full-time – C722
ff: 280 IB: 30

**omedical Sciences (Biochemistry,
ick sandwich)**

unel University B84
(Hons): 4 years sandwich – C723
f: 280 IB: 30

omedical Sciences and Chemistry

rthumbria University N77
(Hons): 3 years full-time or 4 years sandwich – BF11
f: 240 IB: 28

Biomedical Sciences with Diploma in Professional Practice

University of Ulster U20
BSc (Hons): 4 years sandwich – B990 C
Tariff: 280
AMLS, IBMS

Biomedical Sciences (Forensic)

Brunel University B84
BSc (Hons): 3 years full-time – F410
Tariff: 280 IB: 30

Biomedical Sciences (Forensic, thick sandwich)

Brunel University B84
BSc (Hons): 4 years sandwich – F411
Tariff: 280 IB: 30

Biomedical Sciences (Forensic Toxicology)

University of Wales Institute, Cardiff C20
BSc (Hons): 3 years full-time or 4 years sandwich – B9B2
Tariff: 180

Biomedical Sciences (with foundation)

University of Durham D86
BSc (Hons): 5 years sandwich including foundation year – B901
Interview

University of Durham D86
BSc (Hons): 4 years full-time including foundation year – B902
Interview

Biomedical Sciences (with foundation and placement years)

University of Essex E70
BSc (Hons): 5 years sandwich including foundation year – B993
Tariff: 240 IB: 26

Biomedical Sciences (Genetics)

Brunel University B84
BSc (Hons): 3 years full-time – C400
Tariff: 280 IB: 30

Biomedical Sciences (Genetics, thick sandwich)

Brunel University B84
BSc (Hons): 4 years sandwich – C401
Tariff: 280 IB: 30

Biomedical Sciences (Human Biology)

Leeds Metropolitan University L27
BSc (Hons): 3 years full-time or 5 years part-time – C900
Tariff: 160 IB: 24

Biomedical Sciences (Human Health)

Brunel University B84
BSc (Hons): 3 years full-time – B990
Tariff: 280 IB: 30

Biomedical Sciences (Human Health, thick sandwich)

Brunel University B84
BSc (Hons): 4 years sandwich – B991
Tariff: 280 IB: 30

Biomedical Sciences (Immunology)

Brunel University B84
BSc (Hons): 3 years full-time – C550
Tariff: 280 IB: 30

Biomedical Sciences (Immunology, thick sandwich)

Brunel University B84
BSc (Hons): 4 years sandwich – C551
Tariff: 280 IB: 30

Biomedical Sciences (with industrial or professional experience)

University of Manchester M20
BSc (Hons): 4 years sandwich – B941
A2: BBB - AAB BTEC: DDM - DDD SQA: AABBB - AAAAB
ILC: AAABB IB: 32 - 35 Interview

Biomedical Sciences (Microbiology/Molecular Biology)

Leeds Metropolitan University L27
BSc (Hons): 3 years full-time or 5 years part-time – CC57
Tariff: 160 IB: 24

Biomedical Sciences (Molecular Biology)

University of Aberdeen A20
BSc (Hons): 4 years full-time – B9C7
A2: BCC SQA: ABBB ILC: ABBBB IB: 32

University of Wales Institute, Cardiff C20
BSc (Hons): 3 years full-time – B9C7
Tariff: 180
IBMS

Biomedical Sciences (Neuroscience)

Cardiff University C15
BSc (Hons): 3 years full-time – B142
Tariff: 300 - 340 IB: 32

Cardiff University C15
BSc (Hons): 4 years sandwich – B143
Tariff: 300 - 340 IB: 32

Biomedical Sciences and Psychology

University of Strathclyde S78
BSc (Hons): 3 - 4 years full-time – BC98
A2: BBC SQA: BBBB - AAB

Biomedical Studies

De Montfort University D26
BSc: 3 years full-time or 4 years sandwich – B941 Y
Tariff: 180 - 220 IB: 28

Biomedicine

Birkbeck, University of London
BSc: 4 years part-time evening
A2: CC

University of East Anglia E14
BSc (Hons): 3 years full-time – C930
A2: BBB SQA: BBBBB ILC: BBBBBB IB: 31

Biomedicine and Medical Statistics

Lancaster University L14
BSc (Hons): 3 years full-time – BG91
Tariff: 280 IB: 32

Biosciences (Medical Biochemistry and Molecular Biology)

University of Greenwich G70
BSc (Hons): 3 years full-time or 4 years sandwich or 5 years part-time – C700
Tariff: 180

Cancer Biology

University of Bradford B56
BSc (Hons): 3 years full-time or 4 years sandwich – B133
Tariff: 260

Cancer Biology and Immunology

University of Bristol B78
BSc (Hons): 3 years full-time or 4 years sandwich – B131
A2: BBB BTEC: DDM SQA: BBBBB IB: 32

Cancer Biology and Virology

University of Bristol B78
BSc (Hons): 3 years full-time – BCC5
A2: BBB - ABC BTEC: DDM SQA: BBBBB IB: 32

Cellular and Molecular Pathology

University of Bradford B56
BSc (Hons): 3 years full-time or 4 years sandwich – B131
Tariff: 260 IB: 24
HPC

Combined Studies (Biomedical Science/Molecular Medicine/Pharmacology/Psychology/Sport and Exercise Science)

University of Wolverhampton W75
BA (Hons)/BSc (Hons): 3 years full-time or 4 years full-time with time abroad or 4 years sandwich or 5 - 6 years part-time – BCF0
Tariff: 160 - 220 IB: 24 - 28
BPS, RSC

Combined Studies (Biomedical Sciences/Sport and Exercise Science/Psychology)

Napier University N07
BA/BSc: 3 years full-time BA (Hons)/BSc (Hons): 4 years full-time – Y001
Tariff: 200

Genetics Applied to Professional Practice

University of Glamorgan G14
BSc (Hons): 2 - 5 years part-time
HE credits: 120, RN, RM, HP

Genetics and Biomedical Science

Anglia Ruskin University A60
BSc (Hons): 3 years full-time – C4B9
Tariff: 200 IB: 24

Genetics (Immunology)

University of Aberdeen A20
BSc (Hons): 4 years full-time – C450
A2: CDD SQA: BBBB ILC: BCCCC - BBCC IB: 26

Genetics (Immunology, with industrial placement)

University of Aberdeen A20
BSc (Hons): 5 years sandwich – C451
A2: CDD SQA: BBBB ILC: BCCCC - BBCC IB: 26

Immunology

University of Aberdeen A20
BSc (Hons): 4 years full-time – C552
A2: CDD BTEC SQA: BBBB ILC: BCCCC - BBCC IB: 26

University of Bristol B78
BSc (Hons): 3 years full-time – C551
A2: BBB BTEC: DDM SQA: BBBBB IB: 32

University of Edinburgh E56
BSc (Hons): 4 years full-time – C550
A2: BBB SQA: BBBB IB: 30

University of Glasgow G28
BSc (Hons): 4 years full-time – C550
A2: BCC SQA: BBBB ILC: BBBB IB: 28 HND

University of Glasgow G28
MSci (Hons): 5 years full-time – C551
A2: BBB SQA: BBBB ILC: BBBB IB: 28

Immunology with Clinical Science

University of East London E28
BSc (Hons): 3 years full-time – C5BX
Tariff: 160

Immunology with Criminology

University of East London E28
BSc (Hons): 3 years full-time – C5M9
Tariff: 160

Immunology and Early Childhood Studies

University of East London E28
BA (Hons)/BSc (Hons): 3 years full-time – CX53
Tariff: 160

Immunology and Fitness and Health

University of East London E28
BSc (Hons): 3 years full-time – CB59
Tariff: 160

Immunology with Forensic Science

University of East London E28
BSc (Hons): 3 years full-time – C5F4
Tariff: 160

Immunology with History

University of East London E28
BSc (Hons): 3 years full-time – C5V1
Tariff: 160

Immunology with Information Security Systems

University of East London E28
BSc (Hons): 3 years full-time – C5GM
Tariff: 160

Immunology with Medical Microbiology

University of East London E28
BSc (Hons): 3 years full-time – C590
Tariff: 160

Immunology and Microbiology

University of Strathclyde S78
BSc (Hons): 4 years full-time – CC59
A2: BBC SQA: BBB

Immunology and Pharmacology

University of Strathclyde S78
BSc (Hons): 4 years full-time – CB92
A2: BBC SQA: BBB

mmunology and Toxicology

apier University N07
c: 3 years full-time or 4 years part-time BSc (Hons):
years full-time or 6 years part-time – BC29
iff: 200 HND

mmunology with Toxicology

niversity of East London E28
c (Hons): 3 years full-time – C5B2
iff: 160

nfection Biology

niversity of Glasgow G28
c (Hons): 4 years full-time – C930
CCC - BBC SQA: BBB - BBBB ILC: BBBB IB: 28 HND

nfection and Immunity

ston University A80
c (Hons): 3 years full-time or 4 years sandwich – C550
BBC SQA: BBBBB ILC: 420 IB: 30

edical Biochemistry

iversity of Birmingham B32
c (Hons): 3 years full-time – C720
iff: 300 - 320 IB: 32

iversity of Bradford B56
(Hons): 3 years full-time or 4 years sandwich – C740
iff: 260 IB: 24

iversity of Glasgow G28
ci (Hons): 5 years sandwich – C722
BCC SQA: BBBB ILC: BBBB IB: 28 HND

iversity of Glasgow G28
: 3 years full-time BSc (Hons): 4 years full-time –
23
BCC SQA: BBBB ILC: BBBB IB: 28 HND

iversity of Huddersfield H60
(Hons): 3 years full-time or 4 years sandwich – C741
ff: 160 - 280

g's College London (University of ndon) K60
(Hons): 3 years full-time – C721
BBB SQA: ABBBB ILC: AABBBB IB: 32

ngston University K84
(Hons): 3 years full-time – C740
f: 200 - 240

ngston University K84
(Hons): 4 years full-time including foundation year –
3
f: 40 Interview

ngston University K84
(Hons): 4 years sandwich – C741
f: 200 - 240

iversity of Leeds L23
(Hons): 3 years full-time or 4 years full-time with time
ad or 4 years sandwich – C741
f: 320 IB: 32

University of Leicester L34
BSc (Hons): 3 years full-time or 4 years sandwich – C720
Tariff: 320 IB: 32 - 34

Liverpool John Moores University L51
BSc (Hons): 3 years full-time – C741
Tariff: 160

University of Manchester M20
BSc (Hons): 3 years full-time – C724
A2: BBB - AAB BTEC: DDM - DDD SQA: AABBB - AAAAB
ILC: AAABB IB: 32 - 35 Interview

Royal Holloway, University of London R72
BSc (Hons): 3 years full-time – C741
A2: BCC - BBC SQA: ABBBB ILC: ABBBBB IB: 30

University of Sheffield S18
BSc (Hons): 3 years full-time – C741
A2: ABB SQA: AAAB ILC: AABBB IB: 33

University of Sheffield S18
MBioSci: 4 years full-time – C749
A2: ABB SQA: AAAB ILC: AABBB IB: 33

University of Wales, Swansea S93
BSc (Hons): 3 years full-time – C741
Tariff: 280 - 300 IB: 30

Medical Biochemistry (with industrial or professional experience)

University of Manchester M20
BSc (Hons): 4 years full-time – C741
A2: BBB - AAB BTEC: DDM - DDD SQA: AABBB - AAAAB
ILC: AAABB IB: 32 - 35 Interview

Medical Biology

Harlow College [Middlesex University] ▲
FdSc: 2 years full-time or 3 years part-time – C190
Tariff: 120

University of Huddersfield H60
BSc (Hons): 3 years full-time or 4 years part-time – C131
Tariff: 160 - 280

Medical Biosciences

London Metropolitan University L68
BSc (Hons): 3 years full-time or 4 years part-time – C900
Tariff: 200 IB: 28

Medical Engineering

University of Bath B16
MEng (Hons): 4 years full-time – H102
A2: AAB IB: 36

University of Bath B16
MEng (Hons): 5 years sandwich – H103
A2: AAB IB: 36

University of Bradford B56
MEng: 5 years sandwich – HB1C
Tariff: 300

University of Bradford B56
BEng (Hons): 3 years full-time – H1B1
Tariff: 260 IB: 28

University of Bradford B56
MEng: 4 years full-time – HB11
Tariff: 300 IB: 28

University of Bradford B56
BEng (Hons): 4 years sandwich – H1BC
Tariff: 260 IB: 28

Cardiff University C15
BEng (Hons): 3 years full-time – H1B8
Tariff: 240 - 280 Interview

Cardiff University C15
MEng (Hons): 4 years full-time – H1BV
Tariff: 300 - 320 Interview

Cardiff University C15
MEng: 5 years sandwich – HB99
Tariff: 320 IB: 30

Cardiff University C15
BEng (Hons): 4 years sandwich – BH99
Tariff: 280 IB: 28

University of Leeds L23
BEng (Hons): 3 years full-time MEng: 4 years full-time –
HHH6
A2: BBB SQA: BBBBB IB: 32
EC, IMechE

Queen Mary, University of London Q50
MEng: 4 years full-time – HB18
Tariff: 320 - 340 IB: 30 - 32
IMechE

University of Surrey S85
BEng (Hons): 3 years full-time – HB38
Tariff: 280 IB: 30
IMechE

University of Surrey S85
BEng (Hons): 4 years sandwich – HBJ8
Tariff: 280 IB: 30
IMechE

University of Surrey S85
MEng: 4 years full-time – HB3V
Tariff: 320 IB: 32
IMechE

University of Surrey S85
MEng: 5 years sandwich – HBH4
Tariff: 320 IB: 32
IMechE

University of Surrey S85
BEng (Hons): 4 years full-time including foundation year or 5 years sandwich including foundation year – HB3W
A2: CCC
IMechE

Medical Engineering with French

University of Bath B16
MEng: 4 years full-time – H1R1
A2: AAB

University of Bath B16
MEng: 5 years sandwich – H304
A2: AAB

Medical Engineering with German

University of Bath B16
MEng: 4 years full-time – H308
A2: AAB

University of Bath B16
MEng: 5 years sandwich – H305
A2: AAB

Medical Genetics

University of Huddersfield H60
BSc (Hons): 3 years full-time or 4 years sandwich – C440
Tariff: 200 - 280

University of Leicester L34
BSc (Hons): 3 years full-time or 4 years sandwich – C431
Tariff: 320 IB: 32 - 34

University of Sheffield S18
BSc (Hons): 3 years full-time – C431
A2: ABB SQA: AAAB ILC: AABBB IB: 32 - 33

University of Sheffield S18
MBioSci: 4 years full-time – C433
A2: ABB SQA: AAAB ILC: AABBB IB: 32 - 33

University of Wales, Swansea S93
BSc (Hons): 3 years full-time – C431
Tariff: 280 - 300 IB: 30

Medical Microbiology

University of Aberdeen A20
BSc (Hons): 4 years full-time – C521
Tariff: 240 - 300

University of Aberdeen A20
BSc (Hons): 5 years sandwich – C523
Tariff: 240 - 300

University of Bradford B56
BSc (Hons): 3 years full-time or 4 years sandwich – C500
Tariff: 260 IB: 24
HPC

University of Bristol B78
BSc (Hons): 3 years full-time or 4 years sandwich – C521
A2: BBB - ABC BTEC: DDM SQA: BBBBB IB: 32

University of Leeds L23
BSc (Hons): 3 years full-time or 4 years full-time with time abroad or 4 years sandwich – C521
Tariff: 300 IB: 32

University of Reading R12
BSc (Hons): 3 years full-time – C521
Tariff: 280 IB: 32

Medical Microbiology with Biochemistry

University of East London E28
BSc (Hons): 3 years full-time – C5C7
Tariff: 160

Medical Microbiology and Clinical Science

University of East London E28
BSc (Hons): 3 years full-time – CB5X
Tariff: 160

Medical Microbiology with Health Studies

University of East London E28
BSc (Hons): 3 years full-time – C5BY
Tariff: 160

Medical Microbiology with Human Biology

University of East London E28
BSc (Hons): 3 years full-time – C5B1
Tariff: 160

Medical Microbiology and Immunology

University of East London E28
BSc (Hons): 3 years full-time – C591
Tariff: 160

Newcastle University N21
BSc (Hons): 3 years full-time – CC59
A2: ABB ILC: ABBBB IB: 30 - 32

Medical Microbiology with Information Technology

University of East London E28
BSc (Hons): 3 years full-time – C5G5
Tariff: 160

Medical Microbiology with Public Health

University of East London E28
BSc (Hons): 3 years full-time – C5B9
Tariff: 160

Medical Microbiology with Sociology (Professional Development)

University of East London E28
BSc (Hons): 3 years full-time – C5L3
Tariff: 160

Medical Neuroscience

University of Sussex S90
BSc (Hons): 3 years full-time – B142
A2: ABB IB: 34

Medical Science

University of Birmingham B32
BMedSc (Hons): 3 years full-time – B900
Tariff: 300 - 320 IB: 32

Medical Sciences

University of Leeds L23
BSc (Hons): 3 years full-time or 4 years full-time with time abroad or 4 years sandwich – B100
A2: BBB IB: 32

Medical Sciences and Humanities

University of Wales, Swansea S93
BSc (Hons): 3 years full-time – BV95
A2: BBC BTEC: DDM SQA: ABBBB ILC: ABBBBB IB: 30

Medicinal Biochemistry

University of Wolverhampton W75
BSc (Hons): 3 years full-time or 4 years sandwich or 5 - 6 years part-time day and evening – C741
Tariff: 160 - 220 IB: 24

Microbiology (Medical)

University of Surrey S85
BSc (Hons): 3 years full-time or 4 years sandwich – C50
A2: BCC - BBB BTEC: DMM IB: 30 - 36

Molecular Medicine

University of Sussex S90
BSc (Hons): 3 years full-time – C741
A2: BBB - ABB IB: 32 - 34

University of Sussex S90
BSc (Hons): 4 years sandwich – C743
A2: BBB - ABB IB: 32 - 34

University of Wolverhampton W75
BSc (Hons): 3 years full-time or 4 years sandwich or 5 - years part-time – C710
Tariff: 260 - 320 IB: 24

Molecular Medicine and Biochemistry

University of Essex E70
BSc (Hons): 4 years full-time including foundation year – C722
Tariff: 120 IB: 24

University of Essex E70
BSc (Hons): 3 years full-time – C720
Tariff: 240 - 280 IB: 26 - 30

University of Essex E70
BSc (Hons): 4 years sandwich – C721
Tariff: 240 - 280 IB: 26 - 30

Neuroscience

University of Bristol B78
BSc (Hons): 3 years full-time – B140
A2: BBB BTEC: DMM - DDM SQA: AAABB IB: 32

University of Nottingham N84
MSci (Hons): 4 years full-time – B141
A2: ABB

euroscience with Psychology

niversity of Aberdeen A20

c (Hons): 4 years full-time – B170
: CDD **SQA:** BBBB **ILC:** BCCCC - BBCC **IB:** 26

ports Biomedicine

iversity of Dundee D65

c (Hons): 4 years full-time – CB69
iff: 240 **IB:** 26

University of Dundee D65

BSc (Hons): 3 years full-time – C600
Tariff: 300 **IB:** 32

Virology

University of Glasgow G28

MSci (Hons): 5 years sandwich – C541
A2: BCC **SQA:** BBBB **ILC:** BBBB **IB:** 28

University of Glasgow G28

BSc: 3 years full-time BSc (Hons): 4 years full-time – C540
A2: BCC **SQA:** BBBB **ILC:** BBBB **IB:** 28

Virology and Immunology

University of Bristol B78

BSc (Hons): 3 years full-time or 4 years sandwich – C540
A2: BBB - ABC **BTEC:** DDM **SQA:** BBBBB **IB:** 32

Complementary Medicine

Including:
Aromatherapy
Chiropractic
Complementary Medicine
Holistic Therapies
Homeopathy
Osteopathy
Reflexology

The courses in this chapter used to be thought of as on (or even beyond) the fringe of mainstream medicine. They were traditionally offered at private higher education institutions outside the state funding system. Prospective students therefore had to pay their own fees (at commercial rates) and pay for their own accommodation. Nevertheless, the training was good. Students completing the courses went on to work in small practices around the country or became self-employed as osteopaths, chiropractors and so on.

These arrangements still exist – but as the NHS and 'mainstream' medicine come to recognise the benefits of the treatment these professions offer, so 'mainstream' higher education institutions are now offering the courses under the usual state-funded higher education financial arrangements. (For more information on student finance, see the **Fees and funding** section on page xxii.) However, NHS bursaries are not normally available for complementary medicine.

What would you study?

Complementary therapies each have their own traditions, philosophies, theoretical backgrounds and practical treatment strategies, developed over decades. Most general complementary medicine courses provide an overview of the complementary therapy field and include modules on:

- Health and disease
- Health promotion
- Healthcare ethics
- Human biology
- Law and counselling.

They may also offer specialist modules in, for example, aromatherapy or reflexology. However, the bottom line is that courses vary considerably in approach. Most courses with the title 'Complementary Medicine' will give at least an introduction to several different types of therapy and possibly full qualification to practise in some of them.

But these courses will not necessarily cover all the skills needed to practise and you may find that you need further training before you are allowed to. It is important to be aware that permission to use titles such as 'Aromatherapist' or 'Reflexologist' does not come purely as a result of having taken a course at a higher education institution. The recognition you need comes from the relevant professional body. It is important therefore to check that any course you are considering will actually take you as far as possible in the direction you want to go. A good starting point for finding this out is the Institute for Complementary Medicine (ICM – www.i-c-m.org.uk).

Course length varies depending on the complementary therapies covered and on the level. Foundation degrees will normally last two years. Full degree courses normally last three years for general complementary medicine courses, and three or four years for herbal medicine and homeopathic medicine.

Chiropractic and Osteopathy

These courses tend to have a less generalist approach. Courses are specific to each profession – but study topics within both can include:

- Anatomy
- Pathology
- Physiology
- Theory and tradition of the respective profession.

The institutions will normally have their own clinic, staffed by fully qualified and experienced professionals and taking bookings from the public. This facility allows students on the course to have valuable practical work experience under supervision.

Osteopathy is regulated by the General Osteopathic Council and chiropractic by the General Chiropractic Council. You should ensure that, if you are aiming to qualify in one of these professions, the degree course you choose has been approved by the relevant council. After the course, you will still need a period of practical experience before you can be recognised as fully qualified and registered to practise.

Some osteopathy courses are at specialist colleges, which are privately run. Fees can be as high as £7500pa and the institution may not qualify for the standard student financial support package so you need to be especially careful that you have understood the financial arrangements which apply to the institution which interests you.

Other forms of financial assistance may be available, such as career development loans. The colleges involved will offer further advice. If you want to benefit from a course financed in the usual higher education manner, look for those courses which have now been established either in, or in conjunction with, institutions in the state higher education system. The case study at the end of this section shows how one student is qualifying in chiropractic at the University of Glamorgan using normal state financial support.

Getting in

Each university decides on its own entry requirements. You can see the range of UCAS points asked by each one by consulting the course listings on the following pages.

However, many Foundation degree courses exercise a more flexible admissions procedure which enables them to take into account factors such as work experience in their entrance requirements and which cannot therefore be expressed as part of the UCAS tariff framework.

Graduate outlook

Professionals are likely to work as self-employed therapists or in small businesses. Sometimes small groups of different therapists join together in a business or partnership – for example an osteopath might work with an aromatherapist. The osteopath might even take further qualifications and offer therapies such as acupuncture or Bowen technique to complement his or her service to patients. So if you want to practise one of these therapies, it's likely that you will either work as a self-employed consultant or find a job with an established partnership, initially as an employed member of staff but ultimately probably working your way up to partner status. All this means that, in addition to using your professional skills as a therapist, you will also have to get to grips with running a small business, employing staff and dealing with accounting and tax issues.

What would you earn?

The evidence is that public interest in complementary therapies is rising. The numbers in training, particularly for chiropractic and osteopathy, remain fairly restricted although they have been rising in recent years. This situation means that newly qualified practitioners could reasonably expect to earn around £30,000pa.

With experience, qualified chiropractors and osteopaths could earn over £70,000. Complementary therapists' earnings will be lower – an experienced reflexologist for instance might earn from £13,000 to £40,000. Much depends on the number of hours worked and practice overheads since practitioners in the careers covered in this chapter are nearly always self-employed.

Case Study

James Slade

James is in the fourth year of a BSc in Chiropractic at the University of Glamorgan.

'I left school at 16, tried an engineering course, dropped out and worked for a while before going travelling for 18 months. Back home, a friend talked to me about chiropractic and I am really glad he did. I was well short of the qualification requirements for a degree course so I took an Access course at a local college.

'In the first year we had to hit the ground running. It was hard after my unfocused experiences in education. Theory was dominant – subjects like anatomy, biochemistry, biomechanics, physiology, chiropractic assessment techniques and behavioural sciences. We had about 16–18 hours of lectures and tuition per week, leading to several hours more private study, essay and project work and exams at each stage.

'Practical work started in the first year. Essential equipment for that included clean boxer shorts as, within a week, we were all stripped down to our underwear as we used each other to learn about bone structure and chiropractic technique! The practical element increased in the second and third year and we needed a 70% pass mark throughout.

'The fourth year takes us to the university chiropractic clinic. Members of the public book in for diagnosis and treatment from students under the supervision of the staff. By now the course is a full-on working week – no more time for my bar job.

'Each new patient gets an initial session of around two hours. In the first hour we talk about their symptoms, general health, previous medical treatment and lifestyle. I can deduce valuable information from the way they walk in and sit. Chiropractic teaches that symptoms from one part of the body may have a root cause from somewhere completely different. The second hour sees a complete physical examination – a sort of MOT. We discuss the results and I book another appointment. In the meantime, I write detailed notes to share with my clinician supervisor. I make my proposals for treatment. My clinician questions me and may make alternative suggestions. In following patient appointments I can explain the suggested treatment, carry out my part in any manipulation, train patients where exercise or posture change is required, or refer them to another type of medical practitioner if necessary.

'Seeing a patient follow my course of treatment and emerge 80–100% better gives me such a buzz. I also experience the daily tasks of running a chiropractic clinic – maintaining the equipment, reception, stock control. Case notes are vital, not just to ensure that the correct treatment is given but also, in the unusual event that we might be sued, so that we have reliable evidence to put before a court.

'Following graduation I hope to do what most chiropractic graduates do – that is, to go into a job in a chiropractic clinic with a case-load supervised by an experienced clinician for my first year out of university. Then I can decide on any further specialism I would like to follow, such as sports injuries or even chiropractic for animals.'

Acupuncture

University of East London E28
BSc (Hons): 3 years full-time – B343
Tariff: 140

Kingston University K84
BSc (Hons): 3 years part-time
Tariff: 80

University of Lincoln L39
BSc (Hons): 3 years full-time – B343 L
Tariff: 200 Interview
BACU

University Campus Suffolk [University of East Anglia, University of Essex] S82
BSc (Hons): 3 years full-time – B343 I
Tariff: 180 IB: 24

Acupuncture in Practice (top-up)

University of Salford S03
BSc (Hons): 1 year full-time or 2 - 3 years part-time – B343
HND, Fd, HE credits: 240, RN, RM, HP

Animals and Horticulture as Therapy

Myerscough College [University of Central Lancashire] M99
FdSc: 2 years full-time or 3 years part-time – DD43
Tariff: 80

Chiropractic

Anglo-European College of Chiropractic [University of Portsmouth]
MChiro: 5 years full-time
A2: CD - BC
ECCE

University of Glamorgan G14
BSc (Hons): 4 years full-time – B965
Tariff: 300
ECCE

University of Glamorgan G14
BSc (Hons) (Foundation): 1 year full-time – B326
Tariff: 280 Interview

Complementary Approaches to Health (Aromatherapy and Reflexology)

Kingston College [Thames Valley University] ▲
FdA: 2 years full-time or 2 - 4 years part-time – B390 K
Tariff: 40 HP

Stratford upon Avon College [University of London] S74
FdSc: 2 years full-time or 2 - 4 years part-time – B300
Tariff: 120 HP, Interview

Thames Valley University T40
FdSc: 2 years full-time or 2 - 4 years part-time – B390
Tariff: 120 HP

Complementary Body Therapies

Truro College [University of Plymouth]
FdSc: 2 years full-time or 4 years part-time – B300
Tariff: 60

Complementary Health Care Practice

East Berkshire College [Buckinghamshire Chilterns University College]
FdA: 2 years part-time
BTEC: PP - PPP

Complementary Health Sciences

Middlesex University M80
BSc: 3 years full-time or 5 years part-time – B300 E
A2: CC IB: 25

Complementary Health Sciences (Ayurveda)

Middlesex University M80
BSc (Hons): 3 years full-time – B340 E
A2: CC BTEC: PPP

Complementary Health Studies

City College Plymouth [University of Plymouth] ▲
FdSc: 2 years full-time – B301
A2: D BTEC: PPP

Complementary Health Therapies

City of Bristol College [University of Plymouth] B77
FdSc: 2 years full-time – B300 B
Tariff: 80 - 120

Cornwall College [University of Plymouth] C78
FdSc: 2 years full-time or 3 years part-time – B301 C
Tariff: 80

Complementary Healthcare

Sussex Downs College, Lewes Campus [University of Brighton] ▲
FdSc: 2 years full-time – B340 L
Tariff: 100

Complementary Medicine (Aromatherapy)

Anglia Ruskin University A60
BSc (Hons): 3 years full-time – B344
Tariff: 160

Complementary Medicine and Health Sciences

University of Salford S03
BSc (Hons): 3 years full-time or 4 - 6 years part-time – B342
Tariff: 180 IB: 24 HP

Complementary Medicine in Healthcare (top-up)

Thames Valley University T40
BSc (Hons): 1 year full-time or 2 - 7 years part-time day
B300
Fd, Interview

Complementary Medicine (Reflexology)

Anglia Ruskin University A60
BSc (Hons): 3 years full-time – B346
Tariff: 160

Complementary Therapies

Bexley College [University of Greenwic ▲
FdSc: 2 years full-time or 3 - 4 years part-time – B302
Tariff: 40

Bishop Auckland College [University of Teesside] ▲
FdA: 2 years full-time – B300 H
Tariff: 160

University of Wales Institute, Cardiff C2
BSc (Hons): 3 years full-time – B390
Tariff: 180

University of Derby D39
BA (Hons): 3 years full-time – B300
Tariff: 180 - 200

Hartlepool College of Further Educatio [University of Teesside]
FdA: 2 years work-based learning
A2: CC

New College Durham [University of Sunderland] N28
FdSc: 2 years full-time or 3 years part-time – B300
Tariff: 40

Newcastle College [Leeds Metropolitan University] N23
FdSc: 2 years full-time – B390
Tariff: 80

Riverside College Halton [University of Salford] R30
FdA: 2 years full-time – B390
Tariff: 40

Shrewsbury College of Arts and Technology [Staffordshire University] S
FdSc: 3 years part-time
HP

Stockton Riverside College [University Teesside] ▲
FdA: 2 years full-time or 3 - 5 years part-time – B300 F
A2: CC BTEC: PP - PPP

Swansea College [University of Glamorgan] S94
FdSc: 2 years full-time – B300
Tariff: 40 - 80 HP, Interview

Tyne Metropolitan College T90
FdA: 2 years full-time – B300
BTEC: PPP Interview

West Kent College [University of Greenwich] ▲
FdSc: 2 years full-time or 3 years part-time – B302 T
A2: C BTEC: PPP Interview

University of Wolverhampton W75
BSc (Hons): 3 years full-time or 5 - 6 years part-time – B300
Tariff: 140 - 220 IB: 24 HP

Complementary Therapies (Aromatherapy)

Bishop Auckland College [University of Teesside]
FdA: 2 years full-time
A2 Interview

University of Greenwich G70
BSc (Hons): 3 years full-time or 4 - 6 years part-time – B256
Tariff: 160 HP

Leeds Thomas Danby [University of Teesside]
FdSc: 2 years full-time
HP

Complementary Therapies (Aromatherapy and Reflexology)

Abingdon and Witney College [Thames Valley University] ▲
FdSc: 2 years full-time or part-time – B390 T
Tariff: 40

Complementary Therapies (general route)

University of Greenwich G70
BSc (Hons): 3 years full-time or 4 - 6 years part-time – B255
Tariff: 160 HP

Complementary Therapies (Stress Management)

University of Greenwich G70
BSc (Hons): 3 years full-time or 4 - 6 years part-time – B257
Tariff: 160 HP

Complementary Therapy

Barnfield College, Luton [University of Bedfordshire] ▲
FdSc: 2 years full-time – B340 B
Tariff: 120

University of East London E28
BSc (Hons): 3 years full-time or 4 years sandwich – B340
Tariff: 160

St Helens College [University of Salford] S51
FdSc: 2 years full-time or 2 - 4 years part-time – B390
Tariff: 40 - 80

Wigan and Leigh College [University of Salford] W67
FdSc: 2 years full-time or 3 years part-time – B300 W
A2: C BTEC: PP - PPP Interview

Complementary Therapy in Practice (top-up)

University of Salford S03
BSc (Hons): 1 year full-time or 1.5 - 3 years part-time – B390
HND, Fd, HE credits: 240, HP

Health Sciences (Complementary Therapies)

University of Westminster W50
BSc (Hons): 3 years full-time or 5 years part-time – B255
A2: CC BTEC: MM - MPP SQA: CCCCC ILC: CCCCC IB: 24
Interview

Health Sciences (Complementary Therapies, with foundation)

University of Westminster W50
BSc (Hons): 4 years full-time including foundation year – B300
A2: CC

Health Sciences (Herbal Medicine)

University of Westminster W50
BSc (Hons): 4 years full-time including foundation year – B340
A2: CC
NIMH

University of Westminster W50
BSc (Hons): 3 years full-time or 5 years part-time – B342
A2: CC BTEC: MM - MPP SQA: CCCCC ILC: CCCCC IB: 24
Interview
NIMH

Health Sciences (Homeopathy)

University of Westminster W50
BSc (Hons): 3 years full-time or 5 years part-time – B252
A2: CC BTEC: MM - MPP SQA: CCCCC ILC: CCCCC IB: 24
Interview

Health Sciences (Homeopathy, with foundation)

University of Westminster W50
BSc (Hons): 4 years full-time including foundation year – B390
A2: CC BTEC: MM - MPP SQA: CCCC IB: 26

Health Sciences (Therapeutic Bodywork)

University of Westminster W50
BSc (Hons): 4 years full-time including foundation year – B992
A2: CC

University of Westminster W50
BSc (Hons): 3 years full-time or up to 5 years part-time – B991
A2: CC BTEC: MM - MPP SQA: CCCCC ILC: CCCCC IB: 2
Interview

Herbal Medicinal Science

London Metropolitan University L68
BSc (Hons): 3 years full-time or 4 years sandwich or 4 - years part-time day/evening – B342
Tariff: 160 IB: 28

Herbal Medicine

University of Central Lancashire C30
BSc (Hons): 3 years full-time or 5 years part-time – B342
Tariff: 220

University of Lincoln L39
BSc (Hons): 3 years full-time – B342 L
Tariff: 200 Interview
NIMH

Herbal Medicine (Phytotherapy)

University of East London E28
BSc (Hons): 3 years full-time – B347
Tariff: 120

Middlesex University M80
BSc (Hons): 3 years full-time or 6 years part-time day – B342 E
Tariff: 160 - 220
NIMH

Napier University N07
BSc (Hons): 4 years full-time or 8 years part-time – B342
Tariff: 200

Holistic Therapies

Farnborough College of Technology [University of Surrey] F66
FdSc: 2 years full-time – B300
Tariff: 60 - 120

University Campus Suffolk [University of East Anglia, University of Essex] S82
FdSc: 2 years full-time – B390 L
Tariff: 80 - 120 IB: 24

Homeopathic Medicine

University of Central Lancashire C30
BSc (Hons): 3 years full-time or 5 - 8 years part-time – B251
Tariff: 220 IB: 28

Homeopathy

Thames Valley University T40
BSc (Hons): 4 - 7 years part-time
Interview

Homeopathy in Practice (top-up)

University of Salford S03
BSc (Hons): 1 year full-time or 2 - 3 years part-time – B92
HND, Fd, HE credits: 240, RN, RM, HP

Oriental Medicine (Acupuncture)

International College of Oriental Medicine [University of Brighton] ▲
BSc (Hons): 4 years full-time or 6 years part-time – B343 I
Tariff: 200
BACU

Osteopathic Medicine

British College of Osteopathic Medicine [University of Westminster] B81
MOstMed: 5 years full-time – B112
Tariff: 220 - 260 Interview

British College of Osteopathic Medicine [University of Westminster] B81
BSc (Hons): 4 years full-time – B110
Tariff: 220 - 260 Interview
GOSC

NESCOT [Open University] N49
BSc (Hons): 4 years full-time – B991
Tariff: 240

Osteopathy

British School of Osteopathy [Open University] B87
BOst: 4 years full-time or 5 years mixed mode – B110
A2: BBC - CCC BTEC: DM - DDM Interview
GOSC

College of Osteopaths [Middlesex University]
BSc (Hons): 5 years part-time day
A2: CC - CCC

European School of Osteopathy [University of Wales] E80
BSc (Hons): 4 years full-time – B110
Tariff: 160 - 260
GOSC

Traditional Chinese Medicine

Middlesex University M80
BSc (Hons): 4 years full-time or 6 years part-time – BT21 E
Tariff: 160 - 220

North East Wales Institute of Higher Education [University of Wales] N56
BSc (Hons): 3 years full-time or 6 years part-time – B341
Tariff: 140 - 240

Traditional Chinese Medicine (Acupuncture)

University of Westminster W50
BSc (Hons): 3 years full-time or 5 - 6 years part-time – B256
A2: CC BTEC: MM - MPP SQA: CCCCC ILC: CCCCC IB: 24
Interview
BACU

University of Westminster W50
BSc (Hons): 4 years full-time including foundation year – B341
A2: CC
BACU

Dentistry

Including:
Dental Technology

What would you study?

Your degree course will last for five years if you start with science qualifications or six if you are accepted with non-science subjects. The qualification usually offered is a Bachelor of Dental Surgery (BDS) but, as with Medicine courses, Dentistry courses usually offer you the opportunity to take an intercalated degree. The pre-clinical phase will take two years and you will study subjects like:

- Anatomy
- Biochemistry
- Oral anatomy
- Physiology.

Teaching will involve a mixture of techniques such as lectures, tutorials, seminars, lab work and clinical teaching. The clinical phase lasts for the remainder of the course. Have a look at the case study overleaf to see how it works.

Getting in

Entry to dentristry courses is competitive and requirements are high, with science and mathematics featuring strongly. Dentists need to be good with their hands and able to tackle delicate tasks with accuracy and precision – so it will help your application if you can show that you have these skills. There are 14 dental schools in the UK

If you are interested in courses related to dentistry this chapter also lists dental technology and oral medicine courses, for which entry requirements are likely to be more varied.

Admissions tests

For entry to some courses you will be required to take an entry test in addition to examination grades. These tests have been designed to help admissions staff by measuring general and personal skills and abilities not directly assessed in academic examinations. Institutions state clearly in their prospectuses whether or not applicants must take a test, and if so, which one. You may be asked to take one or more of the following:

- **UK Clinical Aptitude Test (UKCAT):** this is a 2 hour paper test consisting of four separate sections. There are a number of test dates, but you must have taken the test by 10 October. The fee for taking the test in 2007 was £60 before 31 August and £75 between 31 August and 10 October. The fee may be waived for candidates receiving certain benefits – such as Educational Maintenance Allowances or Income support. For more information see www.ukcat.ac.uk.
- **BioMedical Admissions Test (BMAT):** this is a 2 hour paper test consisting of multiple choice and essay questions. It costs £26 and takes place at the beginning of November. You have to register by 28 September. For more information, see www.bmat.org.uk.

For entry to shortened degree courses for graduates in other subjects some universities use an Australian aptitude test – GAMSAT, which takes place at the end of November. Others use UKCAT. For further information contact the schools you wish to apply to.

Graduate outlook

Many dentists, after their initial postgraduate training period, are self-employed – either on their own or in partnership with other dentists. That means that they run a small business, employing their own staff such as receptionists, office workers and surgery assistants. There are records ar accounting systems to be kept – normally computerised. They may even be responsible for the maintenance of their own premises. Alternatively, you might want to specialise in a particular branch of dentistry, in which case you would be employed in a hospital – dealing with oral surgery, restorative dentistry, child dentistry or orthodontics.

Standards in the dental profession are the responsibility of the General Dental Council. The British Dental Association (BDA) is the professional body to which dentists and some ancillary staff belong. The following paragraphs give information on some of the possible career paths.

General practice

Your training does not end with graduation. The next phase after your degree is one year's vocational training (VT).

Dr Ann-Marie Potts is sole owner of a Macclesfield dental practic offering treatment to both NHS and private patients.

'My practice is part of the postgraduate VT scheme. We take a newly qualified dentist each year and offer a structured programme of experien in dental procedures. In order to be part of the VT scheme, we have to meet very strict standards and have to demonstrate that we can offer th breadth of work required and use of the full range of dental equipment with which new dentists must be familiar. We have to re-apply every yea and that means that we are inspected every year. It does not just mean helping new dentists, it keeps us on our toes as well!'

After a successful VT period, you are issued with a VT number and have register with the local Primary Care Trust for the area in which you want work. You may then become an 'associate' dentist. This means that you become self-employed and work in an established practice being responsible, by this stage, for the treatment of your own patients. The alternative is to become an 'assistant' dentist, in which case you will be employee of the practice.

Hospital practice

The specialist dentist has the opportunity to work with specialist diagnos facilities and equipment. They work alongside consultants from other specialisms and a range of hospital support workers as part of a treatme team. Working in hospitals means being employed rather than self-employed. There is a more defined career structure. The alternative to th VT training for those who wish to go for hospital work is training delivere by the local 'Postgraduate Deanery'. Deaneries oversee training for those who wish to become specialists rather than general practitioners. Deaneries are also useful points of contact for those who have left the profession for a while and now wish to return to work.

Community dentistry

The Community Dental Service (CDS) offers treatment to particular grour of people in the community such as those with special needs. The traini process is similar to that outlined in the General practice section. Community Dentistry is a salaried rather than a self-employed professio CDS dentists could also become involved in health promotion campaigns and epidemiology.

Armed forces

Servicemen and women obviously need to have their teeth cared for. Th are therefore opportunities for dentists in the armed forces. Dentists hold commissioned rank.

What would you earn?

Dentists in their first year after dental school earn £24,000. Consultant dentists in the NHS earn from £69,991 to £94,706 (April 2006). These xamples are based on April 2006 salary scales. At the time of writing this ook the public sector unions had not accepted the pay increase of around 5%, which had been offered in April 2007.

s most dentists are self-employed, there are no set pay scales. Typical rnings for a general practice dentist are reckoned to be between 5,000 and £90,000pa.

ental hygienists could earn approximately £18,000 to £25,000 if working the NHS and up to £45,000 if self-employed – depending on hours orked and overheads. Dental technologists could earn up to £35,000 plus.

Related courses

Dental technology

This is a three-year degree for people interested in working in the NHS, commercial labs, hospital dental departments, private practice or dental schools. Graduates will have learnt the theory and practice of dental design, making dental appliances such as crowns, bridges or orthodontic appliances.

Case Study

Chris Vermazza

Chris is a fifth-year student on the Bachelor in Dental Surgery (BDS) course at the University of Sheffield.

'I knew in my sixth form that I wanted something medical with a "hands-on" focus to it. I was very impressed by my work experience in a dental surgery so chose dentistry for my UCAS application. I am now in my final year and have thoroughly enjoyed the first four years.

'I found immediately that universities have a way of working which was new. At school I was spoon-fed. The university teaching style puts far more responsibility on the student to learn. Lectures, seminars and practicals cover various topics for us to follow up with individual research. The first year dentistry timetable was fairly full with perhaps only a couple of hours free each day.

'My first-year subjects included anatomy, physiology, biochemistry and oral anatomy. The introduction to clinical work with clinical skills manikins and then observing work with patients was the best part of the year.

'The second year introduced dental diseases and studying dental materials. We often worked on problem-based projects in groups of six. Progression in the clinical work saw me with a patient of my own for the first time. Although I knew in advance that the treatment I had to do was simple, I had to present a cool professional exterior in spite of being inwardly terrified. Second-year practical work was mainly restorative – fillings and dentures.

'The third year saw us getting into the general medical field as we learned about the effect of medical conditions on dental treatment. On the practical side, I now had my own case-load in the university dental clinic – doing my own diagnosis and treatment, and learning about record-keeping – always under strict supervision. I also performed extractions and simple surgery.

'One highlight was a six-week placement in Uganda where we helped doctors (there were no dentists) deal with issues around HIV in relation to dental treatment. It's now pressure time in the final year. We are doing advanced restorative work in the clinic – crowns and bridges. Some clinical work has been off-campus at local community outreach clinics. This year's big thing is obviously the final exams. While we have been examined at the end of every year, these exams cover the whole course from the beginning. We have also been assessed on every piece of practical work throughout the course.

'It has been enjoyable. In spite of the coursework I have found time to help run the social life of the dental school and, significantly, to represent the student body on the Dental School Teaching Committee where I get to comment from the student angle on the way the programme is run.

'After graduation we all have to do at least one year in a training situation. I want to make this as broad as possible so I have set up a two-year period during which I will alternate between a local surgery and a dental hospital. I can thoroughly recommend this course.'

Dental Hygiene

Cardiff University C15
DipHE: 2 years full-time – B750
A2: CC HP

Dental Hygiene and Dental Therapy

University of Portsmouth P80
BSc (Hons): 3 years full-time – B750
Tariff: 240 Interview

Dental Hygiene and Therapy

University of Birmingham B32
BSc: 3 years full-time – B750
A2: BBC IB: 28 - 30

Dental Surgery

University of Birmingham B32
BDS: 5 years full-time – A200
Tariff: 320 - 340 IB: 36 Interview
GDC

University of Liverpool L41
BDS: 5 years full-time – A200
A2: AAB BTEC: DDD SQA: AAAAB ILC: AAAABB IB: 36
GDC

University of Manchester M20
BDS: 6 years full-time including foundation year – A204
A2: ABB BTEC: DDM SQA: AABBB ILC: AAAAB IB: 35
Interview
GDC

University of Manchester M20
BDS: 5 years full-time – A206
A2: AAB SQA: AAAAB IB: 35 Interview
GDC

Newcastle University N21
BDS: 5 years full-time – A206
A2: AAB IB: 35
GDC

Dental Surgery (first BDS entry)

University of Bristol B78
BDS: 6 years full-time including foundation year – A204
A2: AAB BTEC: DDM SQA: AAAAB IB: 36
GDC

Dental Surgery (graduate entry)

University of Central Lancashire C30
BDS: 4 years full-time

University of Liverpool L41
BDS: 4 years full-time – A201

Dental Surgery (second BDS entry)

University of Bristol B78
BDS: 5 years full-time – A206
A2: AAB BTEC: DDM SQA: AAAAB IB: 36
GDC

Dental Technology

University of Wales Institute, Cardiff C20
BSc (Hons): 3 years full-time – B840
Tariff: 120

Castle College Nottingham [De Montfort University] ▲
FdSc: 2 years full-time or 3 years part-time – B840 V
A2: DD BTEC: PP

Lambeth College [De Montfort University]
FdSc: 2 years full-time or 3 years part-time day and evening
A2: DD BTEC: PP

Liverpool Community College [De Montfort University] L43
FdSc: 3 years part-time day
A2: DD BTEC: PP

Manchester Metropolitan University M40
BSc (Hons): 4 years full-time including foundation year – B841
Tariff: 40 - 100

Manchester Metropolitan University M40
BSc (Hons): 3 years full-time – B930
Tariff: 160 - 220 IB: 26

Dental Technology (with study in industry)

Manchester Metropolitan University M40
BSc (Hons): 4 years sandwich – B931
Tariff: 160 - 220 IB: 26

Manchester Metropolitan University M40
BSc (Hons): 5 years sandwich including foundation year – B842
Tariff: 40 - 100

Dental Technology (top-up)

Castle College Nottingham [De Montfort University] C21
BSc (Hons): 2 years part-time
Fd

Dental Therapy

Cardiff University C15
DipHE: 3 years full-time – B751
A2: CC HP

Dentistry

University of Dundee D65
BDS: 5 years full-time – A200
Tariff: 360
GDC

University of Glasgow G28
BDS: 5 years full-time – A200
A2: ABB SQA: AAAAB Interview
GDC

King's College London (University of London) K60
BDS: 5 years full-time – A205
A2: AAB IB: 36

University of Leeds L23
BChD: 5 years full-time – A200
A2: AAB ILC: AAABBB IB: 35
GDC

Queen Mary, University of London Q50
BDS: 5 years full-time – A200 W
A2: AAB IB: 30 - 32
GDC

Queen's University Belfast Q75
BDS: 5 years full-time – A200
A2: AAA SQA: AAABB IB: 35

University of Sheffield S18
BDS: 5 years full-time – A200
A2: AAB SQA: AAAAB ILC: AAAAB IB: 35

Dentistry (conversion)

King's College London (University of London) K60
BDS: 6 years full-time – A203
A2: AAB SQA: AAAAB ILC: AAAAAB IB: 35

Dentistry (first year entry)

Cardiff University C15
BDS: 5 years full-time – A200
Tariff: 340 IB: 32 Interview
GDC

Dentistry (foundation year entry)

Cardiff University C15
BDS: 6 years full-time including foundation year – A204
Tariff: 340 IB: 34 Interview
GDC

Dentistry (graduate entry)

King's College London (University of London) K60
BDS: 4 years full-time – A202

Peninsula Medical School [University of Exeter, University of Plymouth] P37
BDS: 4 years full-time – A201
Interview

Queen Mary, University of London Q50
BDS: 4 years full-time – A201 W

Dentistry (graduate entry, Lancaster

University of Liverpool L41
BDS: 4 years full-time – A202

Dentistry (with pre-dental year)

University of Dundee D65
BDS: 6 years full-time – A204
Tariff: 360
GDC

ral Health Science

niversity of Manchester M20

c (Hons): 3 years full-time – **B840**
: CCC **SQA:** ABCCC **ILC:** ABCCC **Interview**

Oral Health Sciences

University of Dundee D65

BSc (Hons): 3 years full-time – **B750**
Tariff: 240

Dietetics and Nutrition

Including:
Dietetics
Food Science
Food Studies
Nutrition

What do dietitians and nutritionists do?

Dietitians learn about the science of nutrition and apply it for the benefit of their patients. Food scientists include nutrition in their courses but are more likely to go for work in food manufacturing or even retail distribution. More detailed information on what is involved in these two areas of work is given in the Graduate outlook section, below.

What would you study?

These subjects are offered both as single subject degrees and in combination with a huge range of other subjects. Food Science and Food Studies are offered at a range of levels including Foundation degree and three- or four-year degree courses. With any of these courses, biology- and chemistry-based subjects feature strongly. Both Dietetics and Food Science include topics such as:

- Applied nutrition
- Biochemistry
- Health promotion
- Physiology.

Food science as a topic features in both dietetics and nutrition, although the manufacturing aspects feature less strongly in dietetics courses.

If you are going for a food-based course and you know that you want to be a dietitian, you need to take the four-year course accredited by the British Dietetics Association. Clinical experience forms the biggest slice of activity in the extra year. The alternative is to take a related subject and go for an approved postgraduate course afterwards. NHS bursaries are likely to be available for students applying for accredited dietetics courses but not for the others listed in this chapter.

Getting in

There is a preference in all these courses for applicants with biology and chemistry. Each university decides on its own entry requirements. You can see the range of UCAS points asked by each one by consulting the course listings on the following pages.

However, many Foundation degree courses exercise a more flexible admissions procedure which enables them to take into account factors such as work experience in their entrance requirements and which cannot therefore be expressed as part of the UCAS tariff framework.

Graduate outlook

Whilst most dietitians work in the NHS, this is a chapter in which, on the whole, the NHS is not the major employer. For example, many food scientists will find work in the food manufacturing industry.

Dietitian

Graduates from approved dietetics courses will complete their registration with the Health Professions Council (HPC) and the majority will go on to work in the NHS. Their patients will include:

- People with weight problems who need either to reduce weight for the sake of their health, or to increase weight where they may have lost it following illness or medical treatment
- People with allergies to particular types of food
- People with illnesses such as diabetes or heart or kidney problems who need to follow special diets.

Working for the NHS does not necessarily mean working in a hospital all the time. You could be attached to a clinic or health centre for all or part your time, giving advice to individuals or groups – for example:

- At pre-natal classes
- At meetings with elderly people
- Talking to students in schools about healthy eating
- Advising other healthcare professionals on dietary aspects of some of the cases they are dealing with.

Dietitians need to be sensitive to a number of issues that may be importa to patients. For example they may be on low incomes and any dietary recommendations would have to be achievable within a low budget. Religious beliefs may affect the range of food from which the diet has to be constructed. Dietitians must be good motivators, able to interact with wide range of people and capable of contributing to the work of a team other healthcare professionals.

In addition to NHS work, dietitians may also find work opportunities with private organisations such as health clubs, supermarket chains and food and drug companies. Here there is some crossover with the food scienc graduates in that they too will find work in this area.

Food scientist

Food scientists, as the name implies, look at the technology behind producing food and drink. It's all well and good to have a new recipe for dish that tastes good, but how does the manufacturer set about making on an economic scale? How should it be packaged to retain freshness? Will it remain in good condition after being packaged, distributed to wholesale and then retail stores throughout the country, stuck on a supermarket shelf, then transported home by the purchaser before eventual consumption? Is the production process stable in that quality standards are maintained for every batch of production? Does it conforr to the quality standards for that type of product laid down by the Food Standards Agency? Have the ingredients been subject to quality control before being considered for use in manufacturing the product?

While nutrition and dietary issues are common ground between dietitiar and food scientists, dietitians are not likely to concern themselves, like food scientists, with large scale manufacturing plant, chemical engineer production processes or efficient production methods.

Food science and food studies graduates will also be concerned with market research and marketing issues. What is the economic retail pric for a potential new product? Will the company producing it be able to make a profit by selling it at that price? Are members of the public likel be interested in buying such a product in that price range and how sho it be marketed to them? Many food science/studies graduates will deve their careers and become marketing or production specialists.

As well as working for food manufacturers, graduates in these subjects may look for opportunities in the civil service, especially DEFRA, food retailers, universities, consumer protection organisations and local authorities.

What would you earn?

Salary scales for NHS dietitians are on a scale from approximately £19, to £31,000. Promotion could bring salaries of approximately £22,800 t £36,400 and very senior posts are paid up to £61,000.

These examples are based on April 2006 salary scales. At the time of writing this book the public sector unions had not accepted the pay increase of around 2.5%, which had been offered in April 2007.

The food science pay levels are more difficult to pin down as there are nationally agreed pay scales. Generally, lab technicians could expect around £18,500pa while research and development food scientists ma earn around £32,000pa.

Case Study

Tracey Alston

Tracey is in the final year of a BSc in Dietetics at Robert Gordon University, Aberdeen.

'Food and health has always been of interest to me and I wanted a career where I would be working with people and caring for them, so when I discovered a course in Nutrition and Dietetics, I was keen to find out more. After a number of open day visits, I realised that there was a fantastic career opportunity at the end of this degree, where I would be a fully qualified dietitian.

'I chose to study at Robert Gordon University in Aberdeen, which seemed to have a great social scene and an established course structure. The course provides a range of subjects and practical sessions. Practical work includes lab experiments such as titration methods and identifying bacteria sources on contaminated food. Cooking skills are developed, which involves modifying the diet to suit individual requirements, for example reducing the fat content of foods or making meals with gluten-free products to suit coeliac patients. There are also computer lab classes to show you how to work the computer and access information from the library and journals.

'There is a specialised computer programme that calculates all the nutrients within a day's intake and then identifies if there are any nutrient deficits. The course also helps you to develop good communication skills through tutorial sessions, presentations and role-play interviews.

'A huge range of topics is covered throughout the course including biochemistry, physiology, micronutrients, macronutrients, food science, organ systems, diet therapy and dietetic practice – and those are just a select few. Work is assessed through a combination of examinations and coursework.

'During the second year of study, I continued to build on my theoretical knowledge and also had the opportunity finally to put it into practice. During the course I had three practical placements; the first was at the end of the second year and it offered me the chance to shadow dietitians at work and get a feel of the real situations people face. Dietitians have a major role in treating obesity, diabetes, high cholesterol and malnutrition. Those people who are affected are desperate for advice because, untreated, these conditions can have huge implications for health. Individuals who have undergone surgery also need nutritional advice and support to prevent further weight loss and to meet their nutritional needs.

'As I come near to the end of my degree, I can now see how many areas of expertise I can specialise in once qualified. My final qualification will be the degree plus registration with the Health Professions Council (HPC). A dietitian has a well-recognised qualification following a rigorous degree course and has to be state-registered in order to practise.

'I have thoroughly enjoyed my time at university, where I will graduate with a BSc (Hons) in Nutrition and Dietetics. I am also looking forward to the future and will be applying for jobs in April.'

Applied Human Nutrition

University of Wales Institute, Cardiff C20
BSc (Hons): 3 years full-time – B401
Tariff: 200
HPC

Bioscience (Nutrition)

London South Bank University L75
BSc (Hons): 3 years full-time – B400
A2: CC

Diet and Health

Bath Spa University B20
BSc (Hons): 3 years full-time or 5 years part-time – B900
Tariff: 220 - 260

Bath Spa University B20
DipHE: 2 years full-time – B901
Tariff: 80 - 120

Dietetics

Coventry University C85
BSc (Hons): 4 years full-time – B410
Tariff: 240
BDA

University of Hertfordshire H36
BSc (Hons): 3 years full-time – B410
Tariff: 280
HPC

Leeds Metropolitan University L27
BSc (Hons): 4 years sandwich – B410
A2: CCD **IB:** 26
HPC

University of Plymouth P60
BSc (Hons): 3 years full-time – B410
Tariff: 220 - 260

Queen Margaret University, Edinburgh Q25
BSc (Hons): 4 years full-time – B400
Tariff: 180 Interview
HPC

University of Ulster U20
BSc (Hons): 4 years full-time – B460 C
Tariff: 320 **IB:** 35

Food Biochemistry and Health

University of Leeds L23
BSc (Hons): 3 years full-time or 4 years full-time with time abroad or 4 years sandwich – DB69
Tariff: 280 **IB:** 30
IFST

Food Biology

University of Wolverhampton W75
BSc (Hons): 3 years full-time or 4 years sandwich or 5 - 6 years part-time day and evening – C560
Tariff: 160 **IB:** 24
IFST

Food Bioscience

Glasgow Caledonian University G42
BSc: 3 years full-time BSc (Hons): 4 years full-time – D611
A2: DDD - CC **SQA:** BBCC
IFST

Food and Human Nutrition

Newcastle University N21
BSc (Hons): 4 years sandwich – B4D6
A2: ABB **ILC:** AABBB **IB:** 32 - 35
IFST

Food and Nutrition

University of Huddersfield H60
BSc/BSc (Hons): 4 years sandwich – DB64
Tariff: 200
IFST

Liverpool John Moores University L51
BA (Hons): 3 years full-time or 5 years part-time day – D633
Tariff: 160 **IB:** 25
IFST

London South Bank University L75
BSc (Hons): 3 years full-time or 4 years sandwich – BD46
A2: CCD
IFST

Manchester Metropolitan University M40
BSc (Hons): 3 years full-time or 4 years sandwich – BD46
Tariff: 200 **IB:** 28
IFST

Manchester Metropolitan University M40
BSc (Hons): 4 years full-time including foundation year or 5 years sandwich including foundation year – BDK6
Tariff: 40 - 100
IFST

Sheffield Hallam University S21
BSc (Hons): 3 years full-time or 4 years sandwich or 6 years part-time – DB44
Tariff: 200
IFST

University of Ulster U20
BSc (Hons): 4 years full-time – B450 C
Tariff: 240 **IB:** 28

Food, Nutrition and Consumer Protection

Bath Spa University B20
DipHE: 2 years full-time – D6BK
Tariff: 80 - 120

Bath Spa University B20
BSc (Hons): 3 years full-time or 5 years part-time – D6B4
Tariff: 200 - 240

Food, Nutrition and Health

University of Abertay Dundee A30
BSc (Hons): 4 years full-time – BD46
Tariff: 180

College of Agriculture, Food and Rural Enterprise [Queen's University Belfast] A45
FdSc: 2 years full-time or 4 years part-time – BD46
Tariff: 40

University of Huddersfield H60
BSc/BSc (Hons): 4 years sandwich – B4D6
Tariff: 180
IFST

Food, Nutrition and Health Science

University of Teesside T20
BSc (Hons): 3 years full-time or 4 years sandwich – BB4
Tariff: 180 - 240

Food Science

Bournemouth University B50
BSc (Hons): 3 years full-time – D615
Tariff: 80

University of Leeds L23
BSc (Hons): 3 years full-time or 4 years full-time with tim abroad or 4 years sandwich – D610
A2: BBC
IFST, RSC

University of Nottingham N84
BSc (Hons): 3 years full-time – D610
A2: BCD **ILC:** CCCCD **IB:** 24 - 30
IFST

University of Reading R12
BSc (Hons): 3 years full-time – D610
Tariff: 260 - 280 **IB:** 27
IFST

University of Reading R12
BSc (Hons): 4 years sandwich – D611
Tariff: 260 - 280 **IB:** 27
IFST

Food Science with Business

University of Reading R12
BSc (Hons): 3 years full-time – D690
Tariff: 260 - 280 **IB:** 27

University of Reading R12
BSc (Hons): 4 years sandwich – D691
Tariff: 260 - 280 **IB:** 27

Food Science with European Studi (Biosciences)

University of Nottingham N84
BSc (Hons): 4 years full-time with time abroad – D6R9
A2: BCD **ILC:** CCCCD **IB:** 24 - 30
IFST

Food Science and Microbiology

University of Leeds L23
BSc (Hons): 3 years full-time – CD56
A2: BBB

niversity of Surrey S85
c (Hons): 3 years full-time or 4 years sandwich – CD56
: BCC - BBB BTEC: DMM IB: 30 - 32
T

ood Science and Nutrition

orthumbria University N77
c (Hons): 3 years full-time or 4 years sandwich – BD46
iff: 200 IB: 26
H, IFST

ood Science and Technology

iversity of Wales Institute, Cardiff C20
c (Hons): 3 years full-time or 4 years sandwich – D612
ff: 140

ood Science, Technology and anagement

riot-Watt University H24
(Hons): 4 years full-time – C1H8
DDD SQA: BBB ILC: BBCCC IB: 24

ood Studies and Nutrition

iversity of Leeds L23
(Hons): 3 years full-time or 4 years full-time with time
ad or 4 years sandwich – DB64
f: 280 IB: 30

ealth Sciences (Nutritional Therapy)

iversity of Westminster W50
(Hons): 3 years full-time or 5 years part-time – B400
CC BTEC: MM - MPP SQA: CCCCC ILC: CCCCC IB: 24
view

iversity of Westminster W50
(Hons): 4 years full-time including foundation year –
2
CC

uman Nutrition

iversity of Chester C55
(Hons): 3 years full-time – B400
: 240 IB: 30

iversity of Greenwich G70
(Hons): 3 years full-time or 4 years sandwich or 5 years
time day – B401
: 180

don Metropolitan University L68
(Hons): 3 years full-time or 4 years sandwich or 4 - 6
part-time – B400
: 160 IB: 28

nchester Metropolitan University M40
(Hons): 3 years full-time or 4 years sandwich – B400
: 240 IB: 30

nchester Metropolitan University M40
ons): 4 years full-time including foundation year or 5
sandwich including foundation year – B401
: 40 - 100

Northumbria University N77
BSc (Hons): 3 years full-time or 4 years sandwich – B400
Tariff: 220 IB: 28

University of Ulster U20
BSc (Hons): 4 years full-time – B400 C
Tariff: 240 IB: 28

University of Westminster W50
BSc (Hons): 4 years full-time including foundation year – B408
A2: CC BTEC: MM - MPP SQA: CCCC IB: 26

University of Westminster W50
BSc (Hons): 3 years full-time – B401
A2: CC

University of Worcester W80
BSc (Hons): 3 years full-time – B400
Tariff: 120

Human Nutrition with Biology

University of Worcester W80
BA (Hons)/BSc (Hons): 3 years full-time – B4C1
Tariff: 120 IB: 26

Human Nutrition and Dietetics

University of Wales Institute, Cardiff C20
BSc (Hons): 4 years sandwich – B402
A2: CDD SQA: CCCC
HPC

Glasgow Caledonian University G42
BSc (Hons): 4 years full-time – B400
A2: CC SQA: BBCC
BDA

London Metropolitan University L68
BSc (Hons): 4 years full-time – B401
Tariff: 260 IB: 28
HPC

Human Nutrition with Health Studies

University of Worcester W80
BA (Hons)/BSc (Hons): 3 years full-time – B4B9
Tariff: 120 IB: 26

Human Nutrition with Human Biology

University of Worcester W80
BA (Hons)/BSc (Hons): 3 years full-time – B4CC
Tariff: 140 IB: 26

Human Nutrition and Psychology

University of Worcester W80
BA (Hons)/BSc (Hons): 3 years full-time – BC48
Tariff: 160 IB: 26
BPS

Human Nutrition with Psychology

University of Worcester W80
BA (Hons)/BSc (Hons): 3 years full-time – B4C8
Tariff: 140

Human Nutrition and Sports Coaching Science

University of Worcester W80
BA (Hons)/BSc (Hons): 3 years full-time – BC46
Tariff: 200 IB: 26

Human Nutrition with Sports Coaching Science

University of Worcester W80
BA (Hons)/BSc (Hons): 3 years full-time – B4C6
Tariff: 120 IB: 26

Human Nutrition and Sports Science

London Metropolitan University L68
BA (Hons)/BSc (Hons): 3 years full-time – BC46
Tariff: 160 - 240

Human Nutrition and Sports Studies

University of Worcester W80
BA (Hons)/BSc (Hons): 3 years full-time – BC4P
Tariff: 200 IB: 26

Nutrition

Bournemouth University B50
BSc (Hons): 3 years full-time – B400
Tariff: 180

King's College London (University of London) K60
BSc (Hons): 3 years full-time – B400
A2: BCC SQA: BBBBB ILC: BBBBBB IB: 30

Kingston University K84
BSc (Hons): 4 years full-time including foundation year – B401
Tariff: 40 Interview

Kingston University K84
BSc (Hons): 3 years full-time or 6 years part-time – B400
Tariff: 200 - 240

Liverpool John Moores University L51
BSc (Hons): 4 years full-time including foundation year or 5 years sandwich including foundation year – B408
Tariff: 100

Liverpool John Moores University L51
BSc/BSc (Hons): 3 years full-time or 4 years sandwich – B400
Tariff: 180 - 240

Newcastle College [Leeds Metropolitan University] N23
FdSc: 2 years full-time – B400
Tariff: 80

University of Nottingham N84
BSc (Hons): 3 years full-time – B400
A2: CCD - CCC ILC: CCCCD IB: 24 - 30

University of Nottingham N84
MNutr: 4 years full-time – B401
A2: BBC - BBB ILC: CCCCD

Oxford Brookes University O66
BSc (Hons): 3 years full-time or 4 years sandwich – B401
A2: BCC

Queen Margaret University, Edinburgh Q25
BSc: 3 years full-time BSc (Hons): 4 years full-time – B403
Tariff: 156 - 160 HND

Robert Gordon University R36
BSc: 3 years full-time BSc (Hons): 4 years full-time – B400
A2: CC SQA: BBC ILC: BBB

University of Surrey S85
BSc (Hons): 3 years full-time or 4 years sandwich – B400
A2: BBC - BBB BTEC: DMM IB: 30 - 32

University of Surrey S85
BSc (Hons): 4 years full-time including foundation year or 5 years sandwich including foundation year – B405
A2: BCC - BBB

Nutrition and Applied Social Science

University of Chester C55
BA (Hons)/BSc (Hons): 3 years full-time – BL43
Tariff: 240 IB: 30

Nutrition with Applied Social Science

University of Chester C55
BA (Hons)/BSc (Hons): 3 years full-time – B4L3
Tariff: 240 IB: 30

Nutrition and Biology

University of Chester C55
BA (Hons)/BSc (Hons): 3 years full-time – B4C1
Tariff: 240 IB: 30

Nutrition with Biology

University of Chester C55
BSc (Hons): 3 years full-time – B4C1
Tariff: 240 IB: 30

Nutrition and Business

University of Chester C55
BA (Hons): 3 years full-time – BN41
Tariff: 240 IB: 30

Nutrition with Business

University of Chester C55
BA (Hons): 3 years full-time – B4N1
Tariff: 240 IB: 30

Nutrition with Coaching Science

St Mary's University College, Twickenham S64
BA (Hons)/BSc (Hons): 3 years full-time – B4C6
Tariff: 160

Nutrition and Computer Science

University of Chester C55
BA (Hons)/BSc (Hons): 3 years full-time – BG44
Tariff: 240 IB: 30

Nutrition with Computer Science

University of Chester C55
BA (Hons)/BSc (Hons): 3 years full-time – B4G4
Tariff: 240 IB: 30

Nutrition (conversion entry programme)

King's College London (University of London) K60
BSc (Hons): 4 years full-time including foundation year – B490
A2: BCC SQA: BBBBB ILC: BBBBBB IB: 28

Nutrition and Counselling Skills

University of Chester C55
BA (Hons): 3 years full-time – BL4M
Tariff: 240 IB: 30

Nutrition with Counselling Skills

University of Chester C55
BA (Hons): 3 years full-time – B4LN
Tariff: 240 IB: 30

Nutrition and Dietetics

University of Chester C55
BSc (Hons): 3 years full-time – B401
Tariff: 280 IB: 30

King's College London (University of London) K60
BSc (Hons): 4 years full-time – B401
A2: BBB SQA: ABBBB ILC: AABBBB IB: 32
BDA, HPC

Nutrition and Dietetics (with State Registration in Dietetics)

Robert Gordon University R36
BSc (Hons): 4 years full-time – B401
A2: CCC SQA: ABBC ILC: ABBC
BDA, HPC

Nutrition with European Studies (Biosciences)

University of Nottingham N84
BSc (Hons): 4 years full-time with time abroad – B4R9
A2: BCD - BCC ILC: CCCCD IB: 24 - 30

Nutrition, Exercise and Health

London Metropolitan University L68
BSc (Hons): 3 years full-time – B491
Tariff: 160 IB: 28

Nutrition and Food Science

University of Wales Institute, Cardiff C2
BSc (Hons): 3 - 4 years full-time or 4 - 7 years part-time
BD46
Tariff: 140

University of Nottingham N84
BSc (Hons): 3 years full-time – B4D6
A2: BCD - BCC ILC: CCCD IB: 24 - 30

University of Reading R12
BSc (Hons): 3 years full-time – BD46
Tariff: 280 IB: 30

Nutrition and Food Science with European Studies (Biosciences)

University of Nottingham N84
BSc (Hons): 4 years full-time – B4RX
A2: BCD ILC: CCCCD IB: 24 - 30

Nutrition and Food Science (with professional experience)

University of Reading R12
BSc (Hons): 4 years sandwich – BDK6
Tariff: 280 IB: 30

Nutrition, Food Technology and Health

University of Glamorgan G14
BSc (Hons): 3 years full-time or 4 years sandwich – BD
Tariff: 200 - 240

Nutrition with Geography

St Mary's University College, Twickenham S64
BA (Hons)/BSc (Hons): 3 years full-time – B4L7
Tariff: 160

Nutrition and Health

Roehampton University R48
BSc (Hons): 3 years full-time or 4 - 7 years part-time – B400
A2: CCD BTEC: MMM SQA: BCC IB: 26

University Campus Suffolk [University East Anglia, University of Essex] S82
BSc (Hons): 3 years full-time or 5 - 9 years part-time – BB49 I
Tariff: 120 - 180

Nutrition with Health and Exercise

St Mary's University College, Twickenham S64
BA (Hons)/BSc (Hons): 3 years full-time – B4BY
Tariff: 160

Nutrition, Health and Fitness

University of Westminster W50
BSc (Hons): 3 years full-time – BC46
A2: CC BTEC: MMM IB: 26

niversity of Westminster W50
c (Hons): 4 years full-time including foundation year – K6
: CC BTEC: MMM IB: 26

utrition, Health and Lifestyles

heffield Hallam University S21
c (Hons): 3 years full-time or 6 years part-time – L535
iff: 200

utrition and Health with Psychology

eeds, Trinity & All Saints [University of eeds] L24
c (Hons): 3 years full-time – B4C8
iff: 160 - 240

utrition with Human Biology

Mary's University College, ickenham S64
(Hons)/BSc (Hons): 3 years full-time – B4C1
ff: 160

utrition with Japanese

xford Brookes University O66
(Hons)/BSc (Hons): 3 years full-time or 3 years full-time time abroad – B4T2
BCC

utrition with Management Studies

Mary's University College, ickenham S64
(Hons)/BSc (Hons): 3 years full-time – B4NF
ff: 160

utrition and Mathematics

iversity of Chester C55
Hons)/BSc (Hons): 3 years full-time – BG41
f: 240 IB: 30

utrition with Mathematics

iversity of Chester C55
Hons)/BSc (Hons): 3 years full-time – B4G1
f: 240 IB: 30

utrition and Professional and eative Writing

Mary's University College, ickenham S64
Hons)/BSc (Hons): 3 years full-time – BW4V
f: 160 - 200

Nutrition with Professional and Creative Writing

St Mary's University College, Twickenham S64
BA (Hons)/BSc (Hons): 3 years full-time – B4WV
Tariff: 160

Nutrition and Psychology

University of Chester C55
BA (Hons)/BSc (Hons): 3 years full-time – BC48
Tariff: 240 IB: 30

Oxford Brookes University O66
BA (Hons)/BSc (Hons): 3 years full-time or 4 years sandwich – BC48
A2: BCC

Nutrition with Psychology

University of Chester C55
BA (Hons)/BSc (Hons): 3 years full-time – B4C8
Tariff: 240 IB: 30

St Mary's University College, Twickenham S64
BA (Hons)/BSc (Hons): 3 years full-time – B4CV
Tariff: 160

Nutrition and Public Health

University of Huddersfield H60
BSc (Hons): 4 years sandwich – BB4X
Tariff: 200

Nutrition and Retail Management

Oxford Brookes University O66
BA (Hons)/BSc (Hons): 3 years full-time or 4 years sandwich – BNK2
A2: BCC

Nutrition and Sociology

St Mary's University College, Twickenham S64
BA (Hons)/BSc (Hons): 3 years full-time – BL4H
Tariff: 160

Nutrition with Sociology

St Mary's University College, Twickenham S64
BA (Hons)/BSc (Hons): 3 years full-time – B4LH
Tariff: 160 - 200

Nutrition with Spanish

Oxford Brookes University O66
BA (Hons)/BSc (Hons): 3 years full-time or 3 years full-time with time abroad – B4R4
A2: BCC

Nutrition and Sport and Coaching Studies

Oxford Brookes University O66
BA (Hons)/BSc (Hons): 3 years full-time or 4 years sandwich – BC46
A2: BCC

Nutrition and Sport and Exercise Sciences

University of Chester C55
BA (Hons)/BSc (Hons): 3 years full-time – BC4P
Tariff: 240 IB: 30

Nutrition with Sport and Exercise Sciences

University of Chester C55
BA (Hons)/BSc (Hons): 3 years full-time – B4C6
Tariff: 240 IB: 30

Nutrition and Sport Science

St Mary's University College, Twickenham S64
BA (Hons)/BSc (Hons): 3 years full-time – BC4P
Tariff: 160

Nutrition with Sport Science

St Mary's University College, Twickenham S64
BA (Hons)/BSc (Hons): 3 years full-time – B4CP
Tariff: 160

Nutrition and Sports Science

Kingston University K84
BSc (Hons): 3 years full-time – BC4P
Tariff: 200 - 240

Kingston University K84
BSc (Hons): 4 years sandwich – BC46
Tariff: 200 - 240

Nutrition and Tourism Management

Oxford Brookes University O66
BA (Hons)/BSc (Hons): 3 years full-time or 4 years sandwich – BN48
A2: BCC

Nutrition/Dietetics

University of Surrey S85
BSc (Hons): 4 years sandwich – B401
A2: BBC - BBB BTEC: DMM IB: 32
BDA, HPC

Nutrition/Food Science

University of Surrey S85
BSc (Hons): 3 years full-time or 4 years sandwich – BD46
A2: BCC - BBB BTEC: DMM IB: 30 - 32
IFST

Nutritional Biochemistry

University of Nottingham N84
BSc (Hons): 3 years full-time – C770
A2: BCD - BCC ILC: CCCCD IB: 24 - 30

Nutritional Biochemistry with European Studies (Biosciences)

University of Nottingham N84
BSc (Hons): 4 years full-time with time abroad – C7R9
A2: BCD - BCC ILC: CCCCD IB: 24

Nutritional Medicine

Thames Valley University T40
DipHE: 2 years distance learning
Interview

Thames Valley University T40
BSc/BSc (Hons): up to 6 years distance learning
Interview

Nutritional Sciences (top-up)

University of Bedfordshire B22
BSc (Hons): 2 years part-time – B400
Fd

Nutritional Therapy

University of Bedfordshire B22
FdSc: 3 years part-time
A2: CC

Public Health Nutrition

Leeds Metropolitan University L27
BSc (Hons): 3 years full-time or 5 years part-time – LB44
Tariff: 140 IB: 24

Oxford Brookes University O66
BSc (Hons): 3 years full-time – B400
A2: BCC BTEC IB: 28

Sheffield Hallam University S21
BSc (Hons): 3 years full-time or 4 years sandwich or 6 ye
part-time – B400
Tariff: 200

Sport and Exercise Nutrition

Leeds Metropolitan University L27
BSc (Hons): 3 years full-time – CB64
Tariff: 220 - 260 IB: 28

Staffordshire University S72
BSc (Hons): 3 years full-time or 6 years part-time – C60
Tariff: 240 IB: 28

Sports Nutrition

London Metropolitan University L68
BSc (Hons): 3 years full-time – B490
Tariff: 160 IB: 28

Health Studies

Including:
Environmental Health
Exercise Science
Healthcare
Health Education
Health Science
Health Studies
Paramedical Science
Sports Science

What would you study?

The courses listed in this chapter focus on the general healthcare field. A very wide selection of courses is on offer. With the exception of Environmental Health and Paramedical Science, the courses in this chapter are academic degrees to be taken simply because you have an interest in the subject area. They are often offered in combination with other subjects. The common feature of courses listed in this chapter is that they usually include:

- Science-based topics such as nutrition, physiology, aspects of anatomy, and health issues deriving from pollution
- Studies relating to the administration of and policies affecting public healthcare
- Reference to laws related to public health
- A dissertation (usually towards the end of the course) that will require independent research.

Foundation degree courses are on offer in most of the subjects in this chapter. All the courses are widely available within the UK higher education system. They usually last for three or four years and normally result in a BSc. NHS bursaries are not normally available for these degrees.

In addition to the typical 'core' elements common to most, some specific details are discussed below.

Environmental Health

Accredited Environmental Health courses all cover the same basic syllabus although the emphasis may vary from course to course. Subjects covered at a general level include:

- Law
- Public administration
- Science
- Social science
- Statistics
- Technology.

In addition, the following subjects are covered in more depth:

- Food
- Housing issues
- Occupational health
- Pollution.

Laboratory work, case studies, visits, group work and tutorials make the academic studies varied and interesting. Group work is encouraged in all aspects of the course, and students will be expected to work independently.

Environmental Health degrees usually last four years and offer a year out during the course for appropriate work experience to satisfy the requirements of the Chartered Institute of Environmental Health. If you take a three-year version and want to train to be an environmental health officer, you need to get the experience immediately after your degree. You will have to produce a logbook detailing the scope of your work experience and showing that you have covered the areas required for professional qualification.

Health Studies

This subject will tend to deal with topics such as:

- Diet and health
- Drug and alcohol abuse
- Government health policies
- Factors affecting people's health
- Psychological and sociological theories of health
- Specific health issues affecting particular groups in the community.

You could also receive training in statistical analysis, computing and the techniques used to research health issues and people's attitudes to them There will normally be less opportunity to have practical work experience during these courses than on those directed at specific careers such as the EHO degrees in this chapter.

Sports Science

In addition to the 'core' subjects above, sports science takes in the study of the disciplines that underpin success in sport of various types. Anatomy and physiology can feature. There will be a focus on what motivates people to compete and succeed in their chosen sporting field. Conversely you will consider whether there are barriers and inhibitions which affect performance.

As with the other courses in this chapter, some courses pick out discussi of issues such as government policy on sport – both as a leisure activity for the general public and as a specialist activity for elite sports people. Some institutions devote time in the course for students to train and participate in their chosen sport and even learn new ones. It may also be possible to pick up coaching or teaching qualifications specific to your specialist sport.

As sports science students will often have such qualifications before the come to their course, they will often be in a position to find part-time wo in local leisure centres, swimming pools or with clubs – enabling them to earn some money to ease their finances. For further information see www.bases.org.uk.

Paramedical Science

This degree includes skills required for work as an ambulance technicia and paramedic and reflects the trend in healthcare towards higher skills and responsibilities for people working in this field.

Getting in

Required entry grades vary considerably according to the subject and th institution. Science subjects are welcome but not always compulsory.

On the sports science/studies side, institutions vary in the emphasis they place on actually participating in a sport as part of the course. The case study overleaf shows one example of a course that requires little physical involvement in sport. The particular emphasis of the cours you are applying for will be reflected in the level of sporting achievemen you need to show on your application form. Some require a high level of commitment while others are more relaxed. Check prospectuses and websites to find out what the situation is for the courses that interest you.

The courses in this chapter are a fruitful area for mature applicants, eac of whom comes with their own individual mix of previous qualifications and experience. Some courses in health studies recruit high numbers of mature applicants who may already be working in a health-related care and want to improve their existing qualifications. Many institutions offer part-time study courses for this reason.

Each university decides on its own entry requirements. You can see the range of UCAS points asked by each one by consulting the course listing on the following pages. However, many Foundation degree courses exercise a more flexible admissions procedure which enables them to take into account factors such as work experience in their entrance requirements and which cannot therefore be expressed as part of the UCAS tariff framework.

Graduate outlook

Graduates will usually find work in the public or private health sector or use their qualification as a springboard to further training in caree such as nursing or health visiting. With further postgraduate training, ey can also lead to careers in industry or in the NHS for laboratory-sed work. Some of them could lead to one of the fast-track medical grees.

vironmental Health

alifications in this area can lead to a Local Authority-based career as an O. Make sure you check that the course that interests you is accredited the Chartered Institute of Environmental Health if you want to qualify as EHO in the shortest possible time.

orts Science/Exercise Science

ese courses often lead to training for teaching, sports coaching and rk in public and private leisure provision.

Healthcare, Health Studies and Health Education

These courses can lead to a range of jobs or further training in areas such as health promotion. (Although there are opportunities to study these subjects on single-subject courses, most institutions offer them in combination with a wide variety of other subjects.)

What would you earn?

It is difficult to put a figure on this as graduates move into a wide range of different careers with different types of employers. Local government EHOs can expect around £20,000 to start with, increasing to a minimum of £25,000 on final professional qualification. Very senior posts can bring scuaries of up to £70,000. There are no national scales for health studies graduates but, as an example, someone moving into the health promotion area might expect to start at around the £20,000 mark. Go to www.hj-web.co.uk/sheps for further information.

Case Study

Kimberley Mellor

Kimberley is in the final year of a BSc in Sports and Exercise Science at Staffordshire University.

'It's a good job that nobody told me how hard this course was going to be while I was in the sixth form. I might not have applied otherwise! However, I am glad I did because I have enjoyed the course so far and have reached standards, especially in science subjects, of which I was not sure I was capable.

'I was a serious swimmer while I was at school – training with my local club in Cheadle, Staffordshire. I represented Staffordshire and swam in the UK National finals. I took A levels in Art, PE, Media Studies and Psychology. I also qualified as a swimming teacher.

'I wanted a sport-related course and applied to Staffordshire University because it was local. The first thing which hit me when I started was that, on a Sports Science degree, you don't spend all your time playing sport. The first year brought me back to biology-based subjects like physiology, nutrition and biomechanics as well as my choice of theory and practice of badminton. We have to choose from a series of study modules as we go through the course but the Sports Science students have a higher proportion of science-based subjects than those who are on the alternative Sports Studies degree.

'For each module we have a series of lectures and seminars with tutors. They lead to more independent study, on our own or in small groups. We have a mixture of exams and coursework assessment, so we always have some idea of the standard we are working at.

'As the course progressed through the second and into the final year I found that there was increasing emphasis on independent study and less on lectures. You have to have (or learn) self-discipline in order to keep up. There is a dissertation during the final year. I have chosen one based on the subject that has become one of my favourites – nutrition. Competitive swimmers need to understand the value of carbohydrates and I have to research the level of understanding swimmers of different ages have about this aspect of diet. The research has taken me to regional swimming galas to collect the data I need.

'At this stage, I am only in uni for two days per week. I find it easier to work at home. There are fewer distractions than on campus but I live near enough to the library to go there whenever I need to.

'It's been an interesting course. One of the best things has been the friends I have made here. I have eased my financial situation by teaching swimming locally and I am thinking that my next step will be to train as a secondary school PE teacher.'

Acute and Critical Care Practice

University Campus Suffolk [University of East Anglia, University of Essex] S82

BSc: 2 - 3 years part-time
HE credits: 240, RN, RM, HP

Addictions Counselling

University of Bath B16

FdSc: 2 years full-time or 3 years part-time – B940
Tariff: 80

Allied Health Professions

City of Bristol College [Bristol, University of the West of England] ▲

BSc (Hons) (Foundation): 1 year full-time – B900 R
Tariff: 40

Bristol, University of the West of England B80

BSc (Hons) (Foundation): 1 year full-time – B900
Tariff: 40 IB: 24 Interview

Applied Health Studies (post-qualification)

Bournemouth University B50

BSc/Bsc (Hons): 3 years full-time
A2: C

Applied Sport and Exercise Science

Northumbria University N77

BSc (Hons): 3 years full-time – C600
Tariff: 280

Applied Sport Science

University of Edinburgh E56

BSc (Hons): 4 years full-time – C610
A2: BCC SQA: BBBB IB: 32

Applied Sports and Exercise Sciences

North East Wales Institute of Higher Education [University of Wales] N56

BSc (Hons): 3 years full-time – C606
Tariff: 180

Applied Sports Science

University of Salford S03

BSc (Hons): 3 years full-time – C610
Tariff: 240 IB: 29

Applied Sports Science and Coaching with Community Practice

College of St Mark & St John [University of Exeter] M50

BA (Hons): 3 years full-time – C6L5
Tariff: 180 - 240

Applied Sports Science and Coaching with Computing and Information Technology

College of St Mark & St John [University of Exeter] M50

BA (Hons): 3 years full-time – C6G5
Tariff: 180 - 240

Applied Sports Science and Coaching with Education Studies

College of St Mark & St John [University of Exeter] M50

BA (Hons): 3 years full-time – C6X3
Tariff: 180 - 240

Applied Sports Science and Coaching with Geography

College of St Mark & St John [University of Exeter] M50

BA (Hons): 3 years full-time – C6L7
Tariff: 180 - 240

Applied Sports Science and Coaching with Management

College of St Mark & St John [University of Exeter] M50

BA (Hons): 3 years full-time – C6N2
Tariff: 180 - 240

Applied Sports Science and Coaching with Media

College of St Mark & St John [University of Exeter] M50

BA (Hons): 3 years full-time – C6P3
Tariff: 180 - 240

Applied Sports Science and Coaching with Outdoor Adventure

College of St Mark & St John [University of Exeter] M50

BA (Hons): 3 years full-time – C6XH
Tariff: 180 - 240

Applied Sports Science and Coaching with Public Relations

College of St Mark & St John [University of Exeter] M50

BA (Hons): 3 years full-time – C6P2
Tariff: 180 - 240

Applied Sports Science and Coaching with Sociology

College of St Mark & St John [University of Exeter] M50

BA (Hons): 3 years full-time – C6L3
Tariff: 180 - 240

Applied Sports Science (top-up)

Loughborough College [Loughborough University] L77

BSc (Hons): 1 year full-time – C601
HND, Fd, Interview

Applied Sports Studies (Health and Exercise)

Newcastle College [Leeds Metropolitan University] N23

FdSc: 2 years full-time – C604
Tariff: 80

Assisting Professional Practice (Mental Health)

Edge Hill University E42

FdSc: 2 years full-time – B900
Tariff: 40 Interview

Autonomous Emergency Practice

Coventry University C85

BSc (Hons): 1 year full-time or 5 years part-time
RN, RM, HP
NMC

Care, Health and Education (top-up

Bournemouth University B50

BA (Hons): 1 year full-time or 2 years part-time – LX53
Fd

Care of the Older Person

University of Glamorgan G14

BSc (Hons): 2 - 5 years part-time
HE credits: 240

Child and Adolescent Mental Healt Practice

University of Central Lancashire C30

BSc (Hons): part-time
HE credits: 240, RN, HP

Clinical Health Science

University of Portsmouth P80

BSc (Hons): 3 years full-time – B190
Tariff: 140

Clinical Practice

University of Glamorgan G14

BSc (Hons): 1 - 5 years part-time
HE credits: 120, RN, RM, HP

University of Southampton S27

BSc (Hons): 1 year full-time or 2 - 4 years part-time
HE credits: 240, RN, RM, HP

Clinical Practice (post-qualification)

Bournemouth University B50

BSc (Hons): 24 months part-time
HE credits: 240, RN, RM, HP

Clinical Professional Practice

University Campus Suffolk [University of East Anglia, University of Essex] S82

BSc: 1 - 2 years full-time
RN

Clinical Science with Biochemistry

University of East London E28

BSc (Hons): 3 years full-time – B9C7
Tariff: 160

Clinical Science with Education and Community Development

University of East London E28

BA (Hons)/BSc (Hons): 3 years full-time – B9X3
Tariff: 160

Clinical Science and Human Resource Management

University of East London E28

BA (Hons)/BSc (Hons): 3 years full-time – BN96
Tariff: 160

Clinical Science and Immunology

University of East London E28

BSc (Hons): 3 years full-time – BC95
Tariff: 160

Clinical Science (Perfusion)

NESCOT [Open University] N49

BSc (Hons): 4 years part-time block-release
A2: DE

Clinical Science with Psychology

University of East London E28

BSc (Hons): 3 years full-time – B9CV
Tariff: 160

Clinical Science with Public Health

University of East London E28

BSc (Hons): 3 years full-time – B9L4
Tariff: 160

Clinical Sciences

University of Bradford B56

BSc (Hons): 3 years full-time – B990
Tariff: 280

Clinical Sciences/Medicine (foundation)

University of Bradford B56

BSc: 4 years full-time including foundation year – B991
Tariff: 200

Combined Honours (Health Studies/Pharmacology/Psychology/ Sport and Exercise Science)

University of East London E28

BA (Hons)/BSc (Hons): 3 years full-time – Y001
Tariff: 160

Combined Subject Programme (Healing Arts/Psychology)

University of Derby D39

BA (Hons)/BSc (Hons): 3 years full-time or 6 years part-time – Y002
Tariff: 140 - 160

Combined Subject Programme (Psychology/Sports Psychology/Sports Therapy/Strength and Conditioning)

University of Derby Buxton D39

BA (Hons)/BSc (Hons): 3 years full-time or 6 years part-time – Y004 U
Tariff: 140 - 160

Community Health

Manchester Metropolitan University M40

BSc (Hons): 1 year full-time 2 - 3 years part-time
HE credits: 240

University of Sunderland S84

BSc (Hons): 3 years full-time or 4 - 6 years part-time – B910
Tariff: 160

Community Health Care Studies

Northumbria University N77

BSc (Hons): 1 year full-time or 2 years part-time
RN, RM, HP

Community Health Development

Bradford College [Leeds Metropolitan University] B60

FdA: 2 years full-time or 4 years part-time – B710
Tariff: 40 - 80

Community Health and Leadership Studies

Sheffield Hallam University S21

BSc: 3 years full-time – L510
Tariff: 200

Community (Health and Social Care)

South Birmingham College [University of Wolverhampton] ▲

FdA: 2 years full-time or 2 - 3 years part-time – L511 S
Tariff: 80 - 140 IB: 24

Sutton Coldfield College [University of Wolverhampton] ▲

FdA: 2 years full-time or 2 - 3 years part-time – L511 H
Tariff: 80 - 140 IB: 24

Telford College of Arts and Technology [University of Wolverhampton] ▲

FdA: 2 years full-time or 3 years part-time day – L511 I
Tariff: 80 - 140 IB: 24

Walsall College of Arts and Technology [University of Wolverhampton] ▲

FdA: 2 years full-time or 2 - 3 years part-time – L511 J
Tariff: 80 - 140 IB: 24

City of Wolverhampton College [University of Wolverhampton] ▲

FdA: 2 years full-time or 2 - 3 years part-time – L511 K
Tariff: 80 - 140 IB: 24

Community Health and Social Care

University of Wolverhampton W75

FdA: 2 years full-time or 2 - 3 years part-time – L511
Tariff: 60 - 140 IB: 24

Community Health and Wellbeing

University of Bolton B44

BSc (Hons): 3 years full-time – BL95
Tariff: 180

Continuing Professional Developme (Nursing/Health Care)

Northumbria University N77

DipHE: 2 - 5 years part-time
HE credits: 120, RN, HP

Northumbria University N77

BSc (Hons): 2 - 5 years part-time
HE credits: 240, RN, HP

Critical Care

University of Glamorgan G14

BSc (Hons): 2 years part-time
HE credits: 240

Emergency Care (post-qualifying framework)

Bristol, University of the West of Engla B80

BSc (Hons): 1 year full-time or 4 years part-time – B79(
HE credits: 240, RN, HP

mergency and Urgent Care Practice (post-qualification)

ournemouth University B50
c (Hons): 3 years full-time
iff: 120 - 180

nvironmental Health

istol, University of the West of England 30
c (Hons): 3 years full-time or 4 years full-time including ndation year or 4 years sandwich or 5 years sandwich uding foundation year or 4 - 6 years part-time – B910
iff: 180 - 220 IB: 24 - 26
H

iversity of Wales Institute, Cardiff C20
c (Hons): 3 years full-time or 4 years sandwich – B910
iff: 160 - 200 HND
H

anchester Metropolitan University M40
c (Hons): 4 years full-time including foundation year or 5 rs sandwich including foundation year – B918
iff: 40 - 100

anchester Metropolitan University M40
c (Hons): 3 years full-time or 4 years sandwich – N910
ff: 240 IB: 30 Interview
H

ddlesex University M80
c (Hons): 3 years full-time or 4 years sandwich or 5 years -time – B910 E
ff: 160 - 200
H

ddlesex University M80
c (Hons): 4 years full-time including foundation year – 3 E
ff: 160 - 240

rthumbria University N77
(Hons): 3 years full-time or 4 years sandwich – B910
ff: 220 IB: 28

iversity of Salford S03
(Hons): 3 years full-time or 4 years sandwich or 4 - 6 s part-time – F900
ff: 160 IB: 26

iversity of Strathclyde S78
(Hons): 3 - 4 years full-time – CH92
CCC - BCD SQA: BBBB - ABBC
IS

iversity of Ulster U20
(Hons): 4 years sandwich – B910 J
f: 300 IB: 33
H

eston College [Bristol, University of the est of England]
c: 3 years part-time
C BTEC: PP - PPP

quine and Human Sports Science

iversity of Wales, Aberystwyth A40
3 years full-time – CD64
f: 240

Exercise and Fitness Management

Burnley College [University of Central Lancashire] ▲
FdA: 2 years full-time – CNP2 B
Tariff: 80

East Lancashire Institute of Higher Education at Blackburn College [University of Central Lancashire] E25
FdA: 2 years full-time – CN62
Tariff: 80

Exercise and Fitness Practice

University of Bedfordshire B22
BSc (Hons): 3 years full-time or 5 years part-time – BC96
Tariff: 200 - 220

Exercise and Health

Loughborough College [Loughborough University] L77
FdSc: 2 years full-time or 3 years part-time – CN62
Tariff: 140 - 220 Interview

Staffordshire University S72
BSc (Hons): 3 years full-time or 6 years part-time – B991
Tariff: 240 IB: 28

Exercise, Health and Fitness

St Helens College [University of Salford] S51
FdSc: 2 years full-time or 2 - 3 years part-time – C610
Tariff: 40

Exercise and Health Science

University of Chichester C58
BSc (Hons): 3 years full-time – BC96
Tariff: 180 - 220 IB: 28

Exercise and Health Sciences

University of Gloucestershire G50
BSc (Hons): 3 years full-time – C602
Tariff: 240

University of Salford S03
BSc (Hons): 3 years full-time or 3 - 6 years part-time – CB69
Tariff: 180 - 200 IB: 27

Exercise and Health Sciences and Health, Community and Social Care

University of Gloucestershire G50
BA (Hons)/BSc (Hons): 3 years full-time – CL65
Tariff: 200 - 260 IB: 26 - 30

Exercise and Health Sciences and Leisure and Sport Management

University of Gloucestershire G50
BA (Hons)/BSc (Hons): 3 years full-time – CNPF
Tariff: 200 - 260 IB: 26 - 30

Exercise and Health Sciences and Psychology

University of Gloucestershire G50
BA (Hons)/BSc (Hons): 3 years full-time – BC98
Tariff: 200 - 260 IB: 26 - 30
BPS

Exercise and Health (top-up)

University of Paisley P20
BSc: 3 years full-time BSc (Hons): 4 years full-time – CB69
HND

Exercise, Nutrition and Health

University of Central Lancashire C30
BSc (Hons): 3 years full-time – C601
Tariff: 220 - 240

Kingston University K84
BSc (Hons): 4 years full-time including foundation year or 5 years sandwich including foundation year – CB64
Tariff: 40

Kingston University K84
BSc (Hons): 4 years sandwich – BB4X
Tariff: 220 - 260

Kingston University K84
BSc (Hons): 3 years full-time or 6 years part-time – BB49
Tariff: 220 - 260

Oxford Brookes University O66
BSc (Hons): 3 years full-time – CB6K
A2: BCC

Roehampton University R48
BSc (Hons): 3 years full-time – CB64
Tariff: 160

Exercise, Nutrition and Health and Hospitality Management Studies

Oxford Brookes University O66
BA (Hons)/BSc (Hons): 3 years full-time – CNP2
A2: BCC

Exercise, Nutrition and Health and Human Biology

Oxford Brookes University O66
BA (Hons)/BSc (Hons): 3 years full-time – CB6C
A2: BCC

Exercise, Nutrition and Health with Japanese

Oxford Brookes University O66
BA (Hons)/BSc (Hons): 3 years full-time or 3 years full-time with time abroad – B9T2
A2: BCC

Exercise, Nutrition and Health and Leisure Planning

Oxford Brookes University O66
BA (Hons)/BSc (Hons): 3 years full-time – CK6H
A2: BCC

Exercise, Nutrition and Health and Marketing Management

Oxford Brookes University O66
BA (Hons)/BSc (Hons): 3 years full-time – CN6N
A2: BCC

Exercise, Nutrition and Health and Mathematics

Oxford Brookes University O66
BA (Hons)/BSc (Hons): 3 years full-time – CG6D
A2: BCC

Exercise, Nutrition and Health and Nutrition

Oxford Brookes University O66
BA (Hons)/BSc (Hons): 3 years full-time – CB6L
A2: BCC

Exercise, Nutrition and Health and Philosophy

Oxford Brookes University O66
BA (Hons)/BSc (Hons): 3 years full-time – CV6N
A2: BCC

Exercise, Nutrition and Health and Psychology

Oxford Brookes University O66
BA (Hons)/BSc (Hons): 3 years full-time – CC6W
A2: BCC

Exercise, Nutrition and Health and Religion, Culture and Ethics

Oxford Brookes University O66
BA (Hons)/BSc (Hons): 3 years full-time – CV6Q
A2: BCC

Exercise, Nutrition and Health and Sports and Coaching Studies

Oxford Brookes University O66
BA (Hons)/BSc (Hons): 3 years full-time – C605
A2: BCC

Exercise, Nutrition and Health and Tourism Management

Oxford Brookes University O66
BA (Hons)/BSc (Hons): 3 years full-time – CN6W
A2: BCC

Exercise Science

Sheffield Hallam University S21
BSc (Hons): 3 years full-time or 6 years part-time – C601
Tariff: 280

Exercise Science and Cardiac Rehabilitation

Leeds Metropolitan University L27
BSc (Hons): 3 years full-time – C6B8
Tariff: 220 - 260 IB: 28

Exercise Science (Health and Rehabilitation)

Bournemouth University B50
BSc (Hons): 3 years full-time – CB69
Tariff: 160 - 180

Exercise Science and Nutrition

Leeds Metropolitan University L27
BSc (Hons): 3 years full-time – BC46
Tariff: 220 - 260 IB: 28

Exercise Science and Obesity Management

Leeds Metropolitan University L27
BSc (Hons): 3 years full-time – C6B9
Tariff: 220 - 260 IB: 28

Exercise and Sport Sciences

University of Exeter E84
BSc (Hons): 3 years full-time – C602
Tariff: 300 - 320 IB: 32 - 34

Fitness and Community Health

Newman College of Higher Education [University of Leicester] N36
Fd: 3 years part-time
Interview

Fitness and Health

University of East London E28
BSc (Hons): 4 years full-time including foundation year – B997
Tariff: 60

University of East London E28
BSc (Hons): 3 years full-time or 6 years part-time – B992
Tariff: 160

Health

University of Greenwich G70
BSc (Hons): 3 years full-time or 4 years part-time – B990
Tariff: 160 RN, RM, HP

Health Care

University of Bedfordshire B22
BSc (Hons): 1 year full-time or 4 - 5 years part-time
HE credits: 240

Health Care (Acute and Critical Care

University of Bedfordshire B22
BA (Hons): 2 years part-time
HE credits: 240

Health Care (Care Management)

University of Bedfordshire B22
BA (Hons): 2 years part-time
HE credits: 240

Health Care (Health Service Practic

University of Bedfordshire B22
BA (Hons): 2 years part-time
HE credits: 240

Health Care Law and Ethics

Brunel University B84
BSc (Hons): 3 years full-time or 4 - 6 years part-time – L4M1
HE credits: 120 - 240

Health and Care Management

Coleg Sir Gâr [University of Glamorgan C22
FdSc: 2 years full-time – L510
Tariff: 60

Health Care and Management

Thames College of Professional Studie [University of London]
BSc: 3 years full-time

Health Care (Mental Health or Learning Disabilities)

University of Bedfordshire B22
BA (Hons): 2 years part-time
HE credits: 240

Health Care (Palliative Care)

University of Bedfordshire B22
BA (Hons): 2 years part-time
RN, HP

Health and Care Practice

Blackpool and the Fylde College [Lancaster University] B41
FdA: 2 years full-time – L510 C
Tariff: 80 Interview

lth Care Practice

ersity Campus Suffolk [University of Anglia, University of Essex] S82
2 years full-time – BL95 I
60 - 120

ersity of York Y50
: 2 - 5 years part-time

ersity of York Y50
Hons): 2 - 5 years part-time

lth Care Practice (with pathway cific awards)

eorge's, University of London gston University] S49
4 years part-time
M

eorge's, University of London gston University] S49
: 4 years part-time
M

lth Care Sciences

ersity of East London E28
2 years full-time – B900
80

lth Care (Women's Health)

ersity of Bedfordshire B22
ons): 2 years part-time
edits: 240

lth and Child Development

ersity of Greenwich G70
Hons): 3 years full-time – BL95
180 IB: 24

lth and Community Care Services

College [University of Lincoln] H73
years part-time

lth and Community Practice

tol, University of the West of England
Hons): 1 year full-time or 2 - 3 years part-time –
edits: 240, RN, RM, Interview

lth, Community and Social Care

ncester College [University of ucestershire] ▲
up to 3 years part-time – L510 C
80

University of Gloucestershire G50
BSc (Hons): 3 years full-time – L511
Tariff: 120 HP

Gloucestershire College of Arts and Technology [University of Gloucestershire] ▲
FdSc: 2 years full-time or 2 - 3 years part-time – L510 G
Tariff: 80

Health, Community and Social Care and Psychology

University of Gloucestershire G50
BA (Hons)/BSc (Hons): 3 years full-time – LC58
Tariff: 200 - 280
BPS

Health, Community and Social Care and Sociology

University of Gloucestershire G50
BA (Hons)/BSc (Hons): 3 years full-time – LL53
Tariff: 200 - 280 IB: 26

Health, Community and Social Care and Sports Development

University of Gloucestershire G50
BA (Hons)/BSc (Hons): 3 years full-time – LC56
Tariff: 200 - 260

Health and Community Studies

University Centre Barnsley [University of Huddersfield] ▲
BSc (Hons): 3 years full-time – L540 X
Tariff: 200 - 220

Cornwall College [University of Plymouth] C78
FdA: 2 years full-time – L590 C
A2: E

University of Huddersfield H60
BSc/BSc (Hons): 3 years full-time or 5 years part-time – L540
Tariff: 200 - 220

University Centre Oldham [University of Huddersfield] ▲
BSc (Hons): 3 years full-time – L540 Z
Tariff: 200 - 220

Health with Economics

University of Greenwich G70
BSc (Hons): 3 years full-time – B9L1
Tariff: 160

Health and Education

University of Greenwich G70
BSc (Hons): 3 years full-time – BX93
Tariff: 160 IB: 24

Health with Education

University of Greenwich G70
BSc (Hons): 3 years full-time – B9X3
Tariff: 160 IB: 24

Health and Environment

Nottingham Trent University N91
BSc (Hons): 3 years full-time or 4 years sandwich – BF98
Tariff: 240

Health and Exercise

University of Northampton N38
BSc (Hons): 3 year (s) full-time or 5 years part-time – BC96
Tariff: 180 - 220

Trinity College Carmarthen [University of Wales] T80
BA (Hons): 3 years full-time – BC96
Tariff: 140 - 360

Trinity College Carmarthen [University of Wales] T80
FdA: 2 years full-time – B490
Tariff: 100

Health and Exercise with Coaching Science

St Mary's University College, Twickenham S64
BA (Hons)/BSc (Hons): 3 years full-time – B9CQ
Tariff: 160

Health and Exercise with Geography

St Mary's University College, Twickenham S64
BA (Hons)/BSc (Hons): 3 years full-time – B9FV
Tariff: 160

Health and Exercise and Human Biology

St Mary's University College, Twickenham S64
BA (Hons)/BSc (Hons): 3 years full-time – BCY1
Tariff: 160

Health and Exercise with Human Biology

St Mary's University College, Twickenham S64
BA (Hons)/BSc (Hons): 3 years full-time – B9CC
Tariff: 160

Health and Exercise and Management Studies

St Mary's University College, Twickenham S64
BA (Hons)/BSc (Hons): 3 years full-time – BNY2
Tariff: 160

Health and Exercise with Management Studies

St Mary's University College, Twickenham S64
BA (Hons)/BSc (Hons): 3 years full-time – B9NF
Tariff: 160

Health and Exercise and Media Arts

St Mary's University College, Twickenham S64
BA (Hons)/BSc (Hons): 3 years full-time – BPY3
Tariff: 160

Health and Exercise with Media Arts

St Mary's University College, Twickenham S64
BA (Hons)/BSc (Hons): 3 years full-time – B9PH
Tariff: 160

Health and Exercise and Nutrition

St Mary's University College, Twickenham S64
BA (Hons)/BSc (Hons): 3 years full-time – BBY4
Tariff: 160

Health and Exercise with Nutrition

St Mary's University College, Twickenham S64
BA (Hons)/BSc (Hons): 3 years full-time – B9BL
Tariff: 160 - 200

Health and Exercise and Physical Education in the Community

St Mary's University College, Twickenham S64
BA (Hons)/BSc (Hons): 3 years full-time – BCY9
Tariff: 160

Health and Exercise with Physical Education in the Community

St Mary's University College, Twickenham S64
BA (Hons)/BSc (Hons): 3 years full-time – B9CY
Tariff: 160

Health and Exercise and Physical Theatre

St Mary's University College, Twickenham S64
BA (Hons)/BSc (Hons): 3 years full-time – BW94
Tariff: 160

Health and Exercise with Physical Theatre

St Mary's University College, Twickenham S64
BA (Hons)/BSc (Hons): 3 years full-time – B9WL
Tariff: 160

Health and Exercise and Psychology

St Mary's University College, Twickenham S64
BA (Hons)/BSc (Hons): 3 years full-time – BCY8
Tariff: 160

Health and Exercise with Psychology

St Mary's University College, Twickenham S64
BA (Hons)/BSc (Hons): 3 years full-time – B9CV
Tariff: 160

Health and Exercise Science

Thames Valley University T40
FdSc: 2 years full-time or 2 - 5 years part-time – BC96
Tariff: 40

Thames Valley University T40
BSc (Hons): 3 years full-time – B990
Tariff: 180 IB: 30

Health and Exercise Science (Exercise Physiology and Nutrition)

Thames Valley University T40
BSc (Hons): 3 years full-time – BB14
Tariff: 180 IB: 30

Health and Exercise Science (Exercise and Sport Psychology)

Thames Valley University T40
BSc (Hons): 3 years full-time – BC16
Tariff: 180 IB: 30

Health and Exercise Science (Physical Activity and Health)

Thames Valley University T40
BSc (Hons): 3 years full-time – BL95
Tariff: 180 IB: 30

Health and Exercise Science (Sports Science and Medicine)

Thames Valley University T40
BSc (Hons): 3 years full-time – CB6X
Tariff: 180 IB: 30

Health and Exercise and Sport Science

St Mary's University College, Twickenham S64
BA (Hons)/BSc (Hons): 3 years full-time – BCY6
Tariff: 160

Health and Exercise with Sport Science

St Mary's University College, Twickenham S64
BA (Hons)/BSc (Hons): 3 years full-time – B9C6
Tariff: 160 - 200

Health and Exercise and Sports Studies

Trinity College Carmarthen [University o Wales] T80
BA (Hons): 3 years full-time – BC46
Tariff: 180 - 360

Health and Exercise and Tourism

St Mary's University College, Twickenham S64
BA (Hons)/BSc (Hons): 3 years full-time – BNY8
Tariff: 160

Health and Exercise with Tourism

St Mary's University College, Twickenham S64
BA (Hons)/BSc (Hons): 3 years full-time – B9NV
Tariff: 160 - 200

Health and Fitness

Barnet College [Middlesex University]
FdSc: 2 years full-time or 4 years part-time – BC96 V
Tariff: 100 IB: 28

Health, Fitness and Holistic Therapies

University of Wales Institute, Cardiff C
FdSc: 2 years full-time – BC36
Tariff: 80

Health Fitness and Holistic Therap Management (top-up)

University of Wales Institute, Cardiff C
BA/BA (Hons): 1 year full-time – BB39
HND

Health and Fitness Management

Cornwall College [University of Plymouth] C78
FdSc: 2 years full-time – NC26 C
Tariff: 80

Southampton Solent University S30
BA (Hons): 3 years full-time – CBP9
Tariff: 200

Health, Fitness and Personal Train

University of Bedfordshire B22
FdSc: 2 years full-time – C609
Tariff: 80 - 120

ealth with Forensic Biology

verpool Hope University L46

(Hons)/BSc (Hons): 3 years full-time – B9F4
iff: 240

ealth and Human Biology

verpool Hope University L46

(Hons)/BSc (Hons): 3 years full-time – BB19
iff: 180 - 240

ealth and Human Sciences

iversity of Essex E70

(Hons): 3 years full-time – BC98
ff: 260 - 300 IB: 27 - 29

ealth and Illness

ughborough College [Loughborough iversity] L77

c: 3 years full-time – B900
ff: 140

ealth Improvement and Social hange

iversity of Cumbria C99

Hons): 3 years full-time – BL9H
f: 160 IB: 30

alth and Inclusive Education

erpool Hope University L46

Hons)/BSc (Hons): 3 years full-time – XB39
f: 240

alth Informatics (by blended arning)

iversity of Central Lancashire C30

: 2 years full-time or 3 years part-time
f: 80

alth and Information Technology

versity of Greenwich G70

(Hons): 3 years full-time – BG95
f: 160 IB: 24

alth and Internet Technology

erpool Hope University L46

Hons)/BSc (Hons): 3 years full-time – GBM9
: 180 - 240

alth and Irish Studies

erpool Hope University L46

Hons)/BSc (Hons): 3 years full-time – BQ95
: 180 - 240

Health and Law

Liverpool Hope University L46

BA (Hons)/BSc (Hons): 3 years full-time – MB18
Tariff: 180 - 240

Health and Learning Disabilities

University of Greenwich G70

BSc (Hons): 3 years full-time – BB97
Tariff: 160 IB: 24

Health with Learning Disabilities

University of Greenwich G70

BSc (Hons): 3 years full-time – B9B7
Tariff: 160 IB: 24

Health and Leisure

Liverpool Hope University L46

BA (Hons)/BSc (Hons): 3 years full-time – NB29
Tariff: 180 - 240

Health and Leisure Studies

Stranmillis University College [Queen's University Belfast] S79

BSc (Hons): 3 years full-time – LL34
A2: BCC HND

Health and Lifestyle

Bell College [University of Paisley] B26

BSc: 3 years full-time – B901
SQA: CCC

Bell College [University of Paisley] B26

DipHE: 2 years full-time – B900
SQA: CC Interview

Health and Lifestyle Management

University Campus Suffolk [University of East Anglia, University of Essex] S82

BSc (Hons): 3 years full-time – BN92 I
Tariff: 160

Health and Medical Sciences (Paramedic pathway)

Kingston University K84

FdSc: 2 years full-time
A2

Health and Music

Liverpool Hope University L46

BA (Hons)/BSc (Hons): 3 years full-time – BWX3
Tariff: 180 - 240

Health with Nutrition

Liverpool Hope University L46

BA (Hons)/BSc (Hons): 3 years full-time – B9B4
Tariff: 180 - 240

Health, Nutrition and Fitness

Liverpool Hope University L46

BSc (Hons): 3 years full-time or 6 years part-time – B902
Tariff: 220 IB: 25

Health and Philosophy and Ethics

Liverpool Hope University L46

BA (Hons)/BSc (Hons): 3 years full-time – BV95
Tariff: 180 - 240

Health and Physical Activity

Manchester College of Arts and Technology [Manchester Metropolitan University] M10

FdA: 2 years full-time – B900
Tariff: 40

College of St Mark & St John [University of Exeter] M50

BSc (Hons): 3 years full-time – CB69
Tariff: 180 - 240

Health and Politics

Liverpool Hope University L46

BA (Hons)/BSc (Hons): 3 years full-time – LB29
Tariff: 180 - 240

Health Professional Studies

University of Huddersfield H60

BSc (Hons) (Foundation): 1 year full-time or 3 years part-time – B991
Tariff: 120 Interview

University of Hull H72

BSc (Hons): 3 years part-time
HE credits: 240, RN, RM, HP

Health Promotion

University of Aberdeen A20

BSc: 3 years full-time BSc (Hons): 4 years full-time – B901
A2: CCD - BBC SQA: BBCC

Brunel University B84

BSc (Hons): 3 years full-time or 4 - 6 years part-time – L451
HE credits: 120 - 240

University of East London E28

BA (Hons): 4 years full-time including foundation year – B999
A2: DD - CD

University of East London E28

BA (Hons): 3 years full-time or 6 years part-time – B990
Tariff: 160

International Correspondence School [University of East London]
BSc (Hons): distance learning
Tariff: 160 Interview

London Metropolitan University L68
BSc (Hons): 3 years full-time or 4 years sandwich or 4 - 6 years part-time day – B990
Tariff: 160 IB: 28

College of North East London [Middlesex University] ▲
FdSc: 2 years full-time or 3 years part-time – L905 U
Tariff: 100

Health Promotion with Communication Studies

University of East London E28
BA (Hons)/BSc (Hons): 3 years full-time – B9PY
Tariff: 160

Health Promotion with Cultural Studies

University of East London E28
BA (Hons)/BSc (Hons): 3 years full-time – B9LP
Tariff: 160

Health Promotion and Digital Arts with Moving Image

University of East London E28
BA (Hons)/Bsc (Hons): 3 years full-time – BW96
Tariff: 160

Health Promotion with Early Childhood Studies

University of East London E28
BA (Hons)/BSc (Hons): 3 years full-time – B9XH
Tariff: 160

Health Promotion and History

University of East London E28
BA (Hons)/BSc (Hons): 3 years full-time – BV91
Tariff: 120 HP

Health Promotion with Human Biology

University of East London E28
BA (Hons)/BSc (Hons): 3 years full-time – B9B1
Tariff: 160

Health Promotion and Information Technology

University of East London E28
BA (Hons)/BSc (Hons): 3 years full-time – BG95
Tariff: 160

Health Promotion with Marketing

University of East London E28
BA (Hons)/BSc (Hons): 3 years full-time – B9N5
Tariff: 160

Health Promotion with Performing Arts

University of East London E28
BA (Hons)/BSc (Hons): 3 years full-time – B9W4
Tariff: 160

Health Promotion (post-registration)

University of Glamorgan G14
BSc: 1 year part-time BSc (Hons): 1 - 2 years part-time
HE credits: 240, HP

Health Promotion with Psychosocial Studies

University of East London E28
BA (Hons)/BSc (Hons): 3 years full-time – B9CW
Tariff: 160

Health Promotion and Public Health

Thames Valley University T40
DipHE: 3 - 7 years part-time day and evening
HE credits: 120

Thames Valley University T40
BSc (Hons): 2 - 7 years part-time day and evening
HE credits: 120

Health Promotion with Sports Development

University of East London E28
BA (Hons)/BSc (Hons): 3 years full-time – B9C6
Tariff: 160

Health Promotion with Theatre Studies

University of East London E28
BA (Hons)/BSc (Hons): 3 years full-time – B9WK
Tariff: 160

Health Promotion (top-up)

Middlesex University M80
BSc (Hons): 1 year full-time – L900 E
Fd

Health and Psychology

University of Greenwich G70
BSc (Hons): 3 years full-time – BC98
Tariff: 160 IB: 24
BPS

Liverpool Hope University L46
BA (Hons)/BSc (Hons): 3 years full-time – BCX8
Tariff: 180 - 240
BPS

Health with Psychology

University of Greenwich G70
BSc (Hons): 3 years full-time – B9C8
Tariff: 160 IB: 24

Health, Safety and Environment

Bristol, University of the West of Englan
B80
BSc (Hons): 3 years full-time or 4 years full-time including foundation year or 4 years sandwich or 5 years sandwich including foundation year or 4 - 6 years part-time – B91
Tariff: 180 - 220 IB: 24 - 26

Health, Safety and Environmental Management

Aston University A80
BSc (Hons): 3 years full-time or 4 years sandwich – J99
Tariff: 240 - 280

Health Science

Bournemouth University B50
BSc (Hons): 3 years full-time – B900
Tariff: 160

Napier University N07
BSc (Hons): 4 years full-time – B901
A2: CC SQA: BBC

University of Paisley P20
BSc: 3 years full-time BSc (Hons): 4 years full-time – B900
A2: DD SQA: BBC

Health Science (Health Care Suppo Technician)

City University C60
FdA: 2 years full-time – B900
Tariff: 80

Health Science (Pharmacy Practice

University of Greenwich G70
FdSc: 2 years full-time – B231
Tariff: 240

Health Sciences

University of Aberdeen A20
BSc: 3 years full-time BSc (Hons): 4 years full-time – B903
A2: CCD - BBC SQA: BBCC

University of Abertay Dundee A30
BSc (Hons): 4 years full-time – B900
Tariff: 200

ty University C60
: (Hons): 2 - 3 years on-line study
credits: 240, HP

iversity of Glamorgan G14
: (Hons) (Foundation): 1 year full-time – B900
ff: 40

iversity of Salford S03
: (Hons): 3 years full-time or 4 - 6 years part-time –
0
ff: 180 IB: 27

iversity Campus Suffolk [University of st Anglia, University of Essex] S82
c: 2 years full-time or 4 years part-time – B900 I
f: 40

ealth Sciences for Complementary edicine

iversity of Central Lancashire C30
(Hons): 3 years full-time or 5 - 8 years part-time day –
0
f: 200

ealth Sciences (Health and anagement)

iversity of Aberdeen A20
3 years full-time BSc (Hons): 4 years full-time –
2
CCD - BBC SQA: BBCC

ealth Sciences (Health and trition)

versity of Aberdeen A20
3 years full-time BSc (Hons): 4 years full-time –
4
CCD - BBC SQA: BBCC

alth Sciences (Health and Society)

versity of Aberdeen A20
3 years full-time BSc (Hons): 4 years full-time – BL94
CCD - BBC SQA: BBCC

alth Sciences (Health and Sport)

versity of Aberdeen A20
3 years full-time BSc (Hons): 4 years full-time –
6
CCD - BBC SQA: BBCC

alth Sciences (Naturopathy)

versity of Westminster W50
Hons): 3 years full-time or 5 - 6 years part-time –
C BTEC: MPP SQA: CCCC ILC: CCCCC IB: 26
iew

versity of Westminster W50
Hons): 4 years full-time including foundation year –
C BTEC: MPP SQA: CCCC IB: 26 Interview

Health Sciences and Social Policy

University of Salford S03
BSc (Hons): 3 years full-time or 5 years part-time – BL94
Tariff: 180 IB: 27

Health Services Management

International Correspondence School [University of East London]
BSc (Hons): distance learning
Tariff: 160 Interview

Health Services Management with Accounting

University of East London E28
BA (Hons)/BSc (Hons): 3 years full-time – N2N4
Tariff: 160

Health Services Management with Business Studies

University of East London E28
BA (Hons)/BSc (Hons): 3 years full-time – N2N1
Tariff: 160

Health Services Management and Information Technology

University of East London E28
BA (Hons)/BSc (Hons): 3 years full-time – BG9M
Tariff: 160

Health Services Management with Law

University of East London E28
BA (Hons)/BSc (Hons): 3 years full-time – N2M1
Tariff: 160

Health Services Management with Sociology

University of East London E28
BA (Hons)/BSc (Hons): 3 years full-time – N2L3
Tariff: 160

Health Services Management with Third World Development

University of East London E28
BA (Hons)/BSc (Hons): 3 years full-time – N2L9
Tariff: 160

Health Services Research

University of Aberdeen A20
BSc: 3 years full-time BSc (Hons): 4 years full-time –
B900
A2: CCD - BBC SQA: BBCC

Health and Social Care

University of Wales, Bangor B06
BA (Hons): 3 years full-time – L510
Tariff: 220 - 260 IB: 30

Barnfield College, Luton [University of Bedfordshire] ▲
FdA: 2 years full-time – L510 R
Tariff: 80 - 120

University of Bedfordshire B22
BA (Hons): 3 years full-time – L590
Tariff: 160 - 200

University of Bedfordshire B22
FdA: 2 years full-time – L510
Tariff: 160 - 200

University of Bolton B44
FdSc: 2 years full-time – L510
Interview

Bournemouth University B50
FdA: 3 years part-time
A2: C

Bournemouth and Poole College of Further Education [Bournemouth University]
FdA: 2 years part-time
A2: C

University of Bradford B56
FdSc: 2 years full-time or 3 years part-time – L510
Tariff: 120

University of Brighton B72
BA (Hons): 3 years full-time or 4 - 6 years part-time –
L510
Tariff: 280 IB: 28

University of Brighton B72
FdSc: 2 years part-time
HP

Calderdale College [University of Bradford] ▲
FdSc: 2 years full-time – L510
Tariff: 120

University of Central Lancashire C30
FdA: 2 years full-time or 4 years part-time – L511
Tariff: 40

Colchester Institute [University of Essex] C75
FdA: 2 years full-time – L510
Tariff: 80

Colchester Institute [University of Essex] C75
BSc (Hons): 3 years full-time – L511
Tariff: 160 RN, HP

University of Cumbria C99
FdSc: 2 years full-time – L510
A2 Interview

University of Cumbria C99
FdSc: 2 years full-time – L510 L
A2 Interview

University of East London E28
FdSc: 2 years full-time – L510
Tariff: 80

Exeter College [University of Plymouth] E81
FdA: 2 years full-time or 3 years part-time – L510
Tariff: 80

Gateshead College [University of Sunderland] ▲
FdA: 2 years full-time – BL95 G
Tariff: 80

Grimsby Institute of Further and Higher Education [University of Hull] G80
FdA: 2 years full-time or part-time day/evening – L510
Tariff: 40 - 120

Herefordshire College of Technology [University of Worcester] ▲
FdA: 2 years full-time – L511 C
Tariff: 60 IB: 24

Hopwood Hall College [University of Bolton] H54
FdA: 2 years full-time or 3 years part-time – L510
Tariff: 80

International Correspondence School [University of East London]
BA (Hons): distance learning

University of Kent K24
BA (Hons): 3 years full-time – LL45
Tariff: 240 IB: 27

Leeds Thomas Danby [University of Bradford] ▲
FdSc: 2 years full-time or 3 - 4 years part-time – L510
Tariff: 120 Interview

Manchester Metropolitan University M40
FdA: 2 years full-time or 3 years part-time – L512
Tariff: 80

Northumberland College [University of Sunderland] N78
FdSc: 2 years full-time – L510
Tariff: 240 Interview

City College Norwich [University of East Anglia] N82
FdA: 2 years full-time or 3 years part-time – L511
A2: EE BTEC

Roehampton University R48
BSc (Hons): 3 years full-time or 4 - 7 years part-time – L540
A2: CCD BTEC: PPP

Salisbury College [Bournemouth University]
FdA: 2 years part-time
Tariff: 80

Sheffield College [Sheffield Hallam University] S22
FdA: 2 years full-time or 3 years part-time – L510
Tariff: 40 Interview

Shipley College [University of Bradford]
FdSc: 3 years part-time
Interview

South West College [University of Ulster]
BSc (Hons): 2 - 5 years part-time day and evening
HP

University of Southampton S27
FdSc: 2 years full-time or 3 years mixed mode – B900
Tariff: 40

University Campus Suffolk [University of East Anglia, University of Essex] S82
FdA: 2 years full-time – L512 B
Tariff: 60 - 120

University Campus Suffolk [University of East Anglia, University of Essex] S82
FdA: 2 years full-time – L512 Y
Tariff: 80 - 120

University of Sunderland S84
FdSc: 2 years full-time – BL95
Tariff: 80

University of Sunderland S84
BA (Hons): 3 years full-time – L510
Tariff: 160

City of Sunderland College [University of Sunderland] ▲
FdA: 2 years full-time – BL95 K
Tariff: 80

Totton College [University of Southampton] ▲
FdSc: 2 years full-time or 3 years part-time – B900 T
A2: E BTEC: PP

Tyne Metropolitan College [University of Sunderland] ▲
Fd: 2 years full-time – BL95 N
Tariff: 80

West Kent College [University of Greenwich]
FdA: 3 years part-time
Interview

University of Worcester W80
FdA: 2 years full-time – L511
Tariff: 60 IB: 24

Yeovil College [Bournemouth University]
FdA: 3 years part-time
Tariff: 80

Health with Social Care

Warwickshire College, Royal Leamington Spa, Rugby and Moreton Morell [Coventry University] W25
FdA: 2 years full-time or 3 - 4 years part-time – L510
Tariff: 80

Health and Social Care and Advice, Guidance and Counselling

Northumbria University N77
BA (Hons): 3 years full-time – LB59
Tariff: 220 IB: 26

Health and Social Care (Care)

Bromley College of Further and Higher Education [University of Greenwich] ▲
FdSc: 2 years full-time – L510 B
A2: EE Interview

Health and Social Care and Care ar Education (Early Years)

Northumbria University N77
BA (Hons): 3 years full-time – LX5J
Tariff: 220 IB: 26

Health and Social Care (Care Management)

University of Greenwich G70
FdSc: 2 years full-time – LN52
Tariff: 40

Health and Social Care and Childhood Studies

Northumbria University N77
BA (Hons): 3 years full-time – LXMH
Tariff: 220 IB: 26

Health and Social Care and Criminology and Criminal Justice

University of Wales, Bangor B06
BA (Hons): 3 years full-time – LM52
Tariff: 240 - 260 IB: 28

Health and Social Care and Cymrae (Welsh)

University of Wales, Bangor B06
BA (Hons): 3 years full-time – LQ55
Tariff: 220 - 260

Health and Social Care and Disabil Studies

Northumbria University N77
BA (Hons): 3 years full-time – L590
Tariff: 220 IB: 26

Health and Social Care (Early Years Studies)

Bromley College of Further and Highe Education [University of Greenwich] ▲
FdSc: 2 years full-time
A2 BTEC

Health and Social Care (extended degree)

University of Bedfordshire B22
BA (Hons): 4 years full-time including foundation year – L511 D
Interview

lealth and Social Care and History

niversity of Wales, Bangor B06
 (Hons): 3 years full-time – LV51
riff: 220 - 260 IB: 28

lealth and Social Care (Holistic herapies pathway)

urnley College [University of Central ancashire] ▲
: 2 years full-time or 3 years part-time
riff: 80

lealth and Social Care (Learning ifficulties)

omerset College of Arts and echnology [University of Plymouth] S28
Sc: 2 years full-time – LX51
riff: 60 - 150

lealth and Social Care Management

ath Spa University B20
Sc: 2 years full-time or 4 years part-time – L510
: E

ew College, Swindon [Bath Spa niversity] ▲
Sc: 2 years full-time – L510 S
iff: 40 Interview

lealth and Social Care Management op-up)

ornwall College [University of ymouth] C78
 (Hons): 1 year full-time – LL45 C
D

omerset College of Arts and chnology [University of Plymouth] S28
 (Hons): 1 year full-time or part-time day – LL45
D, Fd

ealth and Social Care and laywork/Childhood and Play

rthumbria University N77
(Hons): 3 years full-time – LXMJ
iff: 220 IB: 26

ealth and Social Care Policy

iversity of Ulster U20
 (Hons): 3 years full-time – L510 J
ff: 260 IB: 32

ealth and Social Care (post-ualifying framework)

stol, University of the West of England 0
IE: 1 year full-time or 2 years part-time
credits: 120, HP

Health and Social Care Practice

City of Bristol College [Bristol, University of the West of England] ▲
FdSc: 2 years full-time – L510 R
Tariff: 40

Bristol, University of the West of England B80
FdSc: 2 years full-time – L510
Tariff: 40

Canterbury College [University of Kent] ▲
FdA: 2 years full-time – L511 C
A2: E BTEC: PP

University of Kent K24
BA (Hons): 3 years full-time or part-time – L431 K
Tariff: 200 IB: 27

Mid-Kent College of Higher and Further Education [University of Kent] ▲
BA (Hons): 3 years full-time or 6 years part-time – LLK5 K
Tariff: 200

Sheffield Hallam University S21
BA (Hons): up to 5 years part-time
RN, RM, HP
NMC

Health and Social Care Practice (Mental Health)

Sheffield Hallam University S21
BA (Hons): 3 - 6 years part-time
RN, HP

Health and Social Care and Professional Practice Studies

Northumbria University N77
BA (Hons): 3 years full-time – L592
Tariff: 220 IB: 26

Health and Social Care Professions

Sheffield Hallam University S21
BSc (Hons): 4 years full-time including foundation year – B991
Tariff: 80

Health and Social Care and Social Policy

University of Wales, Bangor B06
BA (Hons): 3 years full-time – LL54
Tariff: 240 - 280 IB: 28

Health and Social Care and Sociology

University of Wales, Bangor B06
BA (Hons): 3 years full-time – LL53
Tariff: 240 - 280 IB: 28

Health and Social Care and Sport Health and Physical Education

University of Wales, Bangor B06
BA (Hons): 3 years full-time – LC56
Tariff: 260 - 280 IB: 28

Health and Social Care and Sports Science

University of Wales, Bangor B06
BA (Hons): 3 years full-time – CL65
Tariff: 260 - 280 IB: 28

Health and Social Care Studies

Somerset College of Arts and Technology [University of Plymouth] S28
FdA: 2 years full-time – L510
Tariff: 60 - 150

Health and Social Care Studies (Counselling Skills)

Somerset College of Arts and Technology [University of Plymouth] S28
FdA: 2 years full-time – LB59
Tariff: 60 - 150

Health and Social Care and Welsh History

University of Wales, Bangor B06
BA (Hons): 3 years full-time – LV52
Tariff: 260 - 280 IB: 28

Health and Social Studies

University of Glasgow G28
MA: 3 years full-time or part-time – LL34 C
A2: BBC SQA: BBBB ILC: BBBB IB: 30 HND

Health and Social Welfare

Bradford College [Leeds Metropolitan University] B60
BA (Hons): 3 years full-time – B900
Tariff: 100 - 140

Burnley College [University of Central Lancashire] ▲
FdA: 2 years full-time – L510 B
A2: EE

University of Central Lancashire C30
FdA: 2 years full-time or 3 years part-time – L510
Tariff: 40 Interview

University of Huddersfield H60
BSc (Hons): 3 years full-time or 5 years part-time – L5L4
Tariff: 200 - 220

Hugh Baird College [University of Central Lancashire] ▲
Fd: 2 years full-time or 3 years part-time – L510 H
Tariff: 80

Kendal College [University of Central Lancashire] ▲
FdSc: 2 years full-time or 3 years part-time – L510 K
Tariff: 80 Interview

Preston College [University of Central Lancashire] ▲
FdSc: 2 years full-time or 3 years part-time – L510 P
A2: E BTEC: PPP Interview

Health and Society

University Campus Suffolk [University of East Anglia, University of Essex] S82
BSc (Hons): 3 years full-time – LL43 I
Tariff: 160

Health and Sociology

University of Greenwich G70
BSc (Hons): 3 years full-time – BL93
Tariff: 160 IB: 24

Health with Sociology

University of Greenwich G70
BSc (Hons): 3 years full-time – B9L3
Tariff: 160 IB: 24

Health and Special Needs

Liverpool Hope University L46
BA (Hons)/BSc (Hons): 3 years full-time – BX91
Tariff: 180 - 240 IB: 25

Health and Sport Studies

Liverpool Hope University L46
BA (Hons)/BSc (Hons): 3 years full-time – CBP9
Tariff: 180 - 240

Health and Sports Development

Liverpool Hope University L46
BA (Hons)/BSc (Hons): 3 years full-time – BC96
Tariff: 240

Health and Sports Studies

University of Huddersfield H60
BSc (Hons): 3 years full-time or 5 years part-time – CL65
Tariff: 200 - 220

Health Studies

University of Bolton B44
BA (Hons): 2 - 8 years part-time day and evening
RN, RM, HP

Brunel University B84
BSc (Hons): 3 years full-time or 4 - 6 years part-time – L450
HE credits: 120 - 240

Canterbury Christ Church University C10
BSc (Hons): 3 years full-time or 5 - 6 years part-time – B900
A2: CC SQA: CCCC ILC: CCCCC IB: 24

University of Central Lancashire C30
BA (Hons): 3 years full-time or 4 - 6 years part-time – LB49
Tariff: 180

Coventry University C85
BSc (Hons): 3 years full-time or up to 5 years part-time – B990
Tariff: 200

De Montfort University D26
BA (Hons): 3 years full-time – B991 Y
A2: CD - CC

International Correspondence School [University of East London]
BSc (Hons): distance learning
Tariff: 160 Interview

Lews Castle College (UHI Millennium Institute) H49
BA: 3 years full-time – L450
A2: DD - AA SQA: BCC

University of Lincoln L39
BSc (Hons): 3 years full-time – L450 L
Tariff: 200 IB: 24

London South Bank University L75
DipHE: 2 - 5 years part-time
HE credits: 120, HP

London South Bank University L75
BSc (Hons): 2 - 5 years part-time
HE credits: 120, HP

City College Norwich [University of East Anglia] N82
FdSc: 2 years full-time – B900
Tariff: 80

Roehampton University R48
BSc (Hons): 3 years full-time or 4 - 7 years part-time – B900
A2: CCD BTEC: MMM SQA: BCC IB: 24

Thames Valley University T40
BSc (Hons): 3 years full-time or 3 - 7 years part-time – L510
Tariff: 160 IB: 29

University of Wolverhampton W75
BSc (Hons): 3 years full-time or 5 - 6 years part-time – B900
Tariff: 160 - 220 IB: 24

University of Worcester W80
BSc (Hons): 3 years full-time – L450
Tariff: 80 IB: 24

Health Studies with Accounting

University of Northampton N38
BA (Hons)/BSc (Hons): 3 years full-time or 4 - 6 years part-time – L4N4
Tariff: 180 - 220

Health Studies with American Studies

University of Northampton N38
BA (Hons)/BSc (Hons): 3 years full-time or 4 - 6 years par time – L4T7
Tariff: 180 - 220

University of Sunderland S84
BA (Hons)/BSc (Hons): 3 years full-time – B9T7
Tariff: 200 - 360

Health Studies with Business Entrepreneurship

University of Northampton N38
BA (Hons)/BSc (Hons): 3 years full-time or 4 - 6 years pa time – L4NF
Tariff: 180 - 220

Health Studies with Business Finance

University of East London E28
BA (Hons)/BSc (Hons): 3 years full-time – B9N3
Tariff: 160

Health Studies with Business and Management

University of Sunderland S84
BA (Hons)/BSc (Hons): 3 years full-time – B9N1
Tariff: 200

Health Studies and Business Studie

University of East London E28
BA (Hons)/BSc (Hons): 3 years full-time – BN91
Tariff: 120 HP

Health Studies with Communicatior Studies

University of East London E28
BA (Hons)/BSc (Hons): 3 years full-time – B9PA
Tariff: 160

Health Studies and Computing

University of Worcester W80
BA (Hons)/BSc (Hons): 3 years full-time – BG95
Tariff: 80

Health Studies with Computing

University of Sunderland S84
BA (Hons)/BSc (Hons): 3 years full-time – B9G4
Tariff: 200

Health Studies with Criminology

University of Northampton N38
BA (Hons)/BSc (Hons): 3 years full-time or 4 - 6 years p time – L4M9
Tariff: 180 - 220

niversity of Sunderland S84
\ (Hons)/BSc (Hons): 3 years full-time – B9M9
riff: 200

lealth Studies with Cultural Studies

niversity of East London E28
\ (Hons)/BSc (Hons): 3 years full-time – B9LQ
riff: 160

lealth Studies with Dance

niversity of Northampton N38
\ (Hons)/BSc (Hons): 3 years full-time or 4 - 6 years part-
ie – L4W5
riff: 180 - 220

niversity of Sunderland S84
(Hons)/BSc (Hons): 3 years full-time – B9W5
riff: 200

lealth Studies and Early Childhood tudies

niversity of Wolverhampton W75
(Hons)/BSc (Hons): 3 years full-time or 4 years
ndwich – BXX3
riff: 160 - 220 IB: 30

ealth Studies with Economics

niversity of Northampton N38
(Hons)/BSc (Hons): 3 years full-time or 4 - 6 years part-
e – L4L1
iff: 180 - 220

ealth Studies with Education

iversity of Sunderland S84
(Hons)/BSc (Hons): 3 years full-time – B9X3
iff: 200

ealth Studies and Education and ommunity Development

iversity of East London E28
(Hons)/BSc (Hons): 3 years full-time – BX93
ff: 120 HP

ealth Studies with English

iversity of Northampton N38
(Hons)/BSc (Hons): 3 years full-time or 4 - 6 years part-
– L4Q3
ff: 180 - 220

ealth Studies with English anguage

iversity of East London E28
(Hons): 3 years full-time – B9Q3
ff: 120 HP

Health Studies with English Studies

University of Sunderland S84
BA (Hons)/BSc (Hons): 3 years full-time – B9Q3
Tariff: 200 - 360

Health Studies with Equine Studies

University of Northampton N38
BA (Hons)/BSc (Hons): 3 years full-time or 4 - 6 years part-time – L4D4
Tariff: 180 - 220

Health Studies with Fine Art Painting and Drawing

University of Northampton N38
BA (Hons)/BSc (Hons): 3 years full-time or 4 - 6 years part-time – L4W1
Tariff: 180 - 220

Health Studies with French

University of Northampton N38
BA (Hons)/BSc (Hons): 3 years full-time or 4 - 6 years part-time – L4R1
Tariff: 180 - 220

Health Studies and Geographic Information Systems

Bath Spa University B20
DipHE: 2 years full-time – FL8K
Tariff: 80 - 120

Health Studies with Geography

University of Sunderland S84
BA (Hons)/BSc (Hons): 3 years full-time – B9L7
Tariff: 200

Health Studies with German

University of Northampton N38
BA (Hons)/BSc (Hons): 3 years full-time or 4 - 6 years part-time – L4R2
Tariff: 180 - 220

Health Studies and History

University of Sunderland S84
BA (Hons)/BSc (Hons): 3 years full-time – BV91
Tariff: 200

University of Worcester W80
BA (Hons)/BSc (Hons): 3 years full-time – BV91
Tariff: 80 IB: 24

Health Studies with History

University of Northampton N38
BA (Hons)/BSc (Hons): 3 years full-time or 4 - 6 years part-time – L4V1
Tariff: 180 - 220

University of Sunderland S84
BA (Hons)/BSc (Hons): 3 years full-time – B9V1
Tariff: 200

Health Studies with History of Art and Design

University of Northampton N38
BA (Hons)/BSc (Hons): 3 years full-time or 4 - 6 years part-time – L4V3
Tariff: 180 - 220

Health Studies and Human Biology

University of Worcester W80
BA (Hons)/BSc (Hons): 3 years full-time – LC51
Tariff: 120

Health Studies with Human Biology

University of Northampton N38
BA (Hons)/BSc (Hons): 3 years full-time or 4 - 6 years part-time – L4B1
Tariff: 180 - 220

Health Studies and Human Biosciences

Roehampton University R48
BA (Hons)/BSc (Hons): 3 years full-time – CB19
Tariff: 120 - 200 IB: 28

Health Studies with Human Geography

University of Northampton N38
BA (Hons)/BSc (Hons): 3 years full-time or 4 - 6 years part-time – L4L7
Tariff: 180 - 220

Health Studies and Human Nutrition

London Metropolitan University L68
BA (Hons)/BSc (Hons): 3 years full-time – LB44
Tariff: 160 - 200 IB: 28

University of Worcester W80
BA (Hons)/BSc (Hons): 3 years full-time – BB94
Tariff: 120 IB: 26

Health Studies and Human Resource Management

Manchester Metropolitan University M40
BA (Hons)/BSc (Hons): 3 years full-time – BN96
Tariff: 200 IB: 28

Health Studies with Human Resource Management

University of Northampton N38
BA (Hons)/BSc (Hons): 3 years full-time or 4 - 6 years part-time – L4N6
Tariff: 180 - 220

Health Studies with Information Communication Technologies

University of Northampton N38
BA (Hons)/BSc (Hons): 3 years full-time or 4 - 6 years part-time – L4G5
Tariff: 180 - 220

Health Studies and Information and Communications Applications Technology

Manchester Metropolitan University M40
BA (Hons)/BSc (Hons): 3 years full-time – GB69
Tariff: 200 IB: 28

Health Studies and Information Technology

University of East London E28
BSc (Hons): 3 years full-time – G5B9
Tariff: 120 HP

Health Studies with Information Technology

University of East London E28
BA (Hons)/BSc (Hons): 3 years full-time – B9GM
Tariff: 160

Health Studies and Interactive Digital Media

University of Worcester W80
BA (Hons)/BSc (Hons): 3 years full-time – BG94
Tariff: 160

Health Studies and International Politics

University of East London E28
BA (Hons)/BSc (Hons): 3 years full-time – LLK2
Tariff: 120 HP

Health Studies and International Relations

University of Lincoln L39
BA (Hons)/BSc (Hons): 3 years full-time – LLK2 L
Tariff: 200

Health Studies with Journalism

University of Sunderland S84
BA (Hons)/BSc (Hons): 3 years full-time – B9P5
Tariff: 200

Health Studies and Law

University of East London E28
BA (Hons)/BSc (Hons): 3 years full-time – BM91
Tariff: 120 RN, RM, HP

London Metropolitan University L68
BA (Hons)/BSc (Hons): 3 years full-time – LM4C
Tariff: 200 - 240 IB: 28

University of Sunderland S84
BA (Hons)/BSc (Hons): 3 years full-time – BM91
Tariff: 200

Health Studies with Law

University of Northampton N38
BA (Hons)/BSc (Hons): 3 years full-time or part-time – L4M1
Tariff: 180 - 220

Health Studies and Leisure Studies

Manchester Metropolitan University M40
BA (Hons)/BSc (Hons): 3 years full-time – BL94
Tariff: 200 IB: 28

Health Studies and Management

University of Lincoln L39
BA (Hons)/BSc (Hons): 3 years full-time – LN42 L
Tariff: 200

London Metropolitan University L68
BA (Hons)/BSc (Hons): 3 years full-time – LN42
Tariff: 160 - 200 IB: 28

Health Studies and Marketing

Manchester Metropolitan University M40
BA (Hons)/BSc (Hons): 3 years full-time – BN95
Tariff: 200 IB: 28

Health Studies with Marketing

University of Northampton N38
BA (Hons)/BSc (Hons): 3 years full-time or part-time – L4N5
Tariff: 180 - 220

Health Studies and Mass Communications

London Metropolitan University L68
BA (Hons)/BSc (Hons): 3 years full-time – LP49
Tariff: 160 - 200

Health Studies with Mathematics

University of Northampton N38
BA (Hons)/BSc (Hons): 3 years full-time or 4 - 6 years part-time – L4G1
Tariff: 180 - 220

Health Studies and Media Communications

Bath Spa University B20
BA (Hons)/BSc (Hons): 3 years full-time – LP49
Tariff: 220 - 260

Bath Spa University B20
DipHE: 2 years full-time – PL94
Tariff: 80 - 120

Health Studies and Media and Cultural Studies

University of Worcester W80
BA (Hons)/BSc (Hons): 3 years full-time – BP93
Tariff: 160 IB: 26

Health Studies and Media Studies

University of Sunderland S84
BA (Hons)/BSc (Hons): 3 years full-time – BP93
Tariff: 200

Health Studies with Media Studies

University of Sunderland S84
BA (Hons)/BSc (Hons): 3 years full-time – B9P3
Tariff: 200

Health Studies and Music

Bath Spa University B20
BA (Hons)/BSc (Hons): 3 years full-time – LW43
Tariff: 200 - 240

Bath Spa University B20
DipHE: 2 years full-time – WL34
Tariff: 80 - 120

Manchester Metropolitan University M4
BA (Hons)/BSc (Hons): 3 years full-time – BW93
Tariff: 200 IB: 28

University of Sunderland S84
BA (Hons)/BSc (Hons): 3 years full-time – BW93
Tariff: 200

Health Studies with Music

University of Sunderland S84
BA (Hons)/BSc (Hons): 3 years full-time – B9W3
Tariff: 200

Health Studies with Performance

University of Northampton N38
BA (Hons)/BSc (Hons): 3 years full-time or part-time – L4W4
Tariff: 180 - 220

Health Studies and Philosophy

Manchester Metropolitan University M4
BA (Hons)/BSc (Hons): 3 years full-time – BV95
Tariff: 200 IB: 28

Health Studies and Philosophy and Ethics

Bath Spa University B20
BA (Hons)/BSc (Hons): 3 years full-time – BV95
Tariff: 200 - 260

ealth Studies and Physical ducation

iversity of Worcester W80
(Hons)/BSc (Hons): 3 years full-time – BX93
ff: 200

ealth Studies with Physical eography

iversity of Northampton N38
(Hons)/BSc (Hons): 3 years full-time or 4 - 6 years part-
– L4F8
ff: 180 - 220

ealth Studies and Plant Science

iversity of Worcester W80
(Hons)/BSc (Hons): 3 years full-time – LC9X
f: 120 IB: 26

ealth Studies and Politics

iversity of Lincoln L39
Hons)/BSc (Hons): 3 years full-time – LL42 L
f: 200

iversity of Sunderland S84
Hons)/BSc (Hons): 3 years full-time – BL92
f: 200

ealth Studies with Politics

iversity of Northampton N38
Hons)/BSc (Hons): 3 years full-time or 4 - 6 years part-
– L4L2
: 180 - 220

iversity of Sunderland S84
Hons)/BSc (Hons): 3 years full-time – B9L2
: 160 - 360 IB: 31

ealth Studies and Psychology

th Spa University B20
Hons)/BSc (Hons): 3 years full-time – LC48
: 200 - 240

th Spa University B20
E: 2 years full-time – CL84
: 80 - 120

Montfort University D26
Hons): 3 years full-time or 4 years sandwich – CL84 Y
: 180 - 200 IB: 24

versity of Lincoln L39
Hons)/BSc (Hons): 3 years full-time or 6 years part-
– CLV4 L
: 200

nchester Metropolitan University
0
Hons)/BSc (Hons): 3 years full-time – LC48
: 200 IB: 28

Roehampton University R48
BA (Hons)/BSc (Hons): 3 years full-time – BC98
Tariff: 160 - 200 IB: 28
BPS

University of Sunderland S84
BA (Hons)/BSc (Hons): 3 years full-time – BC98
Tariff: 200

University of Worcester W80
BA (Hons)/BSc (Hons): 3 years full-time – BC98
Tariff: 160 IB: 26
BPS

Health Studies with Psychology

University of East London E28
BSc (Hons): 3 years full-time – B9C8
Tariff: 120 HP

University of Northampton N38
BA (Hons)/BSc (Hons): 3 years full-time or 4 - 6 years part-time – L4C8
Tariff: 180 - 220

University of Sunderland S84
BA (Hons)/BSc (Hons): 3 years full-time – B9C8
Tariff: 160 - 360

Health Studies and Psychology (Applied)

London Metropolitan University L68
BA (Hons)/BSc (Hons): 3 years full-time – LC48
Tariff: 160 - 200 IB: 28

Health Studies and Psychosocial Studies

University of East London E28
BA (Hons)/BSc (Hons): 3 years full-time – BC98
Tariff: 120 HP

Health Studies with Psychosocial Studies

University of East London E28
BA (Hons)/BSc (Hons): 3 years full-time – B9CA
Tariff: 160

Health Studies and Public Relations

University of Sunderland S84
BA (Hons)/BSc (Hons): 3 years full-time – PB29
Tariff: 200

Health Studies and Science of Sport and Exercise

Roehampton University R48
BA (Hons)/BSc (Hons): 3 years full-time – CB69
Tariff: 120

Health Studies and Social Anthropology

Roehampton University R48
BA (Hons)/BSc (Hons): 3 years full-time – BL96
Tariff: 160 - 200 IB: 28

Health Studies and Social Justice

Manchester Metropolitan University M40
BA (Hons)/BSc (Hons): 3 years full-time – MB29
Tariff: 200 IB: 28

Health Studies and Social Policy

University of Lincoln L39
BA (Hons)/BSc (Hons): 3 years full-time – L451 L
Tariff: 200

Health Studies and Social Welfare

University of Worcester W80
BA (Hons)/BSc (Hons): 3 years full-time – BL95
Tariff: 120 IB: 26

Health Studies with Social Welfare

University of Northampton N38
BA (Hons)/BSc (Hons): 3 years full-time or 4 - 6 years part-time – L4L5
Tariff: 180 - 220

Health Studies and Sociology

Bath Spa University B20
BA (Hons)/BSc (Hons): 3 years full-time – LL43
Tariff: 220 - 260

Bath Spa University B20
DipHE: 2 years full-time – LL34
Tariff: 80 - 120

London Metropolitan University L68
BA (Hons)/BSc (Hons): 3 years full-time – LL43
Tariff: 200 - 240 IB: 28

Manchester Metropolitan University M40
BA (Hons)/BSc (Hons): 3 years full-time – LLK3
Tariff: 200

University of Sunderland S84
BA (Hons)/BSc (Hons): 3 years full-time – BL93
Tariff: 200

University of Wolverhampton W75
BA (Hons)/BSc (Hons): 3 years full-time or 4 years sandwich – BL93
Tariff: 160 - 220 IB: 24

University of Worcester W80
BA (Hons)/BSc (Hons): 3 years full-time – BL93
Tariff: 160 IB: 26

Health Studies with Sociology

University of Sunderland S84
BA (Hons)/BSc (Hons): 3 years full-time – B9L3
Tariff: 160 - 360

Health Studies (with specialist pathways)

UCE Birmingham C25
BSc (Hons): 3 years full-time – BL94
HE credits: 120, HP, Interview

Health Studies (with Specialist Practice Awards)

University of Wales, Bangor B06
BSc (Hons): 1 year full-time or 2 - 5 years part-time
HE credits: 120, RN, RM, HP

Health Studies and Sport

Manchester Metropolitan University M40
BA (Hons)/BSc (Hons): 3 years full-time – CBP9
Tariff: 200 IB: 28

University of Sunderland S84
BA (Hons)/BSc (Hons): 3 years full-time – CB69
Tariff: 200

Health Studies with Sport

University of Sunderland S84
BA (Hons)/BSc (Hons): 3 years full-time – B9C6
Tariff: 200

Health Studies and Sport and Exercise Science

University of Wolverhampton W75
BA (Hons)/BSc (Hons): 3 years full-time or 4 years sandwich – BC96
Tariff: 160 - 220

Health Studies with Sport Studies

University of Northampton N38
BA (Hons)/BSc (Hons): 3 years full-time or 4 - 6 years part-time – L4C6
Tariff: 180 - 220

Health Studies and Sports Coaching Science

University of Worcester W80
BA (Hons)/BSc (Hons): 3 years full-time – BCX6
Tariff: 200 IB: 26

Health Studies and Sports Science

London Metropolitan University L68
BA (Hons)/BSc (Hons): 3 years full-time – LC46
Tariff: 160 - 200 IB: 28

Health Studies and Sports Studies

University of Worcester W80
BA (Hons)/BSc (Hons): 3 years full-time – BC96
Tariff: 240 IB: 26

Health Studies and Studies in English Language/Linguistics

University of Sunderland S84
BA (Hons)/BSc (Hons): 3 years full-time – BQ91
Tariff: 200

Health Studies with Studies in English Language/Linguistics

University of Sunderland S84
BA (Hons)/BSc (Hons): 3 years full-time – B9Q1
Tariff: 160 - 360

Health Studies and Study of Religions

Bath Spa University B20
BA (Hons)/BSc (Hons): 3 years full-time – LV46
Tariff: 200 - 240

Bath Spa University B20
DipHE: 2 years full-time – VL64
Tariff: 80 - 120

Health Studies and Third World Development

University of East London E28
BA (Hons)/BSc (Hons): 3 years full-time – BLXJ
Tariff: 120 HP

Health Studies with Third World Development

University of Northampton N38
BA (Hons)/BSc (Hons): 3 years full-time or 4 - 6 years part-time – L4LX
Tariff: 180 - 220

Health Studies and Time-Based Digital Media

University of Worcester W80
BA (Hons)/BSc (Hons): 3 years full-time – BGX4
Tariff: 160 IB: 26

Health Studies (top-up)

University of Brighton B72
BA (Hons): 1 year full-time or 2 - 4 years part-time day – L511
HE credits: 240

Swansea Institute of Higher Education [University of Wales] S96
BSc (Hons): 1 year full-time
HND, Fd

University of Wolverhampton W75
BSc (Hons): 1 year full-time or 2 years part-time – B902
Tariff: 160 - 220 RN, RM, HP

Health Studies and Tourism

University of Sunderland S84
BA (Hons)/BSc (Hons): 3 years full-time – NB89
Tariff: 200

Health Studies and Visual Arts

University of Worcester W80
BA (Hons)/BSc (Hons): 3 years full-time – BW92
Tariff: 160

Health Studies with Wastes Management

University of Northampton N38
BA (Hons)/BSc (Hons): 3 years full-time or 4 - 6 years pa
time – L4FV
Tariff: 180 - 220

Health Studies and Writing

Manchester Metropolitan University M
BA (Hons)/BSc (Hons): 3 years full-time – BW98
Tariff: 200 IB: 28

Health Studies/Health Science

Isle of Man College [University of Liverpool]
BA (Hons)/BSc (Hons): 3 years full-time or 4 years full-ti
including foundation year
A2: CCC

Health Studies/Nursing

University of Paisley P20
BSc/BSc (Hons): part-time day/evening
RN, HP

Health and Tourism

Liverpool Hope University L46
BA (Hons)/BSc (Hons): 3 years full-time – BN98
Tariff: 180 - 240

Health and War and Peace Studies

Liverpool Hope University L46
BA (Hons)/BSc (Hons): 3 years full-time – BL92
Tariff: 180 - 240

Healthcare

University Campus Suffolk [University East Anglia, University of Essex] S82
DipHE: up to 5 years part-time
HE credits: 120

Healthcare Practice

University of Teesside T20
FdSc: 2 years part-time
HP

Health-Related Exercise and Fitne

Bradford College [Leeds Metropolitan University] ▲
FdSc: 2 years full-time or 3 years part-time – CN6F B
Tariff: 120

hesterfield College C56

Sc: 2 years full-time – C600
riff: 80 - 120

ewsbury College [Leeds Metropolitan niversity] ▲

Sc: 2 years full-time or part-time – CN6F D
riff: 120

ark Lane College [Leeds Metropolitan niversity] L21

Sc: 2 years full-time – BC96
: E BTEC: PPP SQA ILC IB: 20 Interview

akefield College [Leeds Metropolitan niversity] ▲

Sc: 2 years full-time – CN6F W
riff: 120

ealth-Related Exercise and Fitness op-up)

eeds Metropolitan University L27

(Hons): 9 months full-time or 18 months part-time – 01

ealthy Living and Lifestyles

orcester College of Technology niversity of Worcester] W81

c: 2 years full-time – C600
iff: 40

uman and Equine Sports Science

rtpury College [Bristol, University of e West of England] ▲

: 3 years full-time – DC46 A
ff: 200 - 240

tegrated Practice (Early Years and oung People)

rral Metropolitan College W73

2 - 4 years part-time
rview

terprofessional Practice

ll College [University of Paisley] B26

: 1 - 5 years part-time day and evening
credits: 120 - 240

oint Honours (Food Science/Health udies/Human Nutrition/Sports ience)

ndon Metropolitan University L68

Hons)/BSc (Hons): 3 years full-time or 4 years sandwich - 6 years part-time – Y001
f: 160

Lifespan, Exercise and Health

University of Wales, Newport N37

BSc (Hons): 3 years full-time – BC96
Tariff: 240

Lifestyle Management

Leeds Metropolitan University L27

BA (Hons): 3 years full-time or 6 years part-time – N294
Tariff: 180

Managing Pain

University of Glamorgan G14

BSc (Hons): 2 - 6 years distance learning
HE credits, RN, HP

Marine Sports Science

Falmouth Marine School, Cornwall College [University of Plymouth] C78

FdSc: 2 years full-time – CF67
Tariff: 60 - 120

Penwith College [University of Plymouth] ▲

FdSc: 2 years full-time – C607
Tariff: 60

Mental Health and Counselling

University of Abertay Dundee A30

BA (Hons): 4 years full-time – CL85
Tariff: 200

Occupational Health, Safety and Environmental Management

North East Wales Institute of Higher Education [University of Wales] N56

FdSc: 2 years full-time – BFX8
Tariff: 60

North East Wales Institute of Higher Education [University of Wales] N56

BSc (Hons): 3 years full-time – BF98
Tariff: 120

Occupational Health and Safety Management

North East Wales Institute of Higher Education [University of Wales] N56

FdSc: 2 years full-time – B923
Tariff: 60

Occupational Health and Safety Management (top-up)

Middlesex University M80

BSc (Hons): 1 year full-time or 2 years part-time – N620 E
HND, RN

Palliative Care

Oxford Brookes University O66

BA (Hons): 2 years full-time or 2 - 5 years part-time or 2 - 5 years mixed mode – B733
HE credits: 120, RN, HP
NMC

Paramedic Practice

University of Central Lancashire C30

BSc (Hons): 3 years full-time – B780
Tariff: 320

Paramedic Science

Coventry University C85

FdSc: 2 years full-time – B780
Tariff: 100 Interview
NMC

University of East Anglia E14

DipHE: 2 years full-time
Interview

University of Hertfordshire H36

BSc (Hons): 3 years full-time – B780
Tariff: 280 Interview
HPC

University of Portsmouth P80

FdSc: 3 years part-time
A2: C BTEC: PPP Interview

Paramedic Science with Emergency Care Practice

University of Hertfordshire H36

BSc (Hons): part-time
HP

Paramedic Science (with Paramedic Award)

University of Hertfordshire H36

FdSc: 2 years full-time – B781
Tariff: 120 HP

Physical Activity and Community Health

University of East London E28

BSc (Hons): 3 years full-time – CB69
Tariff: 160

Physical Activity, Exercise and Health

Leeds Metropolitan University L27

BSc (Hons): 3 years full-time – CB69
Tariff: 220 - 260 IB: 28

University of Wolverhampton W75

BSc (Hons): 3 years full-time or 4 - 5 years part-time day and evening – CB69
Tariff: 160 - 220 IB: 24

Physical Activity and Health

Canterbury Christ Church University C10
Fd: 2 - 3 years part-time
A2: C IB: 24 Interview

University of Cumbria C99
FdSc: 2 years full-time – C606 L
Tariff: 60

Newcastle College [Leeds Metropolitan University] N23
FdSc: 2 years full-time – C605
Tariff: 80

Post-Registration Framework for Healthcare Professionals

University of Northampton N38
BSc (Hons): 2 - 3 years part-time
RN, RM, HP

Primary Care

University of Reading R12
BA (Hons): 40 weeks full-time – B710
RN, RM, HP
NMC

Primary Health Care

Thames Valley University T40
BSc (Hons): 2 - 7 years part-time day/evening
HE credits: 240

Thames Valley University T40
DipHE: 2 - 7 years part-time day/evening
HE credits: 120

Primary Health Care Practice

University of Wolverhampton W75
BSc (Hons): 1 year full-time or 2 years part-time
RN, RM, HP
NMC

Professional Development

University of Dundee D65
BA: open learning
RN, RM, HP

Glasgow Caledonian University G42
BSc/BSc (Hons): 1 - 4 years part-time
RN, RM, HP

Professional Practice

Canterbury Christ Church University C10
DipHE: 2 - 5 years part-time
HE credits: 120, RN, RM, HP

Canterbury Christ Church University C10
BSc (Hons): 2 - 5 years part-time
HE credits: 240, RN, RM, HP

University of Glamorgan G14
DipHE: 1 - 5 years part-time
HE credits: 120, RN, RM, HP
HPW

Queen Margaret University, Edinburgh Q25
BSc: 1 year full-time
HE credits: 240, RN, RM, HP

Professional Practice with Care of Older People

Thames Valley University T40
BSc (Hons): 3 - 7 years part-time evening
HE credits: 240

Professional Practice with Critical Care

Thames Valley University T40
DipHE: 2 - 7 years part-time day/evening
HE credits: 120

Thames Valley University T40
BSc (Hons): 2 - 7 years part-time day/evening
HE credits: 240

Professional and Practice Development for Health Practitioners

Sheffield Hallam University S21
BSc (Hons): 4 years part-time
RN, RM, HP

Professional Practice in Health Care

University of Bradford B56
DipHE/BSc (Hons): 1 - 5 years part-time
RN, RM, HP

Professional Practice (Mental Health) with Community Mental Health

Thames Valley University T40
DipHE: 2 - 7 years part-time day/evening
HE credits: 120

Thames Valley University T40
BSc (Hons): 2 - 7 years part-time day/evening
HE credits: 240

Professional Practice (Mental Health) with Dementing Illness in a Variety of Settings

Thames Valley University T40
BSc (Hons): 2 - 7 years part-time day/evening
HE credits: 240

Thames Valley University T40
DipHE: 2 - 7 years part-time day/evening
HE credits: 120

Professional Practice (Mental Health with Functional Mental Health Problems in the Older Person

Thames Valley University T40
DipHE: 2 - 7 years part-time day/evening
HE credits: 120

Thames Valley University T40
BSc (Hons): 2 - 7 years part-time day/evening
HE credits: 240

Professional Practice (Mental Health with Mental Health in Secure Environments

Thames Valley University T40
BSc (Hons): 2 - 7 years part-time day/evening
HE credits: 240

Thames Valley University T40
DipHE: 2 - 7 years part-time day/evening
HE credits: 120

Professional Practice (Mental Health with Mental Health Interventions

Thames Valley University T40
DipHE: 2 - 7 years part-time day/evening
HE credits: 120

Thames Valley University T40
BSc (Hons): 2 - 7 years part-time day/evening
HE credits: 240

Professional Practice (Mental Health with Mental Health Promotion in a Public Health Context

Thames Valley University T40
BSc (Hons): 2 - 7 years part-time day/evening
HE credits: 240

Thames Valley University T40
DipHE: 2 - 7 years part-time day/evening
HE credits: 120

Professional Practice with Tissue Viability

Thames Valley University T40
DipHE: 2 - 7 years part-time day/evening or 2 - 7 years distance learning
HE credits: 120, RN

Thames Valley University T40
BSc (Hons): 2 - 7 years part-time day/evening or 2 - 7 years distance learning
HE credits: 240, RN

Professional Studies

University of Huddersfield H60
BSc/BSc (Hons): 1 - 2 years full-time or 2 - 5 years par time
HE credits: 240, HP

iversity of Hull H72
HE: 3 years part-time
ff: 120

ofessional Studies in Healthcare

iversity of Wolverhampton W75
(Hons)/BSc (Hons): 2 - 8 years work-based learning
credits: 240, RN, RM, HP

ychosocial Interventions

eds Metropolitan University L27
HE: 60 weeks part-time day
HP

ychosocial Interventions for ychosis

iversity of Manchester M20
HE: 3 semesters part-time
HP

ychosocial Interventions for ychosis (post-qualification)

urnemouth University B50
(Hons): 1 - 3 years part-time
HP

blic Health

versity of Central Lancashire C30
Hons)/BSc (Hons): 3 years full-time – L490
f: 160 - 180

versity of East London E28
(Hons): 3 years full-time or 4 - 5 years part-time –
0
f: 120 RN, HP

versity of Greenwich G70
(Hons): 3 years full-time or 4 - 6 years part-time –
2
f: 160

rnational Correspondence School
iversity of East London]
(Hons): distance learning
: 160 Interview

erpool John Moores University L51
(Hons): 3 years full-time – B900
: 160 IB: 28

o College [University of Plymouth]
2 years full-time – B910
: 60

blic Health with Communication udies

versity of East London E28
ons): 3 years full-time – B9PX
: 160

Public Health with Cultural Studies

University of East London E28
BA (Hons): 3 years full-time – B9LA
Tariff: 160

Public Health with Education and Community Development

University of East London E28
BA (Hons): 3 years full-time – B9X9
Tariff: 160

Public Health (Environmental Health)

Leeds Metropolitan University L27
BSc (Hons): 3 years full-time or 4 years sandwich – B910
Tariff: 80 - 160 IB: 28
CIEH

Public Health with Health Promotion

University of East London E28
BA (Hons)/BSc (Hons): 3 years full-time – B904
Tariff: 160

Public Health (Health Studies)

Leeds Metropolitan University L27
BSc (Hons): 3 years full-time or 5 years part-time – L431
Tariff: 120 - 160 IB: 24

Public Health and Health Studies

University of East London E28
BA (Hons)/BSc (Hons): 3 years full-time – B902
Tariff: 160

Public Health and Human Resource Management

University of East London E28
BA (Hons)/BSc (Hons): 3 years full-time – BN9P
Tariff: 160

Public Health with Information Technology

University of East London E28
BSc (Hons): 3 years full-time – B9G5
Tariff: 160

Public Health Practice

University of Southampton S27
BSc (Hons): 1 year full-time or 2 - 4 years part-time
RN, HP

Public Health Practice (Health Visiting)

University of Hertfordshire H36
BSc (Hons): part-time
HE credits: 240, RN

Public Health with Psychosocial Studies

University of East London E28
BA (Hons)/BSc (Hons): 3 years full-time – B9CB
Tariff: 160

Public Health and Well-Being

University of Teesside T20
BSc (Hons): 3 years full-time or 4 - 7 years part-time –
L431
Tariff: 180

Science and Management of Exercise and Health

Farnborough College of Technology [University of Surrey] F66
BSc (Hons): 3 years full-time – BN12
A2: CD

Science of Sport and Exercise

Roehampton University R48
BSc (Hons): 3 years full-time – C602
Tariff: 160 - 200

Sport Biomedicine

Middlesex University M80
BSc (Hons): 3 years full-time – CB69 E
Tariff: 160 - 240

Sport and Exercise (Applied Exercise Science)

University of Teesside T20
BSc (Hons): 3 years full-time – C600
Tariff: 240 IB: 26

Sport and Exercise (Applied Sport Science)

University of Teesside T20
BSc (Hons): 3 years full-time – C610
Tariff: 240 IB: 26

Sport and Exercise (Coaching Science)

University of Teesside T20
BSc (Hons): 3 years full-time – C611
Tariff: 240 IB: 26

Sport and Exercise Development

Gateshead College [University of Sunderland]
FdSc: 3 years part-time
Tariff: 40 - 80

Lincoln College [University of Lincoln] ▲
FdSc: 2 years full-time – C601 P
Tariff: 120

City of Sunderland College [University of Sunderland] ▲
FdA: 2 years full-time – C604 K
Tariff: 100

City of Sunderland College [University of Sunderland] ▲
BSc (Hons) (Foundation): 1 year full-time – C603 K
Tariff: 100

Sport and Exercise Psychology

University of Chichester C58
BSc (Hons): 3 years full-time – C841
Tariff: 200 - 260 IB: 24

Sport and Exercise with Psychology

Leeds, Trinity & All Saints [University of Leeds] L24
BSc (Hons): 3 years full-time – C6C8
Tariff: 160 - 240

Sport and Exercise Psychology and English

Canterbury Christ Church University C10
BSc (Hons): 3 years full-time – QC38
Tariff: 160 IB: 24

Sport and Exercise Psychology with Politics

Canterbury Christ Church University C10
BSc (Hons): 3 years full-time – C8L2
Tariff: 160 IB: 24

Sport and Exercise Science

University of Wales, Aberystwyth A40
BSc (Hons): 3 years full-time – C600
Tariff: 240

University of Bath B16
BSc (Hons): 4 years sandwich or 4 years sandwich with time abroad – BCC7
A2: AAB BTEC: DDD IB: 36

University of Bath B16
BSc (Hons): 3 years full-time – BC17
A2: AAB BTEC: DDD IB: 36

University of Bedfordshire B22
BSc (Hons): 3 years full-time or 4 years sandwich – C6N2
Tariff: 160 - 200

University of Bedfordshire B22
FdSc: 2 years full-time – C604
Tariff: 160 - 200

University of Bedfordshire B22
BSc (Hons): 3 years full-time or 5 years part-time – C600
Tariff: 220 - 280 IB

University of Bolton B44
BSc (Hons): 3 years full-time or 5 years part-time – C603
Tariff: 160

University of Brighton B72
BSc (Hons): 3 years full-time – C600
Tariff: 280 IB: 30

University of Wales Institute, Cardiff C20
BSc (Hons): 3 years full-time – C600
A2: BB SQA: BBB

University of Chichester C58
BSc (Hons): 3 years full-time – C604
Tariff: 200 - 260 IB: 24

University of Cumbria C99
BSc (Hons): 3 years full-time – C600
Tariff: 240 IB: 30

University of East London E28
BSc (Hons): 3 years full-time or 4 - 6 years part-time – C600
Tariff: 160

University of East London E28
BSc (Hons): 4 years full-time including foundation year – C601
Tariff: 60

Edge Hill University E42
BSc (Hons): 3 years full-time – C602
Tariff: 220

University of Glamorgan G14
BSc (Hons): 3 years full-time or 4 years sandwich or 6 years part-time – C600
Tariff: 200 - 220

Heriot-Watt University H24
BSc: 3 years full-time BSc (Hons): 4 years full-time – C600
A2: CCC SQA: BBBB ILC: BBBCC IB: 28

University of Hertfordshire H36
BSc (Hons): 3 years full-time – C600
Tariff: 280

University of Hull H72
BSc (Hons): 3 years full-time – C601
Tariff: 240 - 280 IB: 28

Kingston College [Kingston University] ▲
FdSc: 2 years full-time or 4 years part-time – C601 F
Tariff: 40

Leeds Metropolitan University L27
BSc (Hons): 3 years full-time – C600
Tariff: 200 - 280 IB: 28

University of Lincoln L39
BSc (Hons): 3 years full-time – C600 L
Tariff: 200 IB: 24

London South Bank University L75
BSc (Hons): 3 years full-time – C600
A2: CCD

London South Bank University L75
FdSc: 2 years full-time – C601
Tariff: 80

Loughborough University L79
BSc (Hons): 3 years full-time – CX63
Tariff: 360 IB: 34 - 36

Middlesex University M80
BSc (Hons): 3 years full-time – C615 E
Tariff: 160 - 240

Myerscough College [University of Central Lancashire] M99
FdSc: 2 years full-time – C600
Tariff: 80

Napier University N07
BSc (Hons): 4 years full-time – C600
Tariff: 230 HND

University of Wales, Newport N37
BSc (Hons): 3 years full-time – C602
Tariff: 240

University of Northampton N38
BSc (Hons): 3 years full-time or part-time – C600
Tariff: 180 - 220 IB: 24

Nottingham Trent University N91
BSc (Hons): 3 years full-time – C600
Tariff: 240

Runshaw College [University of Centra Lancashire] ▲
FdSc: 2 years full-time or 3 years part-time – C603 R
Tariff: 120

Sheffield Hallam University S21
BSc (Hons): 3 years full-time or 6 years part-time – C6(
Tariff: 280

University of Strathclyde S78
BSc: 3 years full-time BSc (Hons): 4 years full-time – C600
A2: CCC SQA: BBBB

University of Wolverhampton W75
BSc (Hons): 3 years full-time or 4 - 6 years part-time – C604
Tariff: 160 - 220 IB: 24
BASES

University of Wolverhampton W75
FdSc: 2 years full-time – C600
Tariff: 60 - 120

University of Worcester W80
BSc (Hons): 3 years full-time – C600
Tariff: 200 IB: 30

York St John University Y75
BSc (Hons): 3 years full-time or 6 years part-time – C6
Tariff: 220 IB: 24

Sport and Exercise Science (2+2)

Coventry University C85
BSc (Hons): 4 years full-time – C601
Tariff: 60

Sport and Exercise Science and Business

University of Wolverhampton W75
BA (Hons)/BSc (Hons): 3 years full-time or 4 years sandwich – CN61
Tariff: 160 - 220

ort and Exercise Science with omputing

nterbury Christ Church University C10
(Hons): 3 years full-time – G6GK
f: 160 IB: 24

ort and Exercise Science (Golf udies)

iversity of Lincoln L39
(Hons): 3 years full-time – C603 L
f: 200 IB: 24

ort and Exercise Science with ternet Computing

nterbury Christ Church University C10
(Hons): 3 years full-time – C6GL
f: 160 IB: 24

ort and Exercise Science with gal Studies

nterbury Christ Church University C10
(Hons): 3 years full-time – C6M2
: 160 IB: 24

ort and Exercise Science and isure Management

versity of Wolverhampton W75
Hons)/BSc (Hons): 3 years full-time or 4 years wich – CNQ2
: 160 - 220

ort and Exercise Science (with med awards)

entry University C85
Hons): 3 years full-time or 4 years sandwich or 4 years ime – C600
: 240

ort and Exercise Science with ychology

iot-Watt University H24
3 years full-time BSc (Hons): 4 years full-time –
3
CC BTEC SQA: BBBB ILC: BBBCC IB: 28

rt and Exercise Science with orts Development

entry University C85
Hons): 3 years full-time or 4 years part-time – C6N8
240 IB

rt and Exercise Science and rism and Leisure Studies

terbury Christ Church University C10
ons)/BSc (Hons): 3 years full-time or 5 - 6 years part-
- NC86
C BTEC: MM SQA: CCCC ILC: CCCCC IB: 24

Sport and Exercise Sciences

University of Birmingham B32
BSc (Hons): 3 years full-time – BC17
Tariff: 300 IB: 32

University of Chester C55
BSc (Hons): 3 years full-time – C600
Tariff: 260 IB: 30

University of Gloucestershire G50
BSc (Hons): 3 years full-time – C600
Tariff: 240 IB

Roehampton University R48
BSc (Hons): 3 years full-time or 4 - 7 years part-time – C6L3
A2: CCD BTEC: PPP SQA: BBC IB: 30

University of Ulster U20
BSc (Hons): 3 years full-time or 4 years sandwich – C600 J
A2: AAB BTEC: DDD SQA: AAAAB ILC: AAAB IB: 37

Sport and Exercise Sciences and Applied Social Science

University of Chester C55
BSc (Hons): 3 years full-time – LC36
Tariff: 240 IB: 30

Sport and Exercise Sciences with Applied Social Science

University of Chester C55
BSc (Hons): 3 years full-time – C6L3
Tariff: 240 IB: 30

Sport and Exercise Sciences with Biology

University of Chester C55
BSc (Hons): 3 years full-time – C6C1
Tariff: 240 IB: 30

Sport and Exercise Sciences and Business

University of Chester C55
BA (Hons): 3 years full-time – CN61
Tariff: 240 IB: 30

Sport and Exercise Sciences with Communication Studies

University of Chester C55
BA (Hons): 3 years full-time – C6PH
Tariff: 240 IB: 30

Sport and Exercise Sciences with Computer Science

University of Chester C55
BSc (Hons): 3 years full-time – C6G4
Tariff: 240 IB: 30

Sport and Exercise Sciences with Counselling Skills

University of Chester C55
BA (Hons): 3 years full-time – C6L5
Tariff: 240 IB: 30

Sport and Exercise Sciences with Dance

University of Chester C55
BA (Hons): 3 years full-time – C6W5
Tariff: 240 IB: 30

Sport and Exercise Sciences with Drama and Theatre Studies

University of Chester C55
BA (Hons): 3 years full-time – C6W4
Tariff: 240 IB: 30

Sport and Exercise Sciences with Education Studies

University of Chester C55
BA (Hons): 3 years full-time – C6X3
Tariff: 240 IB: 30

Sport and Exercise Sciences with English

University of Chester C55
BA (Hons): 3 years full-time – C6Q3
Tariff: 240 IB: 30

Sport and Exercise Sciences with Events Management

University of Chester C55
BA (Hons): 3 years full-time – C6NV
Tariff: 240 IB: 30

Sport and Exercise Sciences with Fine Art

University of Chester C55
BA (Hons): 3 years full-time – C6W9
Tariff: 240 IB: 30

Sport and Exercise Sciences and French

University of Chester C55
BA (Hons): 4 years full-time with time abroad – CR61
Tariff: 240 IB: 30

Sport and Exercise Sciences with French

University of Chester C55
BSc (Hons): 3 years full-time – C6R1
Tariff: 240 IB: 30

Sport and Exercise Sciences with Geography

University of Chester C55
BSc (Hons): 3 years full-time – C6F8
Tariff: 240 IB: 30

Sport and Exercise Sciences and German

University of Chester C55
BA (Hons): 4 years full-time with time abroad – CR62
Tariff: 240 IB: 30

Sport and Exercise Sciences with German

University of Chester C55
BSc (Hons): 3 years full-time – C6R2
Tariff: 240 IB: 30

Sport and Exercise Sciences with History

University of Chester C55
BA (Hons): 3 years full-time – C6V1
Tariff: 240 IB: 30

Sport and Exercise Sciences with Internet Technologies

University of Chester C55
BSc (Hons): 3 years full-time – C6H6
Tariff: 240 IB: 30

Sport and Exercise Sciences with Law

University of Chester C55
BA (Hons): 3 years full-time – C6M1
Tariff: 240 IB: 30

Sport and Exercise Sciences with Management

University of Chester C55
BA (Hons): 3 years full-time – C6N2
Tariff: 240 IB: 30

Sport and Exercise Sciences with Marketing

University of Chester C55
BA (Hons): 3 years full-time – C6N5
Tariff: 240 IB: 30

Sport and Exercise Sciences with Mathematics

University of Chester C55
BSc (Hons): 3 years full-time – C6G1
Tariff: 240 IB: 30

Sport and Exercise Sciences with Multimedia Technologies

University of Chester C55
BSc (Hons): 3 years full-time – C6PJ
Tariff: 240 IB: 30

Sport and Exercise Sciences with Nutrition

University of Chester C55
BSc (Hons): 3 years full-time – C6B4
Tariff: 240 IB: 30

Sport and Exercise Sciences and Psychology

University of Chester C55
BSc (Hons): 3 years full-time – CC68
Tariff: 240 IB: 30

Sport and Exercise Sciences with Psychology

University of Chester C55
BSc (Hons): 3 years full-time – C6C8
Tariff: 240 IB: 30

Sport and Exercise Sciences and Spanish

University of Chester C55
BA (Hons): 4 years full-time with time abroad – CR64
Tariff: 240 IB: 30

Sport and Exercise Sciences with Spanish

University of Chester C55
BSc (Hons): 3 years full-time – C6R4
Tariff: 240 IB: 30

Sport and Exercise Sciences and Theology and Religious Studies

University of Chester C55
BA (Hons): 3 years full-time – CV66
Tariff: 240 IB: 30

Sport and Exercise Sciences with Theology and Religious Studies

University of Chester C55
BA (Hons): 3 years full-time – C6V6
Tariff: 240 IB: 30

Sport and Exercise (Sport Studies)

University of Teesside T20
BSc (Hons): 3 years full-time – LC36
Tariff: 240 IB: 26

Sport and Exercise Support and Youth and Community Studies

University of Wales, Newport N37
BA (Hons)/BSc (Hons): 3 years full-time or 6 years part-t
Tariff: 240

Sport, Health and Exercise

Anglia Ruskin University A60
BSc (Hons): 3 years full-time – C6XC
Tariff: 220 IB: 24

University Campus Suffolk [University East Anglia, University of Essex] S82
FdSc: 2 years full-time or 3 years part-time – CL65 B
Tariff: 80 - 120

Sport, Health, Exercise and Nutritic

Leeds, Trinity & All Saints [University c Leeds] L24
BSc (Hons): 3 years full-time or 6 years part-time – CB
Tariff: 160 - 240 IB: 24

Sport, Health and Exercise Science

St Mary's University College, Twickenham S64
BSc (Hons): 3 years full-time – CB69
Tariff: 160

Sport, Health and Fitness

Richmond upon Thames College [University of Surrey]
FdA: 2 years full-time or 4 years part-time
A2: C BTEC: PP - PPP

St Mary's University College, Twickenham S64
FdA: 2 years full-time – CB6X
Tariff: 40

Sport, Health and Fitness Management

Thames Valley University T40
FdA: 2 years full-time or 2 - 4 years part-time – CN62
Tariff: 40

Thames Valley University T40
BA (Hons): 3 years full-time – CB69
Tariff: 160

Sport (Health and Fitness Training

City of Bath College [University of Ba ▲
FdSc: 2 years full-time – C600 G
Tariff: 120

Sport, Health and Leisure and Me

Leeds, Trinity & All Saints [University Leeds] L24
BA (Hons): 3 years full-time or 6 years part-time – CP
Tariff: 160 - 240 IB: 24

Sport, Health and Physical Education with Psychology

University of Wales, Bangor B06
BSc (Hons): 3 years full-time – C6C8
Tariff: 260 IB: 30

Sport Science

Burnley College [University of Central Lancashire] ▲
: 2 years full-time – C604 B
Tariff: 120 Interview

Canterbury Christ Church University C10
BSc (Hons): 3 years full-time or 6 years part-time – C600
Tariff: 160 IB: 24

University of Gloucestershire G50
BSc (Hons): 3 years full-time – C603
Tariff: 240

St Mary's University College, Twickenham S64
BSc (Hons): 3 years full-time – C600
Tariff: 160 IB: 28

Sport Science with American Studies

Canterbury Christ Church University C10
BA (Hons)/BSc (Hons): 3 years full-time – C6T7
A2: CC

Sport Science with Applied Criminology

Canterbury Christ Church University C10
BA (Hons)/BSc (Hons): 3 years full-time – C6M9
A2: CC

Sport Science with Art

Canterbury Christ Church University C10
BA (Hons)/BSc (Hons): 3 years full-time – C6W1
A2: CC

Sport Science with Biosciences

Canterbury Christ Church University C10
BSc (Hons): 3 years full-time – C6C1
A2: CC

Sport Science with Business Studies

Canterbury Christ Church University C10
BA (Hons)/BSc (Hons): 3 years full-time – C6N1
A2: CC

Sport Science with Coaching

Sheffield Hallam University S21
BSc (Hons): 3 years full-time or 6 years part-time – C602
Tariff: 280 IB

Sport Science and Cymraeg (Welsh)

University of Wales, Bangor B06
BSc (Hons): 3 years full-time – CQ6M
Tariff: 260 - 280

Sport Science with Digital Culture, Arts and Media

Canterbury Christ Church University C10
BA (Hons)/BSc (Hons): 3 years full-time – C6G4
A2: CC

Sport Science with Early Childhood Studies

Canterbury Christ Church University C10
BA (Hons)/BSc (Hons): 3 years full-time – C6X3
A2: CC

Sport Science with Education and Employment

St Mary's University College, Twickenham S64
BA (Hons)/BSc (Hons): 3 years full-time – C6X3
Tariff: 160

Sport Science with English

Canterbury Christ Church University C10
BA (Hons)/BSc (Hons): 3 years full-time – C6Q3
A2: CC

Sport Science (Equine and Human)

Warwickshire College, Royal Leamington Spa, Rugby and Moreton Morell [Coventry University] W25
Fd: 2 years full-time or 3 years sandwich – DC4P
Tariff: 80

Sport Science (Exercise and Health)

University Campus Suffolk [University of East Anglia, University of Essex] S82
BSc (Hons): 3 years full-time – CB69 I
Tariff: 140 - 200 IB: 24

Sport Science and French

University of Wales, Bangor B06
BSc (Hons): 4 years full-time with time abroad – CR6C
Tariff: 260 - 280

Sport Science with French

Canterbury Christ Church University C10
BA (Hons)/BSc (Hons): 3 years full-time – C6R1
A2: CC

Sport Science with Geography

Canterbury Christ Church University C10
BA (Hons)/BSc (Hons): 3 years full-time – C6L7
A2: CC

University of Hull H72
BSc (Hons): 3 years full-time – C6F8
Tariff: 260

St Mary's University College, Twickenham S64
BA (Hons)/BSc (Hons): 3 years full-time – C6F8
Tariff: 160

Sport Science and German

University of Wales, Bangor B06
BSc (Hons): 4 years full-time – CR6F
Tariff: 260 - 280

Sport Science with Health and Exercise

St Mary's University College, Twickenham S64
BA (Hons)/BSc (Hons): 3 years full-time – C6BY
Tariff: 160

Sport Science with History

Canterbury Christ Church University C10
BA (Hons)/BSc (Hons): 3 years full-time – C6V1
A2: CC

Sport Science with Human Biology

St Mary's University College, Twickenham S64
BA (Hons)/BSc (Hons): 3 years full-time – C6B1
Tariff: 160

Sport Science with Information Technology

Nottingham Trent University N91
BSc (Hons): 3 years full-time or 4 years sandwich – C6G5
Tariff: 220

Sport Science with Irish Studies

St Mary's University College, Twickenham S64
BA (Hons)/BSc (Hons): 3 years full-time – C6Q5
Tariff: 160

Sport Science and Italian

University of Wales, Bangor B06
BSc (Hons): 4 years full-time – BC6J
Tariff: 260 - 280

Sport Science and Linguistics

University of Wales, Bangor B06
BSc (Hons): 3 years full-time – CQ6C
Tariff: 260 - 280

Sport (Science and Management)

Nottingham Trent University N91
BSc (Hons): 3 years full-time – CN62
Tariff: 240

Sport Science with Management Studies

St Mary's University College, Twickenham S64
BA (Hons)/BSc (Hons): 3 years full-time – C6N2
Tariff: 160

Sport Science with Marketing

Canterbury Christ Church University C10
BA (Hons)/BSc (Hons): 3 years full-time – C6N5
A2: CC

Sport Science and Mathematics

Nottingham Trent University N91
BSc (Hons): 3 years full-time or 4 years sandwich – CG6C
Tariff: 200

Sport Science with Media Arts

St Mary's University College, Twickenham S64
BA (Hons)/BSc (Hons): 3 years full-time – C6P3
Tariff: 160

Sport Science with Media and Cultural Studies

Canterbury Christ Church University C10
BA (Hons)/BSc (Hons): 3 years full-time – C6P3
A2: CC

Sport Science with Music

Canterbury Christ Church University C10
BA (Hons)/BSc (Hons): 3 years full-time – C6W3
A2: CC

Sport Science with Nutrition

St Mary's University College, Twickenham S64
BA (Hons)/BSc (Hons): 3 years full-time – C6BK
Tariff: 160

Sport Science with Philosophy

St Mary's University College, Twickenham S64
BA (Hons)/BSc (Hons): 3 years full-time – C6V5
Tariff: 160

Sport Science (Physical Education)

University of Wales, Bangor B06
BSc (Hons): 3 years full-time – CX6H
Tariff: 260

Sport Science with Physical Education in the Community

St Mary's University College, Twickenham S64
BA (Hons)/BSc (Hons): 3 years full-time – C6C9
Tariff: 160

Sport Science with Professional and Creative Writing

St Mary's University College, Twickenham S64
BA (Hons)/BSc (Hons): 3 years full-time – C6W8
Tariff: 160

Sport Science with Psychology

Canterbury Christ Church University C10
BA (Hons)/BSc (Hons): 3 years full-time – C6C8
A2: CC

St Mary's University College, Twickenham S64
BA (Hons)/BSc (Hons): 3 years full-time – C6C8
Tariff: 160

Sport Science and Religious Studies

University of Wales, Bangor B06
BSc (Hons): 3 years full-time – CV6P
Tariff: 260 - 280

Sport Science with Religious Studies

Canterbury Christ Church University C10
BA (Hons)/BSc (Hons): 3 years full-time – C6V6
A2: CC

Sport Science and Social Policy

University of Wales, Bangor B06
BSc (Hons): 3 years full-time – CL6K
Tariff: 260 - 280

Sport Science with Social Science

Canterbury Christ Church University C10
BA (Hons)/BSc (Hons): 3 years full-time – C6L3
A2: CC

Sport Science and Sociology

University of Wales, Bangor B06
BSc (Hons): 3 years full-time – CL6H
Tariff: 260 - 280

Sport Science with Sociology

St Mary's University College, Twickenham S64
BA (Hons)/BSc (Hons): 3 years full-time – C6L3
Tariff: 160

Sport Science and Spanish

University of Wales, Bangor B06
BSc (Hons): 4 years full-time – CR6L
Tariff: 260 - 280

Sport Science (Sport Performance)

University Campus Suffolk [University of East Anglia, University of Essex] S82
BSc (Hons): 3 years full-time – C602 I
Tariff: 140 - 200 IB: 24

Sport Science with Theology

Canterbury Christ Church University C1
BA (Hons)/BSc (Hons): 3 years full-time – C6VP
A2: CC

Sport Science and Tourism

St Mary's University College, Twickenham S64
BA (Hons)/BSc (Hons): 3 years full-time – CN68
Tariff: 160

Sport Science with Tourism

St Mary's University College, Twickenham S64
BA (Hons)/BSc (Hons): 3 years full-time – C6N8
Tariff: 160

Sport Sciences

Brunel University B84
BSc (Hons): 3 years full-time or 5 - 6 years part-time – C600
Tariff: 260 IB: 29

Sport Sciences (Administration and Development)

Brunel University B84
BSc (Hons): 3 years full-time or 5 - 6 years part-time – CN61
Tariff: 260 IB: 29

Sport Sciences (Coaching)

Brunel University B84
BSc (Hons): 3 years full-time or 5 - 6 years part-time – C603
Tariff: 260 IB: 29

Sport Sciences and Education

University of Exeter E84
BSc (Hons): 3 years full-time – CX63
A2: ABB - AAA

port Sciences (Exercise and Fitness)

unel University B84
c (Hons): 3 years full-time or 5 - 6 years part-time – 01
iff: 260 IB: 29

port Sciences (Physical Education)

unel University B84
c (Hons): 3 years full-time or 5 years part-time – C6X9
iff: 260 IB: 29

port (Sports Therapy)

windon College [University of Bath] ▲
Sc: 2 years full-time or 3 years part-time – CB69 E
iff: 80

orts and Exercise Development

ast Durham and Houghall Community ollege [University of Sunderland] ▲
: 2 years full-time – C604 P
ff: 100

iversity of Sunderland S84
: 2 years full-time – C604
ff: 40

iversity of Sunderland S84
(Hons): 3 years full-time – C602
ff: 200

orts and Exercise Performance

ittle College [University of Essex] W85
: 2 years full-time – C601
ff: 60

ittle College [University of Essex] W85
(Hons): 3 years full-time – C600
f: 140 IB: 24

orts and Exercise Rehabilitation

merset College of Arts and chnology [University of Plymouth] S28
: 2 years full-time – C601
: 80

orts and Exercise Science

iversity of Aberdeen A20
(Hons): 4 years full-time – C600
DD SQA: BBBB ILC: BCCCC - BBCC IB: 26

iversity of Derby D39
(Hons): 3 years full-time or 4 - 6 years part-time – 3
: 140 - 200

iversity of Essex E70
(Hons): 4 years full-time including foundation year – 1
: 120 IB: 24

University of Essex E70
BSc (Hons): 3 years full-time – C600
Tariff: 260 - 300 IB: 28 - 32

Robert Gordon University R36
BSc (Hons): 4 years full-time – C600
A2: CCC SQA: BBCC ILC: BBB

University of Stirling S75
BSc (Hons): 3 - 4 years full-time – CC61
A2: BCC SQA: BBBB IB: 30

University of Westminster W50
BSc (Hons): 3 years full-time – C600
A2: CC BTEC: MM - MPP SQA: CCC ILC: CCC

University of Westminster W50
BSc (Hons): 4 years full-time including foundation year – C608
A2: CC

Sports and Exercise Science with Accounting

University of East London E28
BSc (Hons): 3 years full-time – C6N4
Tariff: 160

Sports and Exercise Science and Cultural Studies

University of East London E28
BA (Hons)/BSc (Hons): 3 years full-time – C6L6
Tariff: 160

Sports and Exercise Science with Education and Community Development

University of East London E28
BA (Hons)/BSc (Hons): 3 years full-time – C6X9
Tariff: 160

Sports and Exercise Science with Human Biology

University of East London E28
BSc (Hons): 3 years full-time – C6BC
Tariff: 160

Sports and Exercise Science and Information Technology

University of East London E28
BSc (Hons): 3 years full-time – CG65
Tariff: 160

Sports and Exercise Science with Marketing

University of East London E28
BSc (Hons): 3 years full-time – C6N5
Tariff: 160

Sports and Exercise Science with Psychology

University of East London E28
BSc (Hons): 3 years full-time – C6CV
Tariff: 160

Sports and Exercise Sciences

University of Leeds L23
BSc (Hons): 3 years full-time – C601
Tariff: 300

Staffordshire University S72
BSc (Hons): 3 years full-time or 6 years part-time – C601
Tariff: 240 IB: 28

University of Sunderland S84
BSc (Hons): 3 years full-time – C601
Tariff: 200 IB: 32

Sports Medicine

University of Glasgow G28
BSc (Hons): 4 years full-time – CB69
A2: BCC SQA: BBBB ILC: BBBB IB: 28 HND

University of Glasgow G28
MSci (Hons): 4 years full-time – C601
A2: BCC - BBC SQA: BBBB - ABBB ILC: BBBB IB: 28

Sports Psychology and Outdoor Recreation

University of Derby Buxton D39
BA (Hons): 3 years full-time or 4 - 6 years part-time – CN8G U
Tariff: 140 - 160 IB: 26

Sports Psychology and Travel and Tourism

University of Derby Buxton D39
BA (Hons): 3 years full-time or 4 - 6 years part-time – CN8V U
Tariff: 140 - 160 IB: 26

Sports Science

Anglia Ruskin University A60
BSc (Hons): 3 years full-time – C600
Tariff: 220 IB: 24

University of Wales, Bangor B06
BSc (Hons): 3 years full-time – C600
Tariff: 260 IB: 30

University of Bedfordshire B22
BSc (Hons): 4 years full-time including foundation year – C606
Interview

Bradford College [Leeds Metropolitan University] B60
FdSc: 2 years full-time – C600
Interview

University of Central Lancashire C30
BSc (Hons): 3 years full-time or 5 years part-time – C600
Tariff: 240

University of Glamorgan G14
BSc (Hons) (Foundation): 1 year full-time – C608
Tariff: 40 Interview

University of Glasgow G28
BSc (Hons): 4 years full-time – C600
A2: BCC SQA: BBBB ILC: BBBB HND

University of Greenwich G70
BSc (Hons): 3 years full-time or 4 years sandwich or 5 years part-time – C600
Tariff: 180

Kingston University K84
BSc (Hons): 3 years full-time or 6 years part-time – C600
Tariff: 220 - 260

Kingston University K84
BSc (Hons): 4 years full-time including foundation year – C608
Tariff: 40 Interview

Kingston College [Kingston University] ▲
BSc (Hons) (Foundation): 1 year full-time – C608 K
Tariff: 40

Liverpool John Moores University L51
BSc/BSc (Hons): 3 years full-time – C600
Tariff: 280 IB: 28

London Metropolitan University L68
BSc (Hons): 3 years full-time or 4 years sandwich or 4 - 5 years part-time day – C603
Tariff: 160 IB: 28

Loughborough College [Loughborough University] L77
FdSc: 2 years full-time or 3 years part-time – C600
Tariff: 140 - 200 Interview

University of Portsmouth P80
BSc (Hons): 3 years full-time – C600
Tariff: 260

University Campus Suffolk [University of East Anglia, University of Essex] S82
BSc (Hons): 3 years full-time or 5 - 9 years part-time – C600 I
Tariff: 140 - 200 IB: 24

City of Sunderland College [University of Sunderland] ▲
BSc (Hons) (Foundation): 1 year full-time – C608 K
Tariff: 100

University of Wales, Swansea S93
BSc (Hons): 3 years full-time – C600
Tariff: 280

University of Winchester W76
BSc (Econ): 3 years full-time – C602
Tariff: 220 IB: 24

University of Winchester W76
DipHE: 2 years full-time – C603
Tariff: 80

Sports Science (Adventure Sports) (top-up)

Pembrokeshire College [University of Glamorgan] P35
BSc (Hons): 1 year full-time – C600
HND

Sports Science and Biology

University of Essex E70
BSc (Hons): 4 years full-time including foundation year – CC61
Tariff: 120 IB: 24

University of Essex E70
BSc (Hons): 3 years full-time – CC16
Tariff: 260 - 300 IB: 28 - 32

University of Glamorgan G14
BSc/BSc (Hons): 3 years full-time or part-time – CC61
Tariff: 200 IB: 24

Sports Science with Biology

University of Glamorgan G14
BSc (Hons): 3 years full-time – C6C1
Tariff: 200 IB: 24

Sports Science with Business

Kingston University K84
BSc (Hons): 4 years full-time including foundation year – C6ND
Tariff: 40 Interview

Kingston University K84
BSc (Hons): 3 years full-time – C6NC
Tariff: 220 - 260

Kingston University K84
BSc (Hons): 4 years sandwich – C6N1
Tariff: 220 - 260

Sports Science and Business Management

University Campus Suffolk [University of East Anglia, University of Essex] S82
BSc (Hons): 3 years full-time or 5 - 9 years part-time – CN62 I
Tariff: 120 - 180

Sports Science and Coaching

University of Bolton B44
BSc (Hons): 3 years full-time or 5 years part-time – C600
Tariff: 140
BASES

London Metropolitan University L68
BSc (Hons): 3 years full-time – C601
Tariff: 160 IB: 28

Sports Science with Education

University of Greenwich G70
BSc (Hons): 3 years full-time – C6X3
Tariff: 160 IB: 24

Sports Science with Education Studies

North East Wales Institute of Higher Education [University of Wales] N56
BA (Hons)/BSc (Hons): 3 years full-time – C6X3
Tariff: 120

Sports Science with Entrepreneurship

University of Greenwich G70
BSc (Hons): 3 years full-time – C6N1
Tariff: 160 IB: 24

Sports Science (Equine and Human)

Warwickshire College, Royal Leamingtc Spa, Rugby and Moreton Morell [Coventry University] W25
BSc (Hons): 3 years full-time or 4 years sandwich – DC3
Tariff: 160

Sports Science and French

University of Wales, Bangor B06
BA (Hons): 3 years full-time – CR61
Tariff: 260 - 280 IB: 28

Sports Science with French

University of Greenwich G70
BSc (Hons): 3 years full-time – C6R1
Tariff: 160 IB: 24

Sports Science and German

University of Wales, Bangor B06
BA (Hons): 3 years full-time – CR62
Tariff: 260 - 280 IB: 28

Sports Science and Human Biology

University Campus Suffolk [University East Anglia, University of Essex] S82
BSc (Hons): 3 years full-time or 5 - 9 years part-time – CC6C I
Tariff: 120 - 180

Sports Science with Human Resources Management

University of Greenwich G70
BSc (Hons): 3 years full-time – C6N6
Tariff: 160 IB: 24

Sports Science and Injury Management

Truro College [University of Plymouth]
FdSc: 2 years full-time – C602
Tariff: 60

Sports Science with Leisure Management

University Campus Suffolk [University East Anglia, University of Essex] S82
BSc (Hons): 3 years full-time or 5 - 9 years part-time – C6N2 I
Tariff: 120 - 180

ports Science and Linguistics

iversity of Wales, Bangor B06
(Hons): 3 years full-time – CQ61
iff: 260 - 280 IB: 28

ports Science with Management

ughborough University L79
(Hons): 3 years full-time – CN62
iff: 340 IB: 34

orts Science with Marketing

iversity of Greenwich G70
(Hons): 3 years full-time – C6N5
iff: 160 IB: 24

orts Science and Materials echnology

iversity of Birmingham B32
(Hons): 3 years full-time – CF62
iff: 300 IB: 32

orts Science and Nutrition and ealth

iversity Campus Suffolk [University of st Anglia, University of Essex] S82
(Hons): 3 years full-time or 5 - 9 years part-time –
4 I
f: 120 - 180

orts Science (Outdoor Activities)

iversity of Wales, Bangor B06
(Hons): 3 years full-time – C602
f: 180 - 260

iversity of Leeds L23
(Hons): 3 years full-time – C600
: 300 IB: 32

orts Science (Outdoor tivities/Marine Pursuits)

nbrokeshire College [University of morgan] P35
year work-based learning

orts Science and Physical ography

versity of Glamorgan G14
BSc (Hons): 3 years full-time or part-time – CF68
: 200 IB: 24

orts Science with Physical ography

versity of Glamorgan G14
Hons): 3 years full-time or part-time – C6F8
: 200 IB: 24

Sports Science and Physics

Loughborough University L79
BSc (Hons): 4 years sandwich – CF63
Tariff: 280 IB: 30

Loughborough University L79
BSc (Hons): 3 years full-time – FC36
Tariff: 280 IB: 28 - 30

Sports Science and Physiology

University of Leeds L23
BSc (Hons): 3 years full-time – BC16
Tariff: 300 IB: 32

Sports Science with Professional Football Coaching

University of Greenwich G70
BSc (Hons): 3 years full-time or 4 years sandwich or 5 years part-time – C690
Tariff: 230

Sports Science with Professional Tennis Coaching

University of Greenwich G70
BSc (Hons): 3 years full-time or 4 years sandwich or 5 years part-time – C602
Tariff: 180

Sports Science with Psychology

University of Wales, Bangor B06
BSc (Hons): 3 years full-time – C6CV
Tariff: 260 IB: 30

Sports Science and Religious Studies

University of Wales, Bangor B06
BA (Hons): 3 years full-time – CV66
Tariff: 260 - 280 IB: 28

Sports Science and Social Policy

University of Wales, Bangor B06
BA (Hons): 3 years full-time – CL64
Tariff: 260 - 280 IB: 28

Sports Science and Sociology

University of Wales, Bangor B06
BA (Hons): 3 years full-time – CL63
Tariff: 260 - 280 IB: 28

Sports Science with Spanish

University of Greenwich G70
BSc (Hons): 3 years full-time – C6R4
Tariff: 160 IB: 24

Sports Science with Sports Management

Loughborough College [Loughborough University] L77
FdSc: 2 years full-time or 3 years part-time – N222
Tariff: 140 - 200 Interview

Sports Science (top-up)

Coleg Sir Gâr [University of Glamorgan] C22
BSc/BSc (Hons): 2 years part-time
HND

Sports Therapy

University of Bedfordshire B22
FdSc: 2 years full-time – C605
Tariff: 80 - 120

Substance Misuse

University of Glamorgan G14
DipHE: 1 year full-time – BL23
HE credits: 120

Substance Misuse (post-qualifying framework)

Bristol, University of the West of England B80
BSc (Hons): 1 year full-time or 4 years part-time – B201
RN, RM, HP

Substance Use and Misuse Studies

Thames Valley University T40
BSc (Hons): 2 - 7 years part-time day
HE credits: 240

Thames Valley University T40
DipHE: 2 - 7 years part-time day
HE credits: 120

Therapeutic Interventions for Addictions (post-qualification)

Bournemouth University B50
BSc (Hons): 1 - 3 years part-time
HE credits: 240

Urgent Care

University Campus Suffolk [University of East Anglia, University of Essex] S82
BSc: 5 years part-time
HE credits: 120, RN, RM, HP

Women's Health Studies

UCE Birmingham C25
BSc (Hons): 2 - 4 years part-time
HE credits: 240, Interview

Medical Technology

Including:
Medical Electronics
Medical Imaging
Medical Technology
Radiography (Diagnostic)

What would you study?

Courses in this chapter are based around physics and mathematics and cover topics such as:

- Computing
- Control engineering
- Digital integrated electronics
- Electromagnetism
- Electronic control
- Software engineering.

We have already seen similar course topics covered in the Biomedical Engineering degree in the chapter on **Biomedical Sciences**. The emphasis for that degree was engineering for the design and adaptation of prosthetics – like artificial limbs – or electrical/electronic control devices designed to meet the individual needs of each patient. In this chapter, the engineering is more geared towards assisting with patient diagnosis. That said, however, your initial choice of degree title would not necessarily commit you to one side or the other. That choice may emerge as your course progresses in the light of the topic choices you make in successive years.

The study of radiography features in this group of courses but mainly in its diagnostic form. See the chapter on **Therapies** for further discussion of radiography as part of treatment. Course titles vary but you need to check the content if you have a particular career in mind at the start.

These courses are normally offered by the engineering departments of HE institutions rather than the medical or healthcare departments, but obviously there are close links between the different departments. Foundation degrees are available for some of the courses in this chapter.

Getting in

We are on the fringes of the engineering area here so maths and physics become the dominant subjects and are normally required at high grades. However, you still need an interest in biology-based study and the ability to think across the whole science spectrum.

Each university decides on its own entry requirements. You can see the range of UCAS points asked by each one by consulting the course listings on the following pages. However, many Foundation degree courses exercise a more flexible admissions procedure which enables them to take into account factors such as work experience in their entrance requirements and which cannot therefore be expressed as part of the UCAS tariff framework.

Graduate outlook

Opportunities exist in the NHS, in the private medicine sector and, for the engineers and scientists, with the large manufacturing companies and universities involved in the production and development of equipment.

Radiography

The most familiar career title in this group is that of the radiographer. This career has been around almost since Roentgen discovered X-rays. Most people have an idea of what a diagnostic radiographer does – we have all seen medical programmes on TV where doctors look at X-ray photos of the insides of patients as an aid to helping them decide what is wrong and what the treatment should be. X-rays carry a risk to the patient and the radiographer has to make decisions on the amount of radiation each patient is exposed to and constantly weigh up that risk against the diagnostic benefits to be gained. (The role of diagnostic radiographer is a different one from that of the therapeutic radiographer described in the **Therapies** chapter.)

X-ray photos *are* produced by diagnostic radiographers and the TV image is a fair one. However, there are developments on the way. Photos are static images but it has now become routine for dynamic (moving) image to be made available using ultrasound techniques. Pregnant women will know about this from the scans that show their baby moving around in th womb.

The introduction of computerised tomography (CT) in 1973 began a revolution in the range and complexity of equipment available in this fiel Technology in this area is rapidly advancing both in terms of availability and of sophistication. The latest development is that of Magnetic Resonance Imaging (MRI) which is a powerful tool bringing new professional skills for the radiographer to master.

Engineering

Besides increasing the professional demands placed on the radiographe sophisticated equipment costing millions of pounds has created new job opportunities for other engineers and physicists. There are now opportunities for engineers to maintain the equipment, advise on radiatio issues, develop new applications and work in university teaching, resear and development. Cutting-edge engineering is now right at the heart of medical diagnosis and treatment.

This area of NHS work is covered by the Health Professions Council (HPC so you need to ensure that your course is accredited by them. You will need two years' practical experience in a training situation before you achieve full registration. However, the HPC is not on its own when it com to the engineers and physicists. The Institute of Electrical Engineers (IEE the Institute of Mechanical Engineers (IMechE) and the Institute of Physi and Engineering in Medicine (IPEM) are also accrediting bodies and play their part in developing and maintaining professional standards for engineers in this field.

Clinical technology

Clinical technologists take an approved degree (which would be either i radiation or engineering-based subjects), and follow this with an IPEM training scheme for trainee clinical technologists. Clinical scientists follo their degree with a two-year training place in an appropriate departmen and read for an MSc, or go for the NHS national training scheme. There then opportunities for yet more study and training leading to the award MIPEM or CEng.

What would you earn?

Salary scales for NHS radiographers and medical technologists are on a scale from approximately £19,000 to £31,000. Promotion could bring salaries of approximately £22,800 to £36,400 and very senior posts are paid up to £61,000.

These examples are based on April 2006 salary scales. At the time of writing this book the public sector unions had not accepted the pay increase of around 2.5%, which had been offered in April 2007.

Clinical engineers could earn from approximately £23,000 to £90,000 depending on their level of seniority and where they are employed.

Case Study

Hasina Mohamed

Hasina is in the final year of a BSc in Diagnostic Radiography at the University of Teesside.

'I have done this course as a mother with two young children, so there is not much I don't know about time management – especially as we work for more weeks in the year than the average student. We have to do a required number of clinical placements so we get just three weeks' holiday at Christmas, two at Easter and then ten weeks during the summer.

'I left school with very few qualifications and worked as a care assistant – which I enjoyed. I then had my children and while I was at home with them I decided that I wanted to do more with my life. I saw a careers adviser, did a lot of research on careers websites into adult nursing and other careers related to medicine and finally made up my mind to be a radiographer. It seemed just right – a career with a lot of people contact, using practical and technical skills and one that would offer a variety of specialisms once I was qualified.

'I contacted the admissions officer at Teesside, my nearest university, and was advised to do an Access course in Health* at a local college. I was offered a place for radiography but on the condition that I did a six week summer school programme in mathematics followed by one in physics at the university. These courses had prepared me well for the degree ahead. My Access course finished in June and I did the two summer schools one after the other! I then started the course.

'It was a bit overwhelming at first, learning all the new subjects, but I appreciated the relevance and managed to work my way through them. The lecturers at university were very supportive and were there for me to discuss any personal and professional problems. I also had to work round my family. I couldn't have done it without my husband who has been marvellous. He runs his own business and does all the child care while I'm at university. It is very important to have a good support network while studying at university, particularly if you have a family of your own. Your own personal commitment has to be there too.

'Because we are training for a profession as well as getting a degree the course is a combination of academic and practical work all the way through. We started with all the core subjects that would prepare us for the first 15 week clinical placement, and then went to local hospitals. I got my first choice and it has been my base hospital throughout the course. I then returned to university for more academic modules and did a second placement of six weeks during the summer. I spent a whole year at the university during part of the second year and the beginning of the third, followed by another summer placement. That one was in two different hospitals so that I could work in different settings and also gain experience in electives such as medical ultrasound, vascular imaging and intervention, and MRI work.

'On clinical placement you begin by observing, then do things under supervision and gradually take more responsibility for your work. The only way to learn is to be hands-on but the qualified radiographers are very supportive and aid your professional development. When you say "I feel comfortable doing this procedure now" you are only then allowed to do it on your own. All examinations are authorised by radiographers and the results are discussed with you to see if anything could have been done to improve the outcome. I'm on my last placement now and I am almost working on my own. I have found the clinical placements very useful as they have given me the opportunity to relate my theoretical knowledge to my practical skills.

'I have enjoyed the course very much. I am now at the stage where I am consolidating all my skills. I feel prepared for practice and look forward to starting my new career in radiography.'

* Other entry requirements are between 240 and 300 tariff points from three six-unit awards, including one science subject, or equivalent qualifications. Applicants must have five GCSEs at grade C or above including English language, mathematics and two science subjects, or double co-ordinated science or equivalent.

Applied Medical Technology

University of Portsmouth P80
FdSc: 2 years full-time or 3 years part-time – B800
Tariff: 40 Interview

Biotechnology in Medicine

University of Westminster W50
BSc (Hons): 4 years full-time including foundation year – J709
A2: EE

University of Westminster W50
BSc (Hons): 3 years full-time – J701
A2: CC SQA: CCC IB: 26

Clinical Technology

University of Bradford B56
BSc (Hons): 3 years full-time – H900
Tariff: 200 - 240

University of Bradford B56
BSc (Hons): 4 years sandwich – H901
Tariff: 200 - 240

Castle College Nottingham [De Montfort University] C21
BSc (Hons): 4 years part-time
Tariff: 140

Diagnostic Imaging

Bristol, University of the West of England B80
BSc (Hons): 3 years full-time – B821
Tariff: 180 - 220 IB: 24
HPC, SOR

Diagnostic Imaging (Radiography)

London South Bank University L75
BSc (Hons): 3 years full-time – B821
A2: CDD
HPC, SOR

Diagnostic Imaging Science

Glasgow Caledonian University G42
BSc (Hons): 4 years full-time – B821
Tariff: 144 - 220
HPC, SOR

Diagnostic Radiography

University of Bradford B56
BSc (Hons): 3 years full-time – B821
Tariff: 240
HPC, SOR

University of Cumbria C99
BSc (Hons): 3 years full-time – B811 L
Tariff: 300 IB: 32 Interview

University of Cumbria C99
BSc (Hons): 3 years full-time – B821 F
Tariff: 300 IB: 32 Interview
HPC, SOR

University of Derby D39
BSc (Hons): 3 years full-time – B821
Tariff: 200

University of Liverpool L41
BSc (Hons): 3 years full-time – B821
A2: CCC BTEC: DMM SQA: BBBCC ILC: BBBCC IB: 26
HPC, SOR

Queen Margaret University, Edinburgh Q25
BSc (Hons): 4 years full-time – B821
Tariff: 180 Interview
HPC, SOR

Robert Gordon University R36
BSc (Hons): 4 years full-time – B821
A2: CCC SQA: BBCC ILC: BBCC
HPC, SOR

St George's, University of London S49
BSc (Hons): 3 years full-time – B821
Tariff: 220

University of Salford S03
BSc (Hons): 3 years full-time – B821
Tariff: 280 IB: 29
HPC

Sheffield Hallam University S21
BSc (Hons): 3 years full-time – B821
Tariff: 260
HPC, SOR

University Campus Suffolk [University of East Anglia, University of Essex] S82
BSc (Hons): 3 years full-time – B821 I
Tariff: 160 - 180 IB: 24 Interview
HPC, SOR

University of Teesside T20
BSc (Hons): 3 years full-time – B821
Tariff: 240 - 300 Interview
HPC

UCE Birmingham C25
BSc (Hons): 3 - 5 years full-time or 6 years part-time – B821
Tariff: 220
HPC, SOR

Diagnostic Radiography and Imaging

University of Wales, Bangor B06
BSc (Hons): 3 years full-time – B820
Tariff: 220 - 240 IB: 26
HPC, SOR

University of Hertfordshire H36
BSc (Hons): 3 years full-time – B821
Tariff: 220 IB: 24
HPC, SOR

Health and Medical Technologies

Coventry University C85
BSc (Hons): 3 years full-time or 4 years sandwich – B900
Tariff: 200

Medical Electronics

University of Plymouth P60
BSc (Hons): 3 years full-time – H607
Tariff: 160

Medical Electronics and Instrumentation

University of Liverpool L41
BEng (Hons): 3 years full-time – H673
A2: BBC BTEC: DMM SQA: AAAB ILC: BBBCC IB: 28
EC, IET

University of Liverpool L41
MEng (Hons): 4 years full-time – H675
A2: ABB BTEC: DDM SQA: AAAAB ILC: ABBBB IB: 34

Medical Imaging

University of Portsmouth P80
FdSc: 2 years full-time or 3 years part-time – B801
Tariff: 40 Interview

Medical Imaging (Diagnostic Radiography)

University of Exeter E84
BSc (Hons): 3 years full-time – B821
Tariff: 260 IB: 26 - 28

Medical Imaging (Radiography)

Canterbury Christ Church University C1
BSc (Hons): 3 years full-time – B821
Tariff: 160 IB: 24
HPC, SOR

Medical Product Design

Aston University A80
BSc (Hons): 3 years full-time or 4 years sandwich – H81
Tariff: 240 - 280 IB: 31 - 32

University of Hull H72
BSc (Hons): 3 years full-time – H390
Tariff: 240 IB: 26

Medical Systems Engineering

University of Sheffield S18
BEng: 3 years full-time – H671
A2: BBB SQA: AABB ILC: ABBBB IB: 32

University of Sheffield S18
MEng: 4 years full-time – H670
A2: BBB SQA: AABB ILC: ABBBB IB: 32
IMC, IET

Medical Systems Engineering with Management

University of Sheffield S18
MEng: 4 years full-time – B8N2
A2: BBB SQA: AABB ILC: ABBBB IB: 32

Medical Technology

Liverpool John Moores University L51
BSc (Hons): 3 years full-time or 4 years sandwich – BH11
Tariff: 160 - 300

Staffordshire University S72
FdSc: 2 years full-time – B800
Tariff: 100

Medical Technology in Sport

University of Bradford B56
BSc (Hons): 3 years full-time – BC8P
Tariff: 200

University of Bradford B56
BSc (Hons): 4 years sandwich – BC86
Tariff: 200

Oncology and Radiotherapy Technology

University Campus Suffolk [University of East Anglia, University of Essex] S82
BSc (Hons): 3 years full-time – B822 I
Tariff: 160 - 180

Radiography

University of Ulster U20
BSc (Hons): 4 years full-time – B820 J
A2: AAB BTEC: DDD SQA: AAAAB ILC: AAAB IB: 37
HPC, SOR

Radiography (Diagnostic)

City University C60
BSc (Hons): 3 years full-time – B821
A2: CC IB

University of Leeds L23
BSc (Hons): 3 years full-time – B821
A2: CCC SQA: CCCCC
HPC, SOR

University of Portsmouth P80
BSc (Hons): 3 years full-time – B821
Tariff: 280 - 300 Interview
HPC, SOR

Radiography (Diagnostic, extended)

University of Portsmouth P80
BSc (Hons): 4 years full-time including foundation year – B818
Tariff: 260 Interview
HPC

Radiography (Diagnostic and Imaging)

Cardiff University C15
BSc (Hons): 3 years full-time – B821
Tariff: 260

Medicine

Including:
Clinical Science
Medical Science
Operating Department Practice

What would you study?

Courses normally last five years, at the end of which you should gain provisional registration with the General Medical Council (GMC). In the majority of cases the degree offered by medical schools is a Bachelor of Medicine *and* a Bachelor of Surgery (MB and BS/ChB).

Most medical schools offer the opportunity to extend the course by taking an extra year before your clinical experience in order to gain an extra science degree, referred to as an intercalated degree.

Degrees in Medicine are now taught in 30 schools in the UK with the Peninsula school, Keele, Brighton and Sussex, Durham, Warwick and Hull York being the newest additions as part of an expansion programme aiming to boost the country's capacity to produce newly qualified doctors.

Some medical schools offer a preliminary year for non-science applicants (not the same as applicants who have taken sciences but not done very well!). Alternatively, if you are already a graduate in a relevant subject, you could apply for one of the four-year fast-track courses specifically designed to offer an accelerated route to qualification.

Courses in medicine consist of pre-clinical (classroom and laboratory based) and clinical (hospital based) stages. A few schools separate the two stages very strictly – as was always done traditionally – but many more courses have moved towards a system that provides more integration of the pre-clinical and clinical teaching and introduces students to patients at a much earlier stage, sometimes as early as the first term. If you have a preference for one method over the other you will need to compare course details very carefully before making your application.

Pre-clinical

Pre-clinical studies comprise the familiar groups of subjects such as anatomy, physiology and the like. However, the trend now is towards using a case study approach to acquire this knowledge. The aim is to move away from the teaching of individual subjects in a purely theoretical manner. Students, working in small groups, will be presented with a patient and told something like 'Mr X is experiencing chest pains'. The group, under supervision, take the patient's case history, establish and discuss the symptoms and suggest treatment strategies. This will lead to discussion and exploration of the theoretical issues underlying that patient's condition and in turn to increasing the students' understanding of pre-clinical theory. At the same time, students will, from the outset, be refining their skills of communicating with and relating to patients, and of debating with and using the strengths of fellow professionals.

Pre-clinical studies take two years, by the end of which you will have acquired a considerable grasp of the science at the core of the medical degree. At this point you may decide to extend this phase of your course and take an intercalated degree. The case study overleaf shows an example of a student taking an intercalated BSc in Physiology before continuing to the clinical phase.

Clinical

The clinical stage takes three years. You may find some newcomers arriving on your course at this point. It is now more common for people who started at university on courses such as some of those described in the chapters on **Anatomy and Physiology** and on **Biomedical Sciences** to apply for fast-track postgraduate medical training. Their first degrees will have covered similar ground to the pre-clinical part of the degree in medicine.

This phase allows students, although still closely supervised, to take on increasing levels of responsibility. They begin to perform more routine medical tasks such as catheterisation, taking blood samples or measuring blood pressure, so patient contact skills are constantly being honed.

Your degree will be assessed by exam at regular intervals, by coursework and by assessed observed clinical examination.

Getting in

Competition for places at medical school is fierce. Since the demand for doctors is so high, the vast majority of graduates progress from their degree to the profession – so it is really the medical course admissions tutor who makes judgements about an individual's suitability for a career in medicine. This applies in terms of both academic ability and personalit attributes. (For more detail on the approach of one medical school towar selection, see the quote from Peninsula Medical School in the **Introducti** to this guide.)

In general, you will need to show the following to be a serious contender for a place at medical school:

- **A high level of academic attainment** – including a proven track record in science subjects with predicted grades for your UCAS application suggesting a top grade performance of around 320 to 340 UCAS tariff points. (Non-science students who are likely to notch up a similar level of tariff points are welcomed as applicants for the six yea courses, where the preliminary year will be a science foundation year enable them to continue alongside those with science who enter the five year course the following year.)
- **Fitness to practise**. There is no point in applying to medical school if you are unlikely to be accepted for provisional registration by the General Medical Council (GMC) on graduation. Bars to registration include certain criminal convictions and cautions. As with many of the healthcare professions, health issues are also significant. For example you should declare at the outset any possible infection with blood-bor viruses. Problems such as this will not necessarily prevent you from gaining a place at medical school, but will mean that you could be subject to procedures designed to protect patients and fellow student from exposure to any risk.
- **A degree of understanding about what a career in medicine is al about**. Normally, judgement on this matter will be made on the basis the evidence you provide of appropriate work experience – like volunteer work in a health-related area, or spending gap year time in healthcare environment.

Admissions tests

For entry to some courses you will be required to take an entry test in addition to examination grades. These tests have been designed to help admissions staff by measuring general and personal skills and abilities r directly assessed in academic examinations. Institutions state clearly in their prospectuses whether or not applicants must take a test, and if so, which one. You may be asked to take one or more of the following:

- **UK Clinical Aptitude Test (UKCAT):** this is a 2 hour paper test consisting of four separate sections. There are a number of test dates but you must have taken the test by 10 October. The fee for taking th test in 2007 was £60 before 31 August and £75 between 31 August and 10 October. The fee may be waived for candidates receiving certain benefits – such as Educational Maintenance Allowances or Income support. For more information see www.ukcat.ac.uk.
- **BioMedical Admissions Test (BMAT):** this is a 2 hour paper test consisting of multiple choice and essay questions. It costs £26 and takes place at the beginning of November. You have to register by 29 September. For more information, see www.bmat.org.uk.

For entry to shortened degree courses for graduates in other subjects some universities use an Australian aptitude test – GAMSAT, which tak place at the end of November. Others use UKCAT. For further informatic contact the schools you wish to apply to.

Graduate outlook

Trainee doctors are required to complete a two-year foundation programme in an NHS hospital. Foundation Year 1 (F1) is equivalent to old pre-registration house officer year, and Foundation Year 2 (F2) equa the former first year of employment as a senior house officer. They are titled to full registration with the GMC at the end of their F1 year.

e Foundation Programme acts as the bridge between undergraduate edical training and specialist training (for example in areas like ediatrics, cardiology, gynaecology, ophthalmology and psychiatry) or GP aining. During the programme trainee doctors will gain a grounding in actical medicine and the opportunity to develop their core clinical skills, luding:

Good clinical care

Maintaining good medical practice

Relationships with patients and colleagues.

the end, graduates will be in a position to proceed to training in their ecialism of choice or to general practice.

nployment

e vast majority of medical graduates undertake postgraduate training, rried out in salaried employment within the NHS.

e publication *What do graduates do?* provides statistics for graduates Medicine. Perhaps not surprisingly it showed that of 4565 students o responded to a survey in 2005 (the latest year for which figures available) the vast majority were working or training in the medical d.

- 86.6% were in employment in the UK
- 7.1% were doing full-time further study
- 4.9% were working and studying
- 0.2% were unemployed

… six months after graduation.

(The figures do not total 100% because some graduates answered the survey stating that they were not available for work.)

Of those in employment 99.1% were in the medical field.

What would you earn?

Sample NHS salaries:

- First year out of medical school – £20,741
- Consultant scale from £69,991 to £94,706 Consultants may also receive awards for 'clinical excellence' from £2,817 to £72,210 and most, of course, do private work in addition to NHS work
- Salaried GP scale £50,322–£76,462 plus a range of allowances for meeting targets which can take salaries to well over £100,000. There have been press reports suggesting that some GPs earn over £250,000.

These examples are based on April 2006 salary scales. At the time of writing this book the public sector unions had not accepted the pay increase of around 2.5%, which had been offered in April 2007.

Case Study

Lauretta Chan

Lauretta graduated in 2004 with a BSc, BM in Medicine from the University of Southampton.

'Medicine appealed to me throughout my sixth form at Newcastle Central High School. Unfortunately my UCAS applications to medical schools were unsuccessful – so I buckled down, managed straight A grades in chemistry, physics and maths and found a place through Clearing to read Medicine at Southampton.

'It was my interest in people coupled with my interest in science which made me so keen. It is always hard at school to find work experience in a hospital environment but I found my work as a hospice volunteer useful. I learned that I had the confidence to talk to patients and my communication skills and ability to break bad news improved during my time there.

'Moving so far away from home – Newcastle to Southampton – was hard. I have to admit to early homesickness but I settled in and enjoyed the course. I started with a two-year pre-clinical period working on medical theory. The teaching was different from school. As well as taking broader subjects like physiology and anatomy, we focused on specific medical areas like cardiology (the study of heart problems). We had a volunteer patient with a heart problem and worked from scratch – from taking the patient history through to suggesting treatment strategies. On the way we learned individual science subjects and gained, from the start, patient contact skills.

'The first term established a common level of knowledge across the group. For example, I had not taken A level biology. The Southampton approach helped me through that and enabled us all to progress on an equal footing.

'After the first two years of pre-clinical I had a choice. Most of my fellow students carried on to complete their degree with three years' clinical work. I decided, however, to take an "intercalated" degree course. That meant spending an extra year capitalising on all the theory I had learned, as well as doing a lab-based research project, and making it into a degree in its own right. I was awarded a First Class BSc (Hons) in Physiology before eventually starting clinical studies.

'The clinical period continued to tackle medical theory, but combined this with more practical elements such as learning clinical skills (like taking blood samples) and amassing clinical histories. There was much bedside teaching.

'The degree is a crucial stage in my career but I still have to take further training in order to practise whichever speciality I choose. My next step? A job with The University Hospital of North Durham for the compulsory two-year MMC foundation programme – just introduced as an improved method of training us for the specific branches of medicine in which we want to work.'

Medical Sciences

Bromley College of Further and Higher Education
Fd: 2 years part-time
A2: C BTEC: PPP

University of Edinburgh E56
BSc (Hons): 4 years full-time – B100
A2: BBB SQA: BBBB IB: 30

University of Glamorgan G14
BSc (Hons): 3 years full-time – B901
Tariff: 300 - 340

Medical Sciences (graduate entry)

University of Cambridge C05
MB BChir: 4 years full-time – A101

Medicinal Chemistry

University of Manchester M20
MChem: 4 years full-time – F152
A2: ABB BTEC: DDM SQA: AAABB ILC: AAABB IB: 33
Interview

Medicine

University of Aberdeen A20
MB ChB: 5 years full-time – A100
A2: ABB SQA: AAAAB ILC: AAAAAB IB: 36

University of Birmingham B32
MB ChB: 5 years full-time – A100
Tariff: 340 IB: 36 Interview
GMC

Brighton and Sussex Medical School B74
BMBS: 5 years full-time – A100
Tariff: 340 IB: 37 Interview
GMC

University of Cambridge C05
MB BChir: 16 terms full-time – A100
Tariff: 360 IB: 36 - 40

Cardiff University C15
MB BCh: 5 years full-time – A100
Tariff: 340 IB: 36 Interview
GMC

University of East Anglia E14
MB BS: 5 years full-time – A100
Tariff: 340 IB: 34 - 36 Interview

University of Edinburgh E56
MB ChB: 5 years full-time – A100
A2: AAA SQA: AAAAB IB: 37

University of Glasgow G28
MB ChB: 5 years full-time – A100
A2: AAB SQA: AAAAB Interview

Hull York Medical School H75
MB BS: 5 years full-time – A100
A2: AAB SQA: AAAAB ILC: AAAAAB IB: 36

Imperial College London I50
BSc: 4 years full-time MB BS: 6 years full-time – A100
A2: AAB IB: 32 Interview
GMC

Keele University K12
MB ChB: 5 years full-time – A100
A2: AAB IB: 34

King's College London (University of London) K60
MB BS: 5 years full-time – A100
A2: AAB IB: 32

University of Leeds L23
MB ChB: 5 years full-time – A100
A2: AAB IB: 36

University of Leicester L34
MBChB (Hons): 5 years full-time – A100
A2: AAB IB: 36

University of Manchester M20
MB ChB: 5 years full-time – A106
A2: AAB IB: 35 Interview

University of Manchester M20
MB ChB: 6 years full-time including foundation year – A104
A2: ABB SQA: AAABB ILC: AAAABB Interview

University of Nottingham N84
BM: 3 years full-time BMedSci/BS: 5 years full-time – A100
A2: AAB IB: 38

University of Oxford O33
BCh/BM: 6 years full-time – A100
A2: AAB - AAA SQA: AAAAB - AAAAA IB: 38

Peninsula Medical School P37
BM/BS: 5 years full-time – A100
Tariff: 370 - 400 IB: 36 Interview

Queen Mary, University of London Q50
MB BS: 5 years full-time – A100 W
A2: AAB SQA: AAAAB IB: 34

Queen's University Belfast Q75
MB BCh BAO: 5 years full-time – A100
A2: AAA SQA: AAAAB IB: 35

University of St Andrews S36
BSc (Hons): 3 years full-time – A100
A2: AAB SQA: AAAAB IB: 37

St George's, University of London S49
MB BS: 5 years full-time – A100
A2: ABB IB: 35 Interview
GMC

University of Southampton S27
BM: 5 years full-time – A100
Tariff: 340 IB: 36
GMC

University College London, University of London U80
MB BS: 6 years full-time – A100
A2: AAB IB: 36

Medicine (accelerated/graduate entry)

Newcastle University N21
MB BS: 4 years full-time – A101
GMC

Medicine (conversion)

King's College London (University of London) K60
MB BS: 6 years full-time – A103
A2: AAB ILC: AAAABB IB: 36

Medicine (foundation year)

University of Sheffield S18
MB ChB: 6 years full-time including foundation year – A1
A2: AAB SQA: AAAAB ILC: AAAAAB IB: 34
GMC

Medicine (foundation year entry)

Cardiff University C15
MB ChB: 6 years full-time including foundation year – A1
Tariff: 340 IB: 36 Interview
GMC

Medicine (graduate entry)

University of Birmingham B32
MB ChB: 4 years full-time – A101
GMC

University of Bristol B78
MB ChB: 4 years full-time – A101

King's College London (University of London) K60
MB BS: 4 years full-time – A102
Interview

University of Leicester L34
MBChB (Hons): 4 years full-time – A101

University of Nottingham N84
BMBS: 4 years full-time – A101

University of Oxford O33
BCh/BM: 4 years full-time – A101

Queen Mary, University of London Q50
MB BS: 4 years full-time – A101

St George's, University of London S49
MB BS: 4 years full-time – A101

University of Southampton S27
BM: 4 years full-time – A101
GMC

University of Wales, Swansea S93
MB BCh: 4 years full-time – A101

University of Warwick W20
MBChB (Hons): 4 years full-time – A101

Understanding How To Make The New Medicines – 5th/6th UCAS Choices

The discovery of penicillin was a momentous achievement. However, it took 15 years and an international effort to find a way to produce it in the quantities needed for medical treatment. The subsequent realisation of the lives lost as a result of this delay from discovery to availability set the scene for the birth of the discipline of biochemical engineering.

The medicines of the future — human proteins, therapeutic vaccines, human cells and tissue for repair — are vastly more complex than penicillin. Even the new, small molecule medicines have a far higher degree of complexity. The challenges to biochemical engineers in understanding how to bring the new discoveries to fruition have therefore never been greater, nor the prospects more exciting.

All who apply for a medical place through UCAS are asked to choose additional fifth and sixth places in other fields. Those seeking a professionally recognised qualification in a subject that is demanding, and who want a life at the cutting edge that is highly rewarded, should consider the excitement of biochemical engineering as a degree option.

Details of courses can be found in Trotman's Green Guides, or on the web and visits can be arranged to explore in more detail the A level requirements, the courses and the careers available.

Medicine (with Health foundation year)

Keele University K12
MB ChB: 6 years full-time including foundation year – B900
A2: AAB

Medicine (Maxfax)

King's College London (University of London) K60
MB BS: 4 years full-time – A104
HP

Medicine (with pre-medical year)

University of Edinburgh E56
MB ChB: 6 years full-time – A104
A2: AAA SQA: AAAAB IB: 37

Medicine (stage 1 entry)

University of Durham [Newcastle University] ▲
MB BS: 2 years full-time – A106 D
A2: AAA SQA: AAAAB ILC: AAAAAB

University of Sheffield S18
MB ChB: 5 years full-time – A106
A2: AAB SQA: AAAAB ILC: AAAAAB IB: 34
GMC

Medicine and Surgery

University of Dundee D65
MB ChB: 5 years full-time – A100
Tariff: 336 - 360 IB: 34
GMC

Lancaster University L14
MB ChB (Hons): 5 years full-time
Tariff: 390 IB: 7 7 6

University of Liverpool L41
MB ChB: 5 years full-time – A100
A2: AAB IB: 38 Interview
GMC

Newcastle University N21
MB BS: 5 years full-time – A106
A2: AAA ILC: AAAAAA IB: 38
GMC

Medicine and Surgery (first MB pre-medical)

University of Bristol B78
MB ChB: 6 years full-time including foundation year – A104
A2: AAB BTEC: DDM SQA: AAAAA IB: 36

Medicine and Surgery (graduate entry)

University of Liverpool L41
MB ChB: 4 years full-time – A101

Medicine and Surgery (graduate entry, Lancaster)

University of Liverpool L41
MB ChB: 5 years full-time – A105

Medicine and Surgery (pre-medical year)

University of Dundee D65
MB ChB: 6 years full-time – A104
Tariff: 348 - 360
GMC

Medicine and Surgery (second MB pre-clinical)

University of Bristol B78
MB ChB: 5 years full-time – A100
A2: AAB BTEC: DDM SQA: AAAAA IB: 36

Medicine (widening access)

University of Southampton S27
BM: 6 years full-time – A102
Tariff: 200 Interview
GMC

Medicines Management

University of Portsmouth P80
FdSc: 3 years part-time
HP

Nursing and Midwifery

Including:
Children's Nursing
Learning Disability Studies
Mental Health (Psychiatric Nursing)

What would you study?

Nursing

All higher education courses offer a combination of study and practical experience. All nurses now start with a common foundation programme as part of either a degree or a diploma course before beginning to specialise in one of four branches of the profession (further details below). The common programme takes you through topics such as:

- Applied sciences for health
- Communication
- Foundations of nursing practice
- Introduction to clinical skills
- Principles of professional nursing
- Principles underpinning personal and professional development
- Psychosocial aspects of health.

Don't confuse the 'common foundation programme', the first part of nurse education, with a 'Foundation degree'.

Following the first year and assuming you don't change your mind and change specialisms, you will continue your course focusing on the nursing branch you chose at the outset. The four branches are:

- **Adult nursing** – dealing with adults suffering from acute or chronic illness or those with disabilities, not just in hospital wards and operating theatres, but also in GPs' surgeries, residential homes and health centres
- **Children's nursing** – dealing with children aged up to 16, learning how to provide a safe and secure environment for children who need medical treatment and working with their parents or carers since the wider family will necessarily be part of the rehabilitation
- **Mental health nursing** – working with people with psychological and personality disorders, many of whom could require long-term treatment either in a hospital setting or in the community. There could be opportunities for work in specialist units for those with issues such as drug or alcohol dependency. Much work is done in teams with psychiatrists, psychologists, social workers and counsellors.
- **Learning disability nursing** – working with people of all ages suffering from learning disabilities. Again work in teams is often a key element here as people with learning disabilities have long-term problems which require support to be delivered in settings such as community centres, the family home, schools, colleges and social care residential accommodation. The teams could involve professionals such as youth and social workers, teachers and counsellors and your training course could well include people from these professions.

As your studies continue into the pre-registration phase, you will encounter practical subjects such as:

- Assisting with physical examinations
- Counselling patients and relatives
- Giving drugs, transfusions and drips
- Medical procedures such as checking temperatures and blood pressure
- Observation and assessment of patients in conjunction with doctors
- Taking patients' clinical histories (which presents different challenges according to the branch of nursing for which you are training)
- Writing care plans.

All these topics will be reinforced by ward experience. The higher education institution will also deal with topics such as management of resources, playing a part in a healthcare team and concepts of healthcare leadership.

Midwifery

You can enter midwifery through a diploma course or a degree programme Alternatively, you can qualify as a registered nurse and then take an accelerated course to qualify as a midwife (normally one year to 18 month All routes lead to registered midwife (RM) status and membership of the Nursing and Midwifery Council (NMC). A degree programme will normally b 50% theory, taught in university, and 50% clinical practice in local hospital Course content will include:

- Anatomy and physiology
- Aspects of sociology, psychology, law and ethics
- Behavioural science
- Clinical midwifery skills
- Handling complexities in childbirth
- Infant feeding
- Nutrition.

As a midwife your role will be to care for pregnant women and new mothe You will run checks on pregnant mothers and discuss their needs in antenatal clinics, assist and support them during the birth, and teach them baby care skills after the baby is born.

Getting in

The number of places available in the system reflects the need for increasing numbers of trained nurses in all parts of the UK. Because the are plenty of places available, you should be able to find a course near you, which is particularly important if you are a mature student who ma need to match study location with other commitments.

Owing to the number of mature applicants, admissions tutors can be flexible and work experience can be an important factor.

Applications to most nursing and midwifery programmes are made through UCAS in the normal way – and you may remember from readin the introduction that you may apply to a maximum of five courses: deg and/or diploma courses. **However, there are no diploma courses in Wales.** In Scotland applications to diploma courses are made through a separate organisation CATCH, PO Box 21, Edinburgh EH2 2YS. You wi find a link to CATCH and may order an application form from the follow website: www.nes.scot.nhs.uk

Graduate outlook

Nursing, like most of the other healthcare professions, has changed in recent years. As medical technology advances and treatment become ever more sophisticated, nurses must keep abreast of developments. greater emphasis on higher education qualifications reflects these trends.

Once you have your degree or diploma in Nursing, you need to register with the Nursing and Midwifery Council (NMC): once you have done this you will be allowed to practise. However, your education and training do not stop there. Your initial course will have prepared you for the need fo continuing professional development. As with most healthcare professic techniques are rapidly developing: increasingly sophisticated equipment becoming available – and, in any case, you might want promotion and wish to gain some form of management qualification. For nurses trained the adult branch, there are further related professions such as midwifer health visiting, district nursing and occupational health nursing which c be reached via further courses in the higher education system. So your first degree or diploma qualification will probably not be your last encounter with higher education.

dwives have the opportunity to work in different healthcare settings, ining experience in all aspects of caring for mothers and babies. You uld progress to become a clinical specialist as a consultant midwife, or u could work in management as a head of midwifery services or pervisor of midwives at local authority level. Midwives have developed ovative specialist roles – for example, in ultrasound, foetal medicine, ensive care neonatal units, public health, parenting education and many hers.

e publication *What do graduates do?* provides statistics for graduates in rsing. Of 8370 students who responded to a survey in 2005 (the latest ar for which figures are available) the vast majority were working or ining in the nursing profession.

- 83 % were in employment in the UK
- 0.6% were doing full-time further study
- 11.5% were working and studying
- 0.9% were unemployed

… six months after graduation.

(The figures do not total 100% because some graduates answered the survey stating that they were not available for work.)

Of those in employment 93.6% were in the medical field.

What would you earn?

Salary scales for nurses and midwives are on a scale from approximately £19,000 to £31,000. Promotion could bring salaries of approximately £22,800 to £36,400. More senior posts are paid up to £51,000 and modern matrons can earn over £61,000.

These examples are based on April 2006 salary scales. At the time of writing this book the public sector unions had not accepted the pay increase of around 2.5%, which had been offered in April 2007.

Case Study

Bryony Palmer

Bryony is in her first year of a BSc (Hons) in Nursing (Adult) at the University of Plymouth.

'I'm from a town called Bishops Waltham near Winchester, where I lived with my parents, both radiographers, and two elder brothers. I have come straight from college in Winchester, having done A levels in Chemistry, Psychology and Biology and an AS in Maths.

'The only prior experience I have is through two short work-experience placements. However I spent the summer previous to starting my course in Boston, MA (USA) where I spent time working as a counsellor for an epilepsy camp, providing 24 hour care. These experiences, however short, did help with the theory and practical parts of the course. They also helped me gain a good insight into the wider multi disciplinary team involved in a patient or client's care.

'I have always wanted to be a nurse and have a direct impact on people and their lives. The rewards and fulfilment of providing even the most basic care is unrivalled in any profession; there is also scope to enjoy working across a range of diverse sectors and potential experience of developing a career abroad.

'Plymouth provided me with so much of what I was looking for. I love the coastal vibe and the accessibility to beaches and Dartmoor! The university campus has a relaxed atmosphere, is based in the City Centre with shops, the bus station, the train station and the seafront all close and easily accessible within a 5–10 minute walk. The facilities are wonderful, modern and well placed with a newly developed library, gym and students' union, along with large lecture theatres and well furnished seminar rooms.

'I have enjoyed spending the first year as a "common foundation year", which has enabled me to share in experiences with students from other branches of nursing. This element, I believe, has helped extend my knowledge and encouraged me to look at patients' and clients' situations from alternative therapeutic viewpoints. The lectures and tutor support have helped to ease me into the course, university and student life, tying together theory and its application to nursing.

'The clinical skills labs are well equipped and set up in the style of wards, where the initial practical training is developed. It's safe, hygienic and carefully managed to ensure a safe learning environment – great for making those early mistakes!

'I have also enjoyed my practical placements. Plymouth carefully designs and structures its placements and because of this is now a recognised National Centre of Excellence for practice placement education. The placements are supported with tutors and mentors, providing you with a range of methods and good practice. It has been a real insight into the profession with weekend working and varying shift patterns which start and finish at all times of the day and night. I have also enjoyed undertaking my placements at a variety of locations as this has provided me with different experiences, I even had to relocate for a short duration which was really exciting! The relocation provided me with the very best learning opportunities and was well worth the short term commitment.

'The university is very inviting and I've been able to form many strong relationships in a variety of places. Along with my course mates, the university accommodation halls meant that there was an immediate network of people around me. I also joined the ladies rugby team through the students' union, having never played before, and have been struck by their spirit and immediate support and encouragement. I would urge everyone to join such a group; my experiences with them have been invaluable.

'I hope to graduate in two years' time and am hoping to be accepted into the Queen Alexandra's Royal Army Nursing Corps and undergo basic and officer training, so that I may pursue an even more varied, challenging and rewarding career. Combining the training received on my university course with skills and camaraderie acquired through taking part in the social side of the University of Plymouth I'm looking forward to continuing to develop my personal and professional skills and experiences.'

Acute Child Care

University of Salford S03
BSc (Hons): 2 years part-time
HE credits: 240, RN

Adult Nursing

University of Birmingham B32
RN: 3 years full-time
BTEC: PP - PPP

Bristol, University of the West of England B80
DipHE: 3 years full-time
A2: CC Interview

Bristol, University of the West of England B80
BSc (Hons): 3 years full-time – B701
Tariff: 180 - 220 IB: 24

University of Chester C55
DipHE: 3 years full-time
A2: CC Interview

City University C60
BSc (Hons): 3 years full-time – B701
Tariff: 220

University of Derby D39
DipHE: 3 years full-time
Tariff: 160

Edge Hill University E42
BSc (Hons): 3 years full-time – B740
Tariff: 160 - 220

Keele University K12
BN (Hons): 4 years full-time including foundation year – B742
A2: EE

Keele University K12
BN (Hons): 3 years full-time – B740
A2: CC BTEC: MMM

University of Northampton N38
DipHE: 3 years full-time
Tariff: 180

University of Salford S03
BSc (Hons): 2 years part-time
HE credits: 240, RN

Staffordshire University S72
DipHE: 3 years full-time
A2: C BTEC: PPP

University of Wales, Swansea S93
BN (Hons): 3 years full-time – B740 T
Tariff: 240

Applied Community and Health Studies (District Nursing/Health Visiting/School Nursing/General Practice Nursing/Community Children's Nursing)

North East Wales Institute of Higher Education [University of Wales] N56
BSc (Hons): 1 year full-time or 2 years part-time
HE credits: 240, RN
HPW

Applied Dementia Studies

University of Bradford B56
DipHE: 2 years distance learning
HE credits: 120, HP

Applied Dementia Studies (top-up)

University of Bradford B56
BSc (Hons): 2 - 4 years distance learning
HE credits: 240, HP

Applied Midwifery Studies

University of York Y50
DipHE: 2 - 5 years part-time
RM

University of York Y50
BSc (Hons): 2 - 5 years part-time
RM

Applied Nursing Science

Northumbria University N77
BSc (Hons): 1 year full-time or part-time
HE credits: 240, RN

Applied Nursing and Social Work (Learning Disability)

Sheffield Hallam University S21
BA (Hons): 3 years full-time – B761
Tariff: 180 Interview

Applied Professional Studies

University of Worcester W80
BSc (Hons): 1 year full-time or 3 years part-time
RN, RM, HP
NMC

Cancer Care

University of Glamorgan G14
BSc (Hons): 2 years distance learning
HE credits: 240, RN, HP

UCE Birmingham C25
BSc: 1 - 5 years part-time BSc (Hons): 2 - 5 years part-time
HE credits: 120, RN

Cancer Care for Nurses and Allied Health Professionals

Thames Valley University T40
BSc (Hons): 18 months part-time
HE credits: 240, RN, HP

Cancer Care (post-qualifying framework)

Bristol, University of the West of Engla B80
BSc (Hons): 1 year full-time or 4 years part-time – B772
HE credits: 240, RN, HP

Cancer Care (top-up)

University of Wolverhampton W75
BSc (Hons): 1 year full-time or 2 - 5 years part-time – B742
Fd, HE credits: 240, RN, HP

Cancer Nursing (The Royal Marsder

Thames Valley University T40
DipHE: 1 year full-time
HE credits: 120, RN

Cancer and Palliative Care (Marie Curie Cancer Care)

Thames Valley University T40
BSc (Hons): 2 - 5 years part-time
Tariff: 120

Care of the Older Person

University of Sunderland S84
BSc (Hons): 2 years part-time
RN, HP

Care of the Older Person (post-qualifying framework)

Bristol, University of the West of Engla B80
BSc (Hons): 1 year full-time or 4 years part-time – B74
HE credits: 240, RN

Child Health Nursing

University of Plymouth P60
BSc (Hons): 3 years full-time – B730
Tariff: 180

Child Health (post-qualifying framework)

Bristol, University of the West of Engla B80
BSc (Hons): 1 year full-time or 4 years part-time – B73
HE credits: 240, RN

alt: 700

-100 0 +100

Rise above the rest

4

NURSES WANTED. MUST HAVE A HEAD FOR HEIGHTS.

At 30,000 feet you won't find a hospital for miles. That's why we need nurses specially trained to treat the injured in aeromedical evacuations. On the ground they're just as essential. From military hospitals overseas to selected NHS Trusts in the UK. If you'd like to be an RAF nurse, call our Nursing Liaison Officer.

01400 266 782

rafcareers.com

ROYAL AIR FORCE

The RAF values every individual's unique contribution, irrespective of race, ethnic origin, religion, gender, sexual orientation or social background.

Child Nursing

University of Northampton N38
DipHE: 3 years full-time
Tariff: 180

Children and Young Persons Mental Health (post-qualifying framework)

Bristol, University of the West of England B80
BSc (Hons): 1 year full-time or 4 years part-time – B761
HE credits: 240, RN

Children's Critical Care (post-qualifying framework)

Bristol, University of the West of England B80
BSc (Hons): 1 year full-time or 4 years part-time – B771
HE credits: 240, RN

Children's Nursing

Bristol, University of the West of England B80
BSc (Hons): 3 years full-time – B702
Tariff: 200 - 240 IB: 24 - 28

Bristol, University of the West of England B80
DipHE: 3 years full-time or 4 - 5 years part-time
A2 BTEC: PPP Interview

City University C60
BSc (Hons): 3 years full-time – B703
Tariff: 220

Edge Hill University E42
BSc (Hons): 3 years full-time – B730
Tariff: 160 - 220

Keele University K12
BN (Hons): 3 years full-time – B730
A2: CC BTEC: MMM

Keele University K12
BN (Hons): 4 years full-time including foundation year – B731
A2: EE

Staffordshire University S72
DipHE: 3 years full-time
A2 BTEC: MMM Interview

Children's Nursing (post-experience/qualification)

Oxford Brookes University O66
BSc (Hons): 2 years full-time or 6 years part-time – B741
A2 RN, Interview

Clinical Governance (post-registration)

University of Glamorgan G14
BSc (Hons): 2 - 5 years distance learning
HE credits: 120

Clinical Nursing

University of Central Lancashire C30
DipHE: 2 - 5 years part-time
RN

University of Hertfordshire H36
BSc (Hons): 3 - 6 years part-time
HE credits: 120, RN

Clinical Nursing Studies (with Specialist Practitioner Award)

UCE Birmingham C25
BSc (Hons): 1 year full-time or 2 - 4 years part-time
HE credits: 240, RN, RM

Clinical Practice

University of Wolverhampton W75
BSc (Hons): 2 - 5 years part-time
HE credits: 240, RN

Clinical Practice (post-registration)

Cardiff University C15
BSc (Hons): 1 year full-time or 2 - 5 years part-time
HE credits: 240, RN, RM

Community Children's Nursing

Oxford Brookes University O66
BA/BA (Hons): 1 year full-time or 2 years part-time day – B717
HE credits: 180, RN

Community Health Care Nursing

University of Plymouth P60
BSc (Hons): 1 year full-time or 2 years part-time – B710
HE credits: 120, RN
NMC

Community Health Nursing

New College Durham [University of Durham] N28
BSc (Hons): 1 year full-time or 2 years part-time
HE credits: 240, RN

Queen Margaret University, Edinburgh Q25
BSc: 1 year full-time or 2 - 3 years part-time
HE credits: 240, RN

Community Health Nursing (Community Mental Health Nursing)

Brunel University B84
BSc (Hons): 1 year full-time or 2 years part-time
HE credits: 240, RN
NMC

Community Health Nursing (District Nursing)

Brunel University B84
BSc (Hons): 1 year full-time
RN
NMC

Community Health Nursing (Health Visiting)

Brunel University B84
BSc (Hons): 1 year full-time or 2 years part-time
RN
NMC

Community Health Nursing (Occupational Health Nursing)

Brunel University B84
BSc (Hons): 1 year full-time or 2 years part-time
RN
NMC

Community Health Nursing (School Nursing)

Brunel University B84
BSc (Hons): 1 year full-time or 2 years part-time
RN
NMC

Community Health Nursing (Specialist Practitioner/Existing Practitioner)

UCE Birmingham C25
BSc (Hons): 1 year full-time or 2 - 5 years part-time
HE credits: 240, RN
NMC

Community Health Studies

University of Glamorgan G14
BSc: 2 - 3 years part-time BSc (Hons): 3 - 4 years part-time
HE credits: 180, RN

University of Wales, Swansea S93
BSc (Hons): 1 year full-time or 2 years part-time – B71
HE credits: 240, RN
HPW

Community Health Studies (level 3 entry)

University of Gloucestershire G50
BSc (Hons): 1 year full-time or 2 years part-time – L50
HE credits: 240, RN, Interview

Community Health Studies (post-registration)

Cardiff University C15
BSc (Hons): 1 year full-time or 2 years part-time
HE credits: 240, RN

ommunity Learning Disabilities ursing

xford Brookes University O66

/BA (Hons): 1 year full-time or 2 years part-time day –
12
credits: 180, RN

ommunity Mental Health Nursing

xford Brookes University O66

/BA (Hons): 1 year full-time or 2 years part-time day –
13
credits: 180, RN

ommunity Nursing

asgow Caledonian University G42

:/BSc (Hons): 1 year full-time or 2 years part-time
credits: 240, RN
S

---

iversity of Hull H72

: (Hons): 3 years part-time
credits: 240, RN
C

---

ndon Metropolitan University L68

: (Hons): 1 year full-time or 2 years part-time
credits: 240, RN

Community Nursing (District Nurse, level 3 entry)

University of Gloucestershire G50

BSc (Hons): 1 year full-time or 2 years part-time day and evening – B710
RN, Interview
NMC

Community Nursing (General Practice, level 3 entry)

University of Gloucestershire G50

BSc (Hons): 1 year full-time or 2 years part-time day and evening – B706
RN, Interview
NMC

Community Nursing in the Home (District Nursing)

Oxford Brookes University O66

BA/BA (Hons): 1 year full-time or 2 years part-time day – B711
HE credits: 180, RN

Community Nursing (Public Health, level 3 entry)

University of Gloucestershire G50

BSc (Hons): 1 year full-time or 2 years part-time day and evening – B707
RN, Interview
NMC

Community Nursing (School Nurse, level 3 entry)

University of Gloucestershire G50

BSc (Hons): 1 year full-time or 2 years part-time day and evening – B708
RN, Interview
NMC

Community Nursing Specialist Practice

University Campus Suffolk [University of East Anglia, University of Essex] S82

BSc (Hons): 1 year full-time or 2 years part-time
HE credits: 240, RN
NMC

Community Nursing Specialist Practitioner

University of Central Lancashire C30

BSc (Hons): 1 year full-time or 2 years part-time
HE credits: 180 - 240
NMC

University of Paisley P20

BSc (Hons): 32 weeks full-time or 2 - 3 years part-time
HE credits: 360, RN

Community Specialist Practice

University of Brighton B72
BSc (Hons): 1 year full-time or 2 years part-time
RN
NMC

Sheffield Hallam University S21
BA (Hons): 1 year full-time or 2 years part-time
HE credits: 240, RN
NMC

Community Specialist Practice Primary Care Nursing (District Nursing)

Sheffield Hallam University S21
BA (Hons): 3 years full-time or 6 years part-time
Tariff: 120 RN

Contemporary Midwifery (post-qualifying framework)

Bristol, University of the West of England B80
BSc (Hons): 1 year full-time or 4 years part-time – B720
HE credits: 180, RM

Critical Care

University of Hertfordshire H36
BSc (Hons): 2 - 3 years part-time
HE credits: 240, RN

Critical Care (post-qualifying framework)

Bristol, University of the West of England B80
BSc (Hons): 1 year full-time or 4 years part-time – B771
RN

Diabetes Care

University of Hertfordshire H36
BSc (Hons): part-time
HE credits: 240, RN, HP

Emergency Nursing

University of Hertfordshire H36
BSc (Hons): 3 - 6 years part-time
HE credits: 120, RN

Enrolled Nursing Conversion

Glasgow Caledonian University G42
DipHE: 2 years full-time
HE credits: 120, RN

European Nursing

Middlesex University M80
BSc (Hons): 4 years full-time with time abroad – B701 E
Tariff: 160 - 220

Evidence-Based Nursing Practice (Adult)

University of York Y50
BSc (Hons): 3 years full-time – B740
A2: CCC - BCC

Evidence-Based Nursing Practice (Child)

University of York Y50
BSc (Hons): 3 years full-time – B730
A2: CCC - BCC

Evidence-Based Nursing Practice (Learning Disability)

University of York Y50
BSc (Hons): 3 years full-time – B761
A2: CCC - BCC

Evidence-Based Nursing Practice (Mental Health)

University of York Y50
BSc (Hons): 3 years full-time – B760
A2: CCC - BCC

General Practice Nursing

Oxford Brookes University O66
BA (Hons): 2 years full-time – B718
RN, RM, HP

Haematological Oncology

UCE Birmingham C25
BSc: 1 - 5 years part-time BSc (Hons): 2 - 5 years part-time
HE credits: 120, RN

Infection Control

University of Hertfordshire H36
BSc (Hons): 4 - 6 years part-time
HE credits: 120, RN

Intellectual and Developmental Disabilities

University of Kent K24
BSc (Hons): 3 years full-time or 6 years part-time – L512
Tariff: 200

Learning Disabilities

University of Derby D39
FdSc: 2 years full-time – X160
Tariff: 40

University of Winchester W76
FdA: 3 - 6 years part-time
Interview

University of Wolverhampton W75
DipHE: 2 - 5 years part-time
HE credits: 120, RN, HP

University of Wolverhampton W75
BSc (Hons): 2 - 5 years part-time
HE credits: 120, RN, HP

Learning Disabilities Nursing

Bristol, University of the West of Englar B80
BSc (Hons): 3 years full-time – B703
Tariff: 160 - 200 IB: 24

Bristol, University of the West of Englar B80
DipHE: 3 years full-time
Interview

Edge Hill University E42
BSc (Hons): 3 years full-time – B761
Tariff: 160 - 220

Learning Disability Nursing

University of Bradford B56
DipHE: 3 years full-time
Tariff: 160

Keele University K12
BN (Hons): 4 years full-time including foundation year – B762
A2: EE

Keele University K12
BN (Hons): 3 years full-time – B761
A2: CC BTEC: MMM

University of Northampton N38
DipHE: 3 years full-time
Tariff: 180

Learning Disability Studies

University of Leeds L23
DipHE: 2 - 5 years part-time
Interview

University of Manchester M20
BA (Hons): 3 years full-time – B760
A2: BCC - BBC SQA: BBCCC - BBBBC IB: 28 - 30

Learning Disability Studies (post-qualifying framework)

Bristol, University of the West of Engla B80
BSc (Hons): 1 year full-time or 4 years part-time – B76
RN, HP

Mental Health

Bournemouth University B50
Diploma: 3 years full-time
HP

University of Plymouth P60
BSc (Hons): 3 years full-time – B760
Tariff: 160 - 180

University of Salford S03
BSc (Hons): 2 years part-time
HE credits: 240

York College Y70
FdA: 3 years sandwich – B760
HP

Mental Health (Acute Inpatient Care)

Bristol, University of the West of England B80
BSc (Hons): 1 year full-time or 4 years part-time
HE credits: 240, RN

Mental Health Nursing

Bristol, University of the West of England B80
BSc (Hons): 3 years full-time – B704
Tariff: 160 - 200 IB: 24

Bristol, University of the West of England B80
DipHE: 3 years full-time
A2 BTEC: PP - PPP

University of Chester C55
DipHE: 3 years full-time
A2 BTEC: PP - PPP

City University C60
BSc (Hons)/RN: 3 years full-time – B702
Tariff: 220

University of Derby D39
Diploma: 3 years full-time
A2

Edge Hill University E42
BSc (Hons): 3 years full-time – B760
Tariff: 160

University of Huddersfield H60
BSc (Hons): 3 years full-time – B760
Tariff: 200 - 240

Keele University K12
BN (Hons): 4 years full-time including foundation year – B763
A2: EE

Keele University K12
BN (Hons): 3 years full-time – B760
A2: CC BTEC: MMM

University of Northampton N38
DipHE: 3 years full-time
A2 BTEC: PP

University of Salford S03
BSc (Hons): 3 years full-time – B760
Tariff: 160

Staffordshire University S72
DipHE: 3 years full-time
A2 BTEC: MMM Interview

University of Wales, Swansea S93
BSc (Hons): 3 years full-time – B760 T
Tariff: 240

Mental Health (post-qualifying framework)

Bristol, University of the West of England B80
BSc (Hons): 1 year full-time or 4 years part-time – B764
HE credits: 240, RN

Mental Health Practice

University of Central Lancashire C30
BSc (Hons): 2 years part-time
HE credits: 240, RN, HP

Napier University N07
BSc: 2 - 5 years part-time
HE credits: 200 - 300, RN, HP

University of Wolverhampton W75
BA (Hons): 2 years part-time
HE credits: 240, RN

Mental Health Studies

Coventry University C85
BSc/BSc (Hons): 2 - 5 years part-time
RN, HP

UCE Birmingham C25
BSc (Hons): 1 year full-time or 2 - 5 years part-time day-release
HE credits: 120

Mental Health (Thorn)

London South Bank University L75
BSc (Hons): part-time
RN, RM, HP

Mental Health (top-up)

Middlesex University M80
BSc (Hons): 1 year full-time – B762 E
RN, RM, HP

Midwifery

University of Wales, Bangor B06
BM: 3 years full-time
Tariff: 240

University of Bedfordshire B22
BSc (Hons): 3 years full-time – B711
Tariff: 160 - 200

Bournemouth University B50
BSc (Hons)/RM: 3 years full-time – B720
Tariff: 220

University of Brighton B72
BSc (Hons): 3 years full-time
Tariff: 180

Bristol, University of the West of Englar B80
BSc (Hons): 3 years full-time – B711
Tariff: 200 - 240 IB: 24

Canterbury Christ Church University C1
BSc (Hons): 3 years full-time – B720
Tariff: 160 IB: 24

Cardiff University C15
BMid (Hons): 3 years full-time – B720
Tariff: 240

University of Chester C55
DipHE: 3 years full-time
A2 BTEC: PP - PPP

University of Chester C55
BSc (Hons): 3 years full-time – B720
Tariff: 240 IB: 30

City University C60
BSc (Hons)/RM: 3 years full-time – B715
Tariff: 220

Coventry University C85
BSc (Hons): 3 years full-time or 88 weeks full-time – B7
Tariff: 260 RN

University of Cumbria C99
BSc (Hons): 3 years full-time – B720 F
Tariff: 300

University of Dundee D65
BMid: 3 years full-time
A2: EE SQA: CCC HND

University of East Anglia E14
BSc (Hons): 3 years full-time – B720
A2: BCC Interview

Edge Hill University E42
BSc (Hons): 3 years full-time – B720
Tariff: 160 - 220

University of Glamorgan G14
BMid (Hons): 3 years full-time – B720
Tariff: 240

Glasgow Caledonian University G42
DipHE: 3 years full-time
SQA: CC

University of Greenwich G70
DipHE: 3 years full-time
A2 BTEC: PPP Interview

University of Hertfordshire H36
BSc (Hons): 3 years full-time
Tariff: 200

University of Hertfordshire H36
BSc (Hons): 4 - 5 years part-time
Tariff: 200

University of Huddersfield H60
BSc (Hons): 78 weeks full-time – B721
HE credits: 180, RN

Keele University K12
BMid (Hons): 4 years full-time including foundation year B721
A2: EE

University of Leeds L23
BHSc (Hons): 3 years full-time – B720
A2: BBC

Liverpool John Moores University L51
BA (Hons): 3 years full-time – B720
Tariff: 200 IB: 30 Interview

Liverpool John Moores University L51
DipHE: 3 years full-time
Tariff: 200 IB: 30

University of Manchester M20
BMid: 3 years full-time – B720
A2: BCC BTEC: MMM SQA: BBCCC ILC: BBCCC Interview

Napier University N07
DipHE: 3 years full-time
Tariff: 100

Napier University N07
BM: 3 years full-time
Tariff: 180

University of Northampton N38
BSc (Hons): 3 years full-time or 4 years part-time – B720
Tariff: 220 - 240

University of Northampton N38
DipHE: 3 years full-time or 4 years part-time
A2 BTEC: PP

Oxford Brookes University O66
BSc (Hons): 3 years full-time – B720
A2: CC - BB IB: 26 - 30

University of Paisley P20
DipHE: 3 years full-time
A2 SQA

University of Paisley P20
BSc: 3 years full-time
A2: E BTEC: PP SQA: CC

University of Plymouth P60
BSc (Hons): 3 years full-time – B720
Tariff: 160 - 180

Robert Gordon University R36
DipHE: 3 years full-time
A2: BB SQA: CC ILC: CC RN

University of Salford S03
BSc (Hons): 3 years full-time – B720
Tariff: 240

University of Southampton S27
BMid (Hons): 18 months full-time
HE credits: 240, RN

University of Southampton S27
BMid (Hons): 3 years full-time – B720
Tariff: 330

University of Stirling S75
DipHE: 3 years full-time
A2 SQA

University Campus Suffolk S82
DipHE: 3 years full-time
A2 Interview

University of Wales, Swansea S93
BMid (Hons): 3 years full-time – B720
Tariff: 240

University of Wales, Swansea S93
BSc (Hons): 1 year full-time or 2 - 4 years part-time
HE credits: 120

University of Teesside T20
BSc (Hons): 3 years full-time or 18 months full-time – B720
Tariff: 200 - 360 Interview

UCE Birmingham C25
BSc (Hons): 3 years full-time – B720
Tariff: 220

University of Worcester W80
BSc (Hons)/RM: 3 years full-time – B720
Tariff: 160

Midwifery (accelerated)

City University C60
BSc (Hons): 18 months full-time
HE credits: 240, RN

Midwifery (with BSc pathway)

Middlesex University M80
DipHE: 3 years full-time
A2 BTEC: MM

Midwifery (for registered nurses)

Canterbury Christ Church University C10
BSc (Hons): 18 months full-time
HE credits: 240, RN

Cardiff University C15
BMid (Hons): 18 months full-time
HE credits: 240, RN

University of East Anglia E14
BSc (Hons): 78 weeks full-time
A2: BCC RN

Middlesex University M80
BSc (Hons): 18 months full-time – B716 E
RN

Napier University N07
DipHE: 18 months full-time
RN, Interview

Napier University N07
BM: 18 months full-time
RN, Interview

Oxford Brookes University O66
BSc (Hons): 3 semesters full-time – B716
HE credits: 120, RN

University of Wales, Swansea S93
BMid (Hons): 18 months full-time – B721
HE credits: 240, RN

UCE Birmingham C25
BSc (Hons): 18 months full-time
HE credits: 240, RN

Midwifery (long or shortened)

Glasgow Caledonian University G42
BMid: 3 years full-time or 18 months full-time
SQA: CC RN

Midwifery (long programme)

University of Hull H72
BSc (Hons): 3 years full-time
Tariff: 280

Midwifery (post-registration)

University of Wales, Bangor B06
BM: 18 months full-time
HE credits: 240, RN

University of Bedfordshire B22
BSc (Hons): 18 months full-time
HE credits: 180, RN

University of Dundee D65
BMid: full-time or part-time
RN, Interview

University of Glamorgan G14
BMid (Hons): 18 months full-time
HE credits: 240, RN

Keele University K12
BMid (Hons): 15 months full-time or 2 years part-time
HE credits: 240, RM

Midwifery Practice

Coventry University C85
BSc (Hons): 2 - 5 years part-time
RM

University of Salford S03
BSc (Hons): 4 years part-time
HE credits: 160, RM

University Campus Suffolk S82
BSc (Hons): 2 - 5 years part-time
HE credits: 120, RM

University of York Y50
BA (Hons): 78 weeks full-time
RN

Midwifery Practice (for registered nurses)

Thames Valley University T40
DipHE: 2 - 7 years part-time day and evening
HE credits: 120, RN

Thames Valley University T40
BSc (Hons): 18 months full-time or 2 - 7 years part-tim
day and evening
HE credits: 120, RN

idwifery Practice (post-ualification)

ournemouth University B50
c (Hons): 2 - 5 years part-time
credits: 240, RM

idwifery Practice (pre-registration)

affordshire University S72
c (Hons): 3 years full-time – B720
iff: 200 IB: 24

idwifery Practice (registered urses)

affordshire University S72
c (Hons): 18 months full-time
credits: 180, RN

idwifery Practice with Registration

ng's College London (University of ndon) K60
(Hons): 18 months full-time
credits: 240, RN

ng's College London (University of ndon) K60
IE: 3 years full-time
CC - CCC

dwifery (pre-registration)

Montfort University D26
E: 3 years full-time
CC

Montfort University D26
(Hons): 3 years full-time – B720 Y
: 260

versity of Greenwich G70
(Hons): 3 years full-time – B710
: 160 Interview

ele University K12
(Hons): 3 years full-time – B720
CC BTEC: MMM HND

ndon South Bank University L75
(Hons): 18 months full-time
redits: 120, RN

ndon South Bank University L75
E: 18 months full-time
: 220 RN

versity of Nottingham N84
Hons): 3 years full-time – B721
CC

versity of Salford S03
Hons): 18 months full-time
edits: 160, RN

University of Teesside T20
BSc (Hons): 18 months full-time
RN, HP, Interview
NMC

Thames Valley University T40
BSc (Hons): 3 years full-time
Tariff: 120

Midwifery (pre-registration programme, long)

University of Central Lancashire C30
BA (Hons): 4 years sandwich – B720
Tariff: 240 Interview

Midwifery (pre-registration programme, shortened)

University of Central Lancashire C30
BA (Hons): 18 months full-time – B711
RN, Interview

Midwifery (with registration)

University of Hertfordshire H36
BSc (Hons): 18 months full-time
HE credits: 120, RN

Midwifery Sciences

Queen's University Belfast Q75
BSc (Hons): 3 years full-time
A2: BCC - AB Interview

Midwifery (short)

University of Brighton B72
BSc (Hons): 18 months full-time
HE credits: 180, RN

Midwifery (short programme for Registered Nurses)

University of Hull H72
BSc (Hons): 2 years full-time
HE credits: 40, RN

Midwifery (shortened)

Bristol, University of the West of England B80
BSc (Hons): 18 months full-time
HE credits: 180, RN

De Montfort University D26
BSc (Hons): 78 weeks full-time
HE credits: 60, RN

University of Nottingham N84
BSc (Hons): 2 years full-time
HE credits, RN, HP

University of Paisley P20
DipHE: 18 months full-time
RN

Midwifery Studies

University of Central Lancashire C30
BSc (Hons): part-time
HE credits: 240, RM

University of Huddersfield H60
BSc (Hons): 3 years full-time – B720
A2: CCC SQA: BBBBC IB: 28

Robert Gordon University R36
BA: 1 - 3 years part-time or 1 - 3 years distance learning
RM

Sheffield Hallam University S21
BSc (Hons): 3 years full-time – B720
Tariff: 180

Staffordshire University S72
BSc (Hons): 2 - 4 years part-time
HE credits: 240, RM

Midwifery Studies (Registered Midwife)

University of Surrey S85
BSc (Hons): 3 years full-time – B711
A2: BCC BTEC: DMM IB: 30

University of Surrey S85
DipHE: 3 years full-time
A2 Interview

Midwifery Studies (top-up)

University of Stirling S75
BSc (Hons): 18 month(s) full-time – B720
RN

Midwifery Studies/Registered Midwife

University of Bradford B56
BSc (Hons): 3 years full-time – B720
Tariff: 240 Interview

Northumbria University N77
BSc (Hons): 3 years full-time – B720
Tariff: 240

Midwifery Studies/Registered Midwife (shortened)

University of Bradford B56
BSc (Hons): 78 weeks full-time
HE credits: 180, RM

Northumbria University N77
BSc (Hons): 80 weeks full-time
HE credits: 60, RN

Midwifery (top-up)

University of Portsmouth P80
BSc (Hons): 2 years part-time
RN, RM, HP

Midwifery and Women's Health Studies

Anglia Ruskin University A60
BA (Hons): part-time
Tariff: 200 IB: 26

Midwifery/Registered Midwife (for registered nurses)

Kingston University K84
DipHE: 18 months full-time
HE credits: 240, RN, Interview

St George's, University of London S49
DipHE: 18 months full-time
RN

Midwifery/Registered Midwife (with top-up to BSc)

Kingston University K84
DipHE: 3 years full-time
A2: CC RN, Interview

St George's, University of London S49
DipHE: 3 years full-time
A2: EE

Neonatal Practice

University of Central Lancashire C30
BSc (Hons): part-time
HE credits: 240, RN

Nurse Practitioner

University of Central Lancashire C30
BSc (Hons): 2 years part-time
RN

University of East Anglia E14
BSc (Hons): 2 years part-time
RN

London Metropolitan University L68
BSc (Hons): 1 year full-time or 2 years part-time
HE credits: 240, RN

Nurse Practitioner (Primary Health Care)

London South Bank University L75
BSc (Hons): 2 - 3 years part-time
HE credits, RN

Nurse Practitioner with RCN Accreditation

University Campus Suffolk [Royal College of Nursing] S82
BSc: 1 year full-time or 2 years full-time
RN, RM, HP

Nursing

University of Bedfordshire B22
DipHE: 3 years full-time
A2

University of Birmingham B32
BNurs (Hons): 3 years full-time – B700
Tariff: 240 - 260 IB: 28 - 30

University of Brighton B72
BSc (Hons): 3 years full-time – B700
Tariff: 220 IB: 28

Buckinghamshire Chilterns University College B94
DipHE: 3 years full-time – B700
A2 SQA: CCC ILC: CCC

Buckinghamshire Chilterns University College B94
BSc (Hons): 3 years full-time – B701
A2: CC SQA: CCCC IB: 27

De Montfort University D26
DipHE: 3 years full-time
A2: CC

University of Edinburgh E56
BN (Hons): 4 years full-time – B700
A2: BBB SQA: BBBB IB: 34

University of Huddersfield H60
BSc (Hons): 3 years full-time – B700
Tariff: 200 - 240

University of Liverpool L41
BN (Hons): 3 years full-time – B700
A2: BCC BTEC: DMM SQA: BBBCC ILC: BBBBC IB: 30

University of Manchester M20
BNurs: 3 years full-time – B701
A2: BCC BTEC: DDM SQA: BBCCC ILC: BBBCCC

Manchester Metropolitan University M40
BSc (Hons): 3 years full-time – B700
Tariff: 160

University of Nottingham N84
MN (Hons): 4 years full-time – B700
A2: BCC ILC: BBBCC IB: 30

University of Portsmouth P80
BSc (Hons): 2 - 3 years part-time
HE credits: 240

Queen Margaret University, Edinburgh Q25
BSc (Hons): 4 years full-time – B740
Tariff: 216 - 220 Interview

Robert Gordon University R36
BA: 3 years full-time
A2: C SQA: C ILC: C

Robert Gordon University R36
DipHE: 3 years full-time
A2: C SQA: C ILC: C

Staffordshire University S72
DipHE: 4 years part-time
A2 BTEC: PP

University Campus Suffolk [University of East Anglia, University of Essex] S82
DipHE: 3 years full-time
A2

University of Sunderland S84
BSc (Hons): 2 years full-time – B700

University of Wales, Swansea S93
BSc (Hons): 1 year full-time or 2 - 5 years part-time
HE credits: 120, RM

Nursing (Adult)

Anglia Ruskin University A60
BSc (Hons): 3 years full-time – B706
Tariff: 160 IB: 24

University of Wales, Bangor B06
BN (Hons): 3 years full-time – B740
Tariff: 200 IB: 26

University of Bedfordshire B22
BSc (Hons): 3 years full-time – B740
Tariff: 160 - 200

University of Bedfordshire B22
DipHE: 3 years full-time
A2

Bell College [University of Paisley] B26
BSc: 3 years full-time
A2: C SQA: CC Interview

Bell College [University of Paisley] B26
DipHE: 3 years full-time
A2: C SQA: CC Interview

Canterbury Christ Church University C
BSc (Hons): 3 years full-time – B740
Tariff: 160 IB: 24

Cardiff University C15
BN (Hons): 3 years full-time – B740
Tariff: 240 IB: 26

University of Chester C55
BSc (Hons): 3 years full-time – B740
Tariff: 240 IB: 30

Coventry University C85
BSc (Hons): 3 years full-time – B740
Tariff: 240

University of Cumbria C99
BSc (Hons): 3 years full-time – B701 C
Tariff: 300 IB: 28

University of Cumbria C99
DipHE: 3 years full-time
A2 BTEC: PP Interview

University of Cumbria C99
BSc (Hons): 3 years full-time – B700
Tariff: 300 IB: 28

University of East Anglia E14
BSc (Hons): 3 years full-time – B701
A2: BCC

iversity of East Anglia E14
HE: 3 years full-time
BTEC: PP Interview

lge Hill University E42
HE: 3 years full-time

iversity of Glamorgan G14
: (Hons): 3 years full-time – B701
iff: 240 Interview

iversity of Glamorgan G14
: (Hons): 3 years full-time – B740
ff: 240 Interview

iversity of Glasgow G28
3 years full-time BN (Hons): 4 years full-time – B700
CCC SQA: BBBBC

iversity of Hertfordshire H36
IE: 3 years full-time
BTEC: PP

iversity of Huddersfield H60
IE: 3 years full-time
BTEC: PP

iversity of Leeds L23
c (Hons): 3 years full-time – B700
CCC

iversity of Lincoln L39
(Hons): 3 years full-time – B710 L
f: 200 IB: 24 Interview

erpool John Moores University L51
Hons): 3 years full-time – B740
f: 200

pier University N07
E: 2 years full-time or 3 years full-time
f: 100

pier University N07
2 years full-time or 3 years full-time
f: 100

ford Brookes University O66
(Hons): 3 years full-time or 4 - 6 years part-time –

CC IB: 26 - 30

ord Brookes University O66
E: 3 years full-time or 4 - 6 years part-time

versity of Plymouth P60
Hons): 3 years full-time – B740
160 - 180

versity of Plymouth P60
: 2 years full-time – 3060
TEC: PP

versity Campus Suffolk [University of
t Anglia, University of Essex] S82
Hons): 3 years full-time – B700 I
160

versity of Wales, Swansea S93
ons): 3 years full-time – B702
240 HND

Nursing (Adult/Child/Learning Disabilities/Mental Health)

University of Dundee D65
DipHE: 3 years full-time
A2 SQA

University of Dundee D65
BN: 3 years full-time
A2 SQA

Nursing (Adult/Children's/Mental Health)

Robert Gordon University R36
BSc (Hons): 4 years full-time – B700
A2: CCC SQA: BBCC ILC: BBCC Interview

Nursing (Adult/Learning Disability/Mental Health)

University of Stirling S75
DipHE: 3 years full-time
A2 SQA

Nursing (Adult/Mental Health)

North East Wales Institute of Higher Education N56
BN (Hons): 3 years full-time – B700
Tariff: 160

Nursing (Adult, accelerated programme for graduates)

St George's, University of London S49
DipHE: 27 months full-time

Nursing (Adult Branch)

University of Southampton S27
BN (Hons): 3 years full-time – B730
Tariff: 310

Nursing (Adult Care)

University of Hertfordshire H36
BSc (Hons): 3 years full-time – B700
Tariff: 200 IB: 26

Nursing (Adult, Children's, Mental Health)

Middlesex University M80
DipHE: 3 years full-time
A2

Middlesex University M80
BSc (Hons): 3 years full-time – B700 E
Tariff: 160 - 240

Nursing (Adult, Children's, Mental Health, shortened for qualified nurses)

Middlesex University M80
DipHE: 18 months full-time
RN

Nursing (Adult Health)

Leeds Metropolitan University L27
BSc (Hons): 3 years full-time – B740
Tariff: 200 - 220 IB: 28 Interview

Nursing (Adult Health Nursing)

Thames Valley University T40
BSc (Hons): 3 years full-time
A2 BTEC: PP

Thames Valley University T40
DipHE: 3 years full-time
A2 BTEC: PP

Nursing (Adult and Mental Health)

Bournemouth University B50
DipHE: 3 years full-time
A2

Nursing (Adult Nursing)

De Montfort University D26
BSc/BSc (Hons): 3 years full-time – B700 Y
A2: CC - CCD BTEC: MMM ILC: BBCC

University of Hull H72
BSc (Hons): 3 years full-time – B740
Tariff: 240

University of Hull H72
DipHE: 3 years full-time
A2

University of Surrey S85
DipHE: 3 years full-time
A2

Nursing (Adult Nursing, conversion)

Robert Gordon University R36
DipHE: 68 weeks full-time
RN

Nursing (Adult or Mental Health)

Manchester Metropolitan University M40
DipHE: 3 years full-time
Tariff: 80

University of Paisley P20
BSc: 3 years full-time
A2 SQA

University of Paisley P20
DipHE: 3 years full-time
A2 SQA

Nursing (Adult, pre-registration)

University of Greenwich G70
BSc (Hons): 3 years full-time – B730
Tariff: 160 Interview

Nursing (Adult, Swindon)

Oxford Brookes University O66
BSc (Hons): 3 years full-time – B700
A2: CCC IB: 26 - 30

Nursing (Adult, with top-up to BSc)

Kingston University K84
DipHE: 3 years full-time
A2: EE

St George's, University of London S49
DipHE: 3 years full-time
A2: EE

Nursing (Cancer Nursing with Specialist Care)

Robert Gordon University R36
BA: 1 - 4 years full-time or 1 - 4 years part-time or 1 - 4 years distance learning
HE credits: 240, RN

Nursing (Child)

Anglia Ruskin University A60
BSc (Hons): 3 years full-time – B707
Tariff: 180 IB: 24

University of Wales, Bangor B06
BN (Hons): 3 years full-time – B731
Tariff: 200 IB: 26

University of Bedfordshire B22
DipHE: 3 years full-time
A2

University of Bedfordshire B22
BSc (Hons): 3 years full-time – B730
Tariff: 160 - 200

Canterbury Christ Church University C10
BSc (Hons): 3 years full-time – B730
Tariff: 160 IB: 24

Coventry University C85
BSc (Hons): 3 years full-time – B730
Tariff: 260

University of Cumbria C99
DipHE: 3 years full-time
A2 BTEC: PP Interview

University of East Anglia E14
BSc (Hons): 3 years full-time – B730
A2: BCC Interview

University of East Anglia E14
DipHE: 3 years full-time
A2 BTEC: PP Interview

Edge Hill University E42
DipHE: 3 years full-time
A2

University of Glamorgan G14
BSc (Hons): 3 years full-time – B702
Tariff: 240 Interview

University of Hertfordshire H36
DipHE: 3 years full-time
A2 BTEC: PP

University of Huddersfield H60
DipHE: 3 years full-time
A2 BTEC: PP

University of Leeds L23
BHSc (Hons): 3 years full-time – B730
Tariff: 240

Liverpool John Moores University L51
BA (Hons): 3 years full-time – B730
Tariff: 200

University of Wales, Swansea S93
BN (Hons): 3 years full-time – B703
Tariff: 240 HND

Nursing (Child Branch)

University of Southampton S27
BN (Hons): 3 years full-time – B721
Tariff: 310

Nursing (Child Health)

Cardiff University C15
BN (Hons): 3 years full-time – B730
Tariff: 240 IB: 26

University of Chester C55
BSc (Hons): 3 years full-time – B730
Tariff: 240 IB: 30

University of Chester C55
DipHE: 3 years full-time
A2 BTEC

De Montfort University D26
BSc/BSc (Hons): 3 years full-time – B702 Y
A2: CC - CCD BTEC: MMM ILC: BBCCC

Napier University N07
BN: 2 years full-time or 3 years full-time
Tariff: 100

Napier University N07
DipHE: 2 years full-time or 3 years full-time
Tariff: 100

Nursing (Child Health Nursing)

Thames Valley University T40
BSc (Hons): 3 years full-time
A2 BTEC: PP

Thames Valley University T40
DipHE: 3 years full-time
A2 BTEC: PP

Nursing (Child Nursing)

University of Surrey S85
DipHE: 3 years full-time
A2

Nursing (Child, with top-up to BSc)

Kingston University K84
DipHE: 3 years full-time
A2: EE

St George's, University of London S49
DipHE: 3 years full-time
A2: EE

Nursing (Children)

University of Hull H72
BSc (Hons): 3 years full-time – B730
Tariff: 240

University of Plymouth P60
DipHE: 3 years full-time
A2 BTEC: PP

Nursing (Children's)

Oxford Brookes University O66
DipHE: 3 years full-time or 4 - 6 years part-time
A2

Oxford Brookes University O66
BSc (Hons): 3 years full-time or 4 - 6 years part-time – B704
A2: CCC IB: 26 - 30

Nursing (Children's Nursing)

University of Hertfordshire H36
BSc (Hons): 3 years full-time – B702
Tariff: 200 IB: 26

University of Hull H72
DipHE: 3 years full-time
A2

Nursing (Children's Nursing, conversion)

Robert Gordon University R36
DipHE: 68 weeks full-time
RN

Nursing (graduate entry)

Napier University N07
BSc (Hons): 2 years full-time

Nursing (Learning Beyond Registration Programme)

University of Nottingham N84
BSc (Hons): 3 - 5 years full-time
RN, RM, HP

ursing (Learning Disabilities)

glia Ruskin University A60
c (Hons): 3 years full-time – B709
iff: 160 IB: 24

iversity of Cumbria C99
HE: 3 years full-time
BTEC: PP Interview

iversity of East Anglia E14
c (Hons): 3 years full-time – B761
BCC Interview

iversity of East Anglia E14
HE: 3 years full-time
BTEC: PP Interview

iversity of Glamorgan G14
c (Hons): 3 years full-time – B703
ff: 240 Interview

iversity of Glamorgan G14
c (Hons): 3 years full-time – B761
ff: 240 Interview

iversity of Hull H72
c (Hons): 3 years full-time – B761
f: 240

ford Brookes University O66
(Hons): 3 years full-time or 4 - 6 years part-time –
3
CD IB: 24 - 28

ursing (Learning Disabilities ursing)

iversity of Hull H72
HE: 3 years full-time

ames Valley University T40
(Hons): 3 years full-time
BTEC: PP

ames Valley University T40
HE: 3 years full-time
BTEC: PP

rsing (Learning Disability)

iversity of Wales, Bangor B06
Hons): 3 years full-time – B761
f: 200 IB: 26

iversity of Bedfordshire B22
E: 3 years full-time

versity of Chester C55
(Hons): 3 years full-time – B761
: 240 IB: 30

versity of Chester C55
E: 3 years full-time
TEC

ge Hill University E42
E: 3 years full-time

University of Hertfordshire H36
DipHE: 3 years full-time
A2 BTEC: PP HP

University of Huddersfield H60
DipHE: 3 years full-time
A2 BTEC: PP

Napier University N07
BN: 2 years full-time or 3 years full-time
Tariff: 100

Napier University N07
DipHE: 2 years full-time or 3 years full-time
Tariff: 100

Oxford Brookes University O66
DipHE: 3 years full-time or 4 - 6 years part-time
A2

Nursing (Learning Disability Branch)

University of Southampton S27
BN (Hons): 3 years full-time – B761
Tariff: 310

Nursing (Learning Disability) and Social Work

University of Hertfordshire H36
BSc: 3 years full-time BSc (Hons): 10 semesters mixed mode – BL75
Tariff: 200 IB: 26

Nursing (Learning Disability, with top-up to BSc)

Kingston University K84
DipHE: 3 years full-time
A2: EE

St George's, University of London S49
DipHE: 3 years full-time
A2: EE

Nursing (Mental Health)

Anglia Ruskin University A60
BSc (Hons): 3 years full-time – B708
Tariff: 160 IB: 24 HND

University of Wales, Bangor B06
BN (Hons): 3 years full-time – B760
Tariff: 200 IB: 26

University of Bedfordshire B22
DipHE: 3 years full-time
A2

University of Bedfordshire B22
BSc (Hons): 3 years full-time – B760
Tariff: 160 - 200

Bell College [University of Paisley] B26
DipHE: 3 years full-time
A2: C SQA: CC Interview

Bell College [University of Paisley] B26
BSc: 3 years full-time
A2: C SQA: CC Interview

Canterbury Christ Church University C10
BSc (Hons): 3 years full-time – B760
Tariff: 160 IB: 24

Cardiff University C15
BN (Hons): 3 years full-time – B760
Tariff: 240 IB: 26

University of Chester C55
BSc (Hons): 3 years full-time – B760
Tariff: 240 IB: 30

Coventry University C85
BSc (Hons): 3 years full-time – B760
Tariff: 240

University of Cumbria C99
BSc (Hons): 3 years full-time – B760
Tariff: 200 IB: 28 Interview

University of Cumbria C99
DipHE: 3 years full-time
A2 BTEC: PP Interview

De Montfort University D26
BSc/BSc (Hons): 3 years full-time – B701 Y
A2: CC - CCD BTEC: MMM ILC: BBCC

University of East Anglia E14
DipHE: 3 years full-time
A2 BTEC: PP Interview

University of East Anglia E14
BSc (Hons): 3 years full-time – B760
A2: BCC Interview

Edge Hill University E42
DipHE: 3 years full-time
A2

University of Glamorgan G14
BSc (Hons): 3 years full-time – B704
Tariff: 240 Interview

University of Glamorgan G14
BSc (Hons): 3 years full-time – B760
Tariff: 240 Interview

University of Hertfordshire H36
BSc (Hons): 3 years full-time – B701
Tariff: 200 IB: 26

University of Hertfordshire H36
DipHE: 3 years full-time
A2 BTEC: PP HP

University of Huddersfield H60
DipHE: 3 years full-time
A2 BTEC: PP

University of Hull H72
BSc (Hons): 3 years full-time – B760
Tariff: 240

Leeds Metropolitan University L27
BSc (Hons): 3 years full-time – B760
Tariff: 200 - 220 IB: 28 Interview

Liverpool John Moores University L51
BA (Hons): 3 years full-time – B760
Tariff: 200

Napier University N07
DipHE: 2 years full-time or 3 years full-time
Tariff: 100

Napier University N07
BN: 2 years full-time or 3 years full-time
Tariff: 100

Oxford Brookes University O66
BA (Hons): 3 years full-time or 4 - 6 years part-time – B702
A2: CD IB: 24 - 28

Oxford Brookes University O66
DipHE: 3 years full-time or 4 - 6 years part-time
A2

University of Plymouth P60
DipHE: 3 years full-time
A2 BTEC: PP

University of Wales, Swansea S93
BN (Hons): 3 years full-time – B704
Tariff: 240 HND

University of Ulster U20
BSc/BSc (Hons): 3 years full-time – B760 M
Tariff: 280 IB: 32

Nursing (Mental Health, accelerated programme for graduates)

St George's, University of London S49
DipHE: 27 months full-time

Nursing (Mental Health Branch)

University of Southampton S27
BN (Hons): 3 years full-time – B760
Tariff: 310

University of Southampton S27
DipHE: 3 years full-time
A2 BTEC: PP

Nursing (Mental Health, Learning Disabilities, Children, Adult)

Glasgow Caledonian University G42
BN: 3 years full-time
SQA: CC

Glasgow Caledonian University G42
DipHE: 3 years full-time
SQA: CC

Nursing (Mental Health Nursing)

University of Hull H72
DipHE: 3 years full-time
A2

University of Surrey S85
DipHE: 3 years full-time
A2

Thames Valley University T40
BSc (Hons): 3 years full-time
A2 BTEC: PP

Thames Valley University T40
DipHE: 3 years full-time
A2 BTEC: PP

Nursing (Mental Health Nursing, conversion)

Robert Gordon University R36
DipHE: 68 weeks full-time
RN, HP

Nursing (Mental Health, pre-registration)

University of Greenwich G70
BSc (Hons): 3 years full-time – B760
Tariff: 160 Interview

Nursing (Mental Health, with top-up to BSc)

Kingston University K84
DipHE: 3 years full-time
A2: EE

St George's, University of London S49
DipHE: 3 years full-time
A2: EE

Nursing (Midwifery)

Bell College [University of Paisley] B26
DipHE: 3 years full-time
A2: C SQA: CC Interview

Bell College [University of Paisley] B26
BSc: 3 years full-time
A2: C SQA: CC Interview

Nursing and Midwifery (second registration shortened programme)

University of Chester C55
DipHE: 18 months full-time
Tariff: 240 - 260 IB: 30

Nursing and Midwifery Studies (top-up)

University of Stirling S75
BSc (Hons): 1 year full-time – B741
RN, RM

Nursing (post-registration)

University of Cumbria C99
BSc (Hons): 1 year full-time – B702
HE credits: 240, RN, Interview

University of Dundee D65
BN: full-time or part-time
RN

Middlesex University M80
BSc (Hons): 1 year full-time or 2 years part-time – B720 E
HE credits: 240, RN

Napier University N07
BSc (Hons): 2 - 5 years part-time
RN

Nursing Practice

University of Bradford B56
BSc (Hons): part-time
RN, HP

Coventry University C85
BSc (Hons): 2 - 5 years part-time
HE credits: 120 - 240, RN

University of East Anglia E14
DipHE: part-time
HE credits: 120, RN

University of East Anglia E14
BSc (Hons): part-time
HE credits: 240, RN

Nursing Practice (Adult)

Staffordshire University S72
BSc (Hons): 3 years full-time – B740
Tariff: 200

Nursing Practice (Child)

Staffordshire University S72
BSc (Hons): 3 years full-time – B730
Tariff: 200

Nursing Practice (Mental Health)

Staffordshire University S72
BSc (Hons): 3 years full-time – B760
Tariff: 200

Nursing (pre-registration)

University of Abertay Dundee A30
BSc (Hons): 4 years full-time – B700
Tariff: 180

University of Central Lancashire C30
BSc (Hons): 3 years full-time or 5 years part-time – B74
Tariff: 220 Interview

University of Central Lancashire C30
DipHE: 3 years full-time or 5 years part-time
A2 Interview

Nursing (pre-registration, alternati route)

University of Central Lancashire C30
DipHE: 18 months mixed mode

University of Central Lancashire C30
BSc (Hons): 1 year full-time or 18 months part-time
HE credits: 240

ursing (professional development)

outh Eastern Regional College
HE: part-time
: DD

ursing (with professional egistration)

ournemouth University B50
c (Hons): 3 years full-time – B700
iff: 180

ournemouth University B50
HE: 2 years full-time
C

ursing (Registered Midwife)

lge Hill University E42
HE: 3 years full-time

ursing (Registered Nurse)

ngston University K84
c (Hons): 3 years full-time – B700
ff: 210

ursing (Registered Nurse, with oecialist pathway awards)

CE Birmingham C25
HE: 3 years full-time
HP

CE Birmingham C25
(Hons): 3 years full-time – B700
f: 200

ursing Science

rthumbria University N77
(Hons): 1 year full-time or 2 years part-time
credits: 240, RN

ursing Sciences

een's University Belfast Q75
: 3 years full-time
CCC - BB

uth West College
(Hons): 2 - 5 years part-time
credits: 240, RN

ursing and Social Work Studies earning Disabilities)

ndon South Bank University L75
(Hons)/DipSW: 3 years full-time – BL75
f: 160

Nursing (Specialist Practitioner, Infection Control Nursing)

University of Dundee D65
BN: 2 - 5 years part-time
RN

Nursing (with specialist practitioner qualification)

Buckinghamshire Chilterns University College B94
BSc (Hons): 2 - 5 years part-time
HE credits: 240, RN, HP

Nursing Studies

University of Abertay Dundee A30
BA: 6 months full-time or 1 year part-time
HE credits: 240, RN

Canterbury Christ Church University C10
DipHE: 3 years full-time or 5 years part-time
A2

Coventry University C85
BSc/BSc (Hons): 2 - 5 years part-time
HE credits: 120 - 240, RN

University of Salford S03
BSc (Hons): 1 year full-time or 2 - 5 years part-time
HE credits: 240, RN

University of York Y50
DipHE: 3 years full-time
A2 BTEC: PP - PPP

Nursing Studies (Adult)

University of Greenwich G70
DipHE: 3 years full-time
A2 BTEC: PPP

Liverpool John Moores University L51
DipHE: 3 years full-time
A2

London South Bank University L75
DipHE: 3 years full-time
A2

London South Bank University L75
BSc (Hons): 3 years full-time – B700
Tariff: 160

University of Northampton N38
BSc (Hons): 3 years full-time – B700
Tariff: 180 - 200

University of Teesside T20
BSc (Hons): 3 years full-time or 4 - 5 years part-time – B700
Tariff: 200 Interview

Nursing Studies (Adult Care)

Sheffield Hallam University S21
BA (I lons): 4 years full-time – B701
Tariff: 180

Nursing Studies (Child)

London South Bank University L75
BSc (Hons): 3 years full-time – B702
Tariff: 160

London South Bank University L75
DipHE: 3 years full-time
A2 BTEC: PPP

University of Northampton N38
BSc (Hons): 3 years full-time – B702
Tariff: 180 - 200

University of Teesside T20
BSc (Hons): 3 years full-time or 4 - 5 years part-time – B701
Tariff: 200 Interview

Nursing Studies (Child Care)

Sheffield Hallam University S21
BA (Hons): 4 years full-time – B702
Tariff: 180

Nursing Studies (Learning Disabilities)

University of Greenwich G70
DipHE: 3 years full-time
A2 BTEC: PPP

University of Northampton N38
BSc (Hons): 3 years full-time – B703
Tariff: 180 - 200

Nursing Studies (Mental Health)

University of Greenwich G70
DipHE: 3 years full-time
A2 BTEC: PPP

Liverpool John Moores University L51
DipHE: 3 years full-time
A2

London South Bank University L75
DipHE: 3 years full-time
A2

London South Bank University L75
BSc (Hons): 3 years full-time – B701
Tariff: 160

University of Northampton N38
BSc (Hons): 3 years full-time – B710
Tariff: 180 - 200

University of Teesside T20
BSc (Hons): 3 years full-time or 4 - 5 years part-time – B702
Tariff: 200 Interview

Nursing Studies (Mental Health Care)

Sheffield Hallam University S21
BA (Hons): 4 years full-time – B703
Tariff: 180

Nursing Studies (post-registration)

University of Central Lancashire C30
BSc (Hons): 1 year full-time or part-time or on-line study
HE credits: 240, RN

North East Wales Institute of Higher Education N56
BSc (Hons): 1 year full-time or part-time
HE credits: 240, RN

Nursing Studies (Registered Nurse)

Glasgow Caledonian University G42
BA (Hons): 4 years full-time – B700
A2: CC SQA: BBCC - BBB

Nursing Studies (Registered Nurse, Adult Nursing)

University of Surrey S85
BSc (Hons): 3 years full-time – B744
A2: BCC BTEC: DMM IB: 30

Nursing Studies (Registered Nurse, Child Nursing)

University of Surrey S85
BSc (Hons): 3 years full-time – B745
A2: BCC BTEC: DMM IB: 30

Nursing Studies with Registration (Adult)

King's College London (University of London) K60
BSc (Hons): 3 years full-time – B740
A2: CCC SQA: BBCCC ILC: BBCCC IB: 28

King's College London (University of London) K60
DipHE: 3 years full-time
A2

Nursing Studies with Registration (Adult, for graduates)

King's College London (University of London) K60
DipHE: 2 years full-time
A2

Nursing Studies with Registration (Child)

King's College London (University of London) K60
DipHE: 3 years full-time
A2

King's College London (University of London) K60
BSc (Hons): 3 years full-time – B730
A2: CCC SQA: BBCCC ILC: BBCCC IB: 28

Nursing Studies with Registration (Child, for graduates)

King's College London (University of London) K60
DipHE: 2 years full-time
A2

Nursing Studies with Registration (Mental Health)

King's College London (University of London) K60
DipHE: 3 years full-time
A2

King's College London (University of London) K60
BSc (Hons): 3 years full-time – B760
A2: CCC SQA: BBCCC ILC: BBCCC IB: 28

Nursing Studies with Registration (Mental Health, for graduates)

King's College London (University of London) K60
DipHE: 2 years full-time
A2

Nursing Studies (with Specialist Practitioner Award)

University of Abertay Dundee A30
BA: 1 year full-time or 2 years part-time day
HE credits: 240, RN
NES

Nursing Studies (top-up)

University of Stirling S75
BSc (Hons): 1 year full-time – B740
RN

Nursing Studies/Registered Nurse

Northumbria University N77
DipHE: 3 years full-time
A2 BTEC: PPP

Nursing Studies/Registered Nurse (Adult)

Northumbria University N77
BSc (Hons): 3 years full-time – B700
Tariff: 240 IB: 26

Nursing Studies/Registered Nurse (Child)

Northumbria University N77
BSc (Hons): 3 years full-time – B701
Tariff: 240 IB: 26

Nursing Studies/Registered Nurse (Learning Disability)

Northumbria University N77
BSc (Hons): 3 years full-time – B741
Tariff: 240 IB: 26

Nursing Studies/Registered Nurse (Mental Health)

Northumbria University N77
BSc (Hons): 3 years full-time – B740
Tariff: 240 IB: 26

Nursing/Health Studies (Specialist Practitioner Gerontological Nursing)

University of Paisley P20
BSc (Hons): 1 year full-time or 2 - 3 years part-time
RN

Nursing/Registered Nurse (Adult)

University of Salford S03
BSc (Hons): 3 years full-time – B701
Tariff: 160

Nursing/Registered Nurse (Child)

University of Salford S03
BSc (Hons): 3 years full-time – B702
Tariff: 160

Occupational Health Nursing

London South Bank University L75
BSc (Hons): 1 year full-time or 2 years part-time
RN

Oncology Nursing

University of Hertfordshire H36
BSc (Hons): 4 years part-time
HE credits: 120, RN

Operating Department Practice

Anglia Ruskin University A60
DipHE: 2 years full-time – B990
Tariff: 120 - 160 IB: 24

University of Bedfordshire B22
DipHE: 2 years full-time
A2 Interview

Bournemouth University B50
DipHE: 2 years full-time – B991
A2 Interview

Cardiff University C15
DipHE: 2 years full-time – B990
Tariff: 160

Cardiff University C15
BSc (Hons): 3 years part-time
Tariff: 160

niversity of Central Lancashire C30
›HE: 3 years full-time
Interview

niversity of East Anglia E14
HE: 2 years full-time
BTEC: PPP Interview

dge Hill University E42
HE: 3 years full-time – B990
Interview

iversity of Huddersfield H60
HE: 2 years full-time – B990
: DD BTEC: PPP Interview

iversity of Hull H72
HE: 2 years full-time
ff: 120

iversity of Leicester L34
HE: 2 years full-time
Interview

orthumbria University N77
HE: 2 years full-time
BTEC: PP - PPP Interview

iversity of Plymouth P60
HE: 2 years full-time – B990
BTEC: PPP Interview

effield Hallam University S21
HE: 2 years full-time
ff: 140

affordshire University S72
HE: 2 years full-time – B901
BTEC: PPP Interview

iversity Campus Suffolk [University of
st Anglia, University of Essex] S82
HE: 2 years full-time or 4 - 9 years part-time –
91 I
ff: 40

iversity Campus Suffolk [University of
st Anglia, University of Essex] S82
: 1 year full-time or 2 years full-time
RM, HP

iversity of Surrey S85
HE: 2 years full-time – B990
Interview

iversity of Teesside T20
HE: 2 years full-time – B991
ff: 160 Interview

ames Valley University T40
HE: 2 - 7 years part-time day
E HE credits: 120

ames Valley University T40
(Hons): 2 - 7 years part-time day
credits: 240

E Birmingham C25
HE: 2 years full-time
f: 160

Operating Department Practitioner

Glasgow Caledonian University G42
DipHE: 2 years full-time – B990
A2: DD - BB SQA: CC

Palliative Care

University of Glamorgan G14
DipHE: 2 - 5 years distance learning
HE credits: 120, RN, RM

University of Hertfordshire H36
BSc (Hons): 4 - 6 years part-time
HE credits: 120, RN

Sheffield Hallam University S21
BA (Hons): 1 - 5 years part-time
HE credits: 240, RN, HP

UCE Birmingham C25
BSc: 1 - 5 years part-time BSc (Hons): 2 - 5 years part-time
HE credits: 240, RN, RM

University of Wolverhampton W75
BSc (Hons): 2 - 5 years part-time
HE credits: 120, RN, HP

Palliative Care and Cancer Care (Marie Curie Cancer Care)

Thames Valley University T40
DipHE: 2 - 7 years distance learning
HE credits: 120, RN, HP

Thames Valley University T40
BSc (Hons): 2 - 7 years distance learning
HE credits: 240, RN, HP

Palliative Care (post-qualifying framework)

Bristol, University of the West of England B80
BSc (Hons): 1 year full-time or 4 years part-time – B706
HE credits: 240, RN, HP

Palliative Care and Publishing

Oxford Brookes University O66
BA (Hons)/BSc (Hons): 3 years full-time – BP74
RN, HP

Perioperative Care

University of Portsmouth P80
BA: 2 years part-time
HE credits: 240

Primary and Community Health Care

Oxford Brookes University O66
BA/BA (Hons): 1 year full-time or 2 years part-time day – B715
HE credits: 120, RN

Professional Midwifery Practice

London South Bank University L75
DipHE: 2 - 5 years part-time
HE credits: 120, RM

London South Bank University L75
BSc (Hons): 2 - 5 years part-time
HE credits: 120, RM

Professional Nursing Practice

London South Bank University L75
BSc (Hons): 2 - 5 years part-time
HE credits: 120, RN

London South Bank University L75
DipHE: 2 - 5 years part-time
HE credits: 120, RN

Professional Practice (Acute and Critical Care)

University of Bedfordshire B22
DipHE: 6 months part-time day and evening BA (Hons): 1 year part-time day and evening
HE credits: 240, RN

Professional Practice (Adult Health)

University of Central Lancashire C30
BSc (Hons): 2 - 5 years part-time
HE credits: 240, RN

Professional Practice with Cardio-Respiratory Care

Thames Valley University T40
BSc (Hons): 2 - 7 years part-time day/evening
HE credits: 240, HP

Thames Valley University T40
DipHE: 2 - 7 years part-time day/evening
HE credits: 120, HP

Professional Practice (Child Health with Neonatal Nursing)

Thames Valley University T40
DipHE: 2 - 7 years part-time day/evening
HE credits: 120, RN, RM

Thames Valley University T40
BSc (Hons): 2 - 7 years part-time day/evening
HE credits, RN, RM

Professional Practice with Clinical Haematology

Thames Valley University T40
DipHE: 2 - 7 years part-time day/evening
HE credits: 120, HP

Thames Valley University T40
BSc (Hons): 2 - 7 years part-time day/evening
HE credits: 240, HP

Professional Practice (Clinical Nursing)

University of Brighton B72
BSc (Hons): 5 years part-time
RN

Professional Practice with Contemporary Issues in Child Health

Thames Valley University T40
DipHE: 2 - 7 years part-time day/evening
HE credits: 120, RN

Thames Valley University T40
BSc (Hons): 2 - 7 years part-time day/evening
HE credits: 240, RN

Professional Practice (Critical Care, Child Health)

Thames Valley University T40
BSc (Hons): 1 - 7 years part-time day/evening
HE credits: 240, RN

Thames Valley University T40
DipHE: 1 - 7 years part-time day/evening
HE credits: 120, RN

Professional Practice for Nurses, Midwives or Health Visitors (post-registration)

University of Glamorgan G14
BSc: 1 - 4 years part-time BSc (Hons): 2 - 5 years part-time
HE credits: 120, RN, RM, HP

Professional Practice (Gerontology)

University of Brighton B72
BSc (Hons): up to 6 years part-time
HE credits: 120, RN

Professional Practice (Mental Health)

University of Brighton B72
BSc (Hons): up to 6 years part-time
RN

Professional Practice (Midwifery)

University of Brighton B72
BSc (Hons): 1 - 5 years part-time
RM

Professional Practice (Nursing, Midwifery and Health Visiting)

Pembrokeshire College [University of Glamorgan] P35
BSc (Hons): 2 - 5 years part-time
HE credits: 240, RN, RM, HP

Professional Practice (Nursing/Midwifery)

University of Bedfordshire B22
BSc (Hons): 1 year full-time or 2 years part-time day
RN, RM

Professional Practice with Ophthalmic Nursing

Thames Valley University T40
DipHE: 2 - 7 years part-time day/evening
HE credits: 120, HP

Thames Valley University T40
BSc (Hons): 2 - 7 years part-time day/evening
HE credits: 240, HP

Professional Practice (Palliative Care)

University of Bedfordshire B22
DipHE: 6 months part-time day and evening BA (Hons): 1 year part-time day and evening
RN, HP

Professional Practice with Peripheral Vascular Nursing

Thames Valley University T40
BSc (Hons): 1 - 7 years part-time day/evening
HE credits: 240, RN

Professional Practice with Renal Nursing

Thames Valley University T40
DipHE: 2 - 7 years part-time day/evening
HE credits: 120, RN

Professional Studies in Nursing and Social Work

University of Salford S03
BSc (Hons): 3 years full-time – BL75
Tariff: 120 - 180

Professional Studies (post-qualifying framework)

Bristol, University of the West of England B80
BSc (Hons): 1 year full-time or 4 years part-time – B999
HE credits: 240, RN, RM, HP

Promoting Practice Effectiveness

University of Teesside T20
BSc (Hons): 2 - 5 years part-time
HE credits: 240

Promoting Practice Effectiveness (Cancer and Palliative Care)

University of Teesside T20
BSc (Hons): 2 - 5 years part-time
HE credits: 240

Promoting Practice Effectiveness (Child)

University of Teesside T20
BSc (Hons): 2 - 5 years part-time
HE credits: 240

Promoting Practice Effectiveness (Complementary Therapies)

University of Teesside T20
BSc (Hons): 2 - 5 years part-time
HE credits: 240

Promoting Practice Effectiveness (Critical Care)

University of Teesside T20
BSc (Hons): 2 - 5 years part-time
HE credits: 240

Promoting Practice Effectiveness (District Nursing)

University of Teesside T20
BSc (Hons): 2 - 5 years part-time
HE credits: 240

Promoting Practice Effectiveness (Emergency Care Practitioner)

University of Teesside T20
BSc (Hons): 2 - 5 years part-time
HE credits: 240

Promoting Practice Effectiveness (General Practice Nursing)

University of Teesside T20
BSc (Hons): 2 - 5 years part-time
HE credits: 240

Promoting Practice Effectiveness (Generic)

University of Teesside T20
BSc (Hons): 2 - 5 years part-time
HE credits: 240

Promoting Practice Effectiveness (Helicopter Emergency Medical Services)

University of Teesside T20
BSc (Hons): 2 - 5 years part-time
HE credits: 240

Promoting Practice Effectiveness (Leadership and Management)

University of Teesside T20
BSc (Hons): 2 - 5 years part-time
HE credits: 240

romoting Practice Effectiveness lurse Practitioner)

iversity of Teesside T20

: (Hons): 2 - 5 years part-time
credits: 240

romoting Practice Effectiveness)ccupational Health Nursing)

iversity of Teesside T20

: (Hons): 2 - 5 years part-time
credits: 240

romoting Practice Effectiveness)lder People)

iversity of Teesside T20

: (Hons): 2 - 5 years part-time
credits: 240

romoting Practice Effectiveness ublic Health or Health Visiting)

iversity of Teesside T20

: (Hons): 2 - 5 years part-time
credits: 240

ıblic Health

stol, University of the West of England
0

: (Hons): 1 year full-time or 2 years part-time – B912
Interview

ıblic Health Nursing (District ırsing)

bert Gordon University R36

1 - 4 years full-time or 1 - 4 years part-time or 1 -
ars distance learning

, NMC

ıblic Health Nursing (Health siting)

ford Brookes University O66

3A (Hons): 1 year full-time or 2 years part-time day –
4

ıblic Health Nursing (Health Visiting th Specialist Practice)

bert Gordon University R36

1 - 4 years full-time or 1 - 4 years part-time or 1 - 4
s distance learning

NMC

Public Health Nursing (Occupational Health Nursing)

Robert Gordon University R36

BA: 1 - 4 years full-time or 1 - 4 years part-time or 1 -
4 years distance learning
RN
NES, NMC

Public Health Nursing (Occupational Health Nursing with Specialist Practice)

Robert Gordon University R36

BA: 1 - 4 years part-time or 1 - 4 years distance learning
RN
NES, NMC

Registered Midwifery

University of Wolverhampton W75

BSc (Hons): 3 years full-time – B720
Tariff: 200 - 260 IB: 24

Registered Midwifery (shortened)

University of Wolverhampton W75

BSc (Hons): 1 - 2 years full-time
HE credits: 180, RN

Registered Nurse (Adult/Child/ Learning Disabilities/Mental Health)

Anglia Ruskin University A60

DipHE: 2 years full-time
Interview

Respiratory Care

University of Hertfordshire H36

BSc (Hons): 4 - 6 years part-time
HE credits: 240, HP

School Nursing

Oxford Brookes University O66

BA/BA (Hons): 1 year full-time or 2 years part-time – B719
RN

Sexual and Reproductive Health

University of Central Lancashire C30

BSc (Hons): 2 - 5 years part-time
HE credits: 240, RN, RM

University of Central Lancashire C30

DipHE: 2 - 5 years part-time
RN, RM

Social Work/Learning Disabilities Nursing

University of Teesside T20

BSc (Hons): 3 years full-time – LB57
Tariff: 200 Interview

Social Work/Mental Health Nursing

University of Teesside T20

BSc (Hons): 3 years full-time – BL75
Tariff: 200 Interview

Specialist Community Nursing Practice

University of Hertfordshire H36

BSc (Hons): 1 year full-time or 2 years part-time
HE credits: 120, RN
NMC

Specialist Community Practice

University of Bedfordshire B22

BA (Hons): 1 year full-time or 2 years part-time
HE credits: 60, RN, RM

Specialist Community Practice (Community Learning Disabilities)

University of Bedfordshire B22

BA (Hons): 1 year full-time or 2 years part-time
HE credits: 60, RN, RM

Specialist Community Practice (Community Mental Health)

University of Bedfordshire B22

BA (Hons): 1 year full-time or 2 years part-time
HE credits: 60, RN, RM

Specialist Community Practice (General Practice Nursing)

University of Bedfordshire B22

BA (Hons): 1 year full-time or 2 years part-time
HE credits: 60, RN, RM

Specialist Community Practice (Nursing in the Home, District Nurse)

University of Bedfordshire B22

BA (Hons): 1 year full-time or 2 years part-time
HE credits: 60, RN, RM

Specialist Community Practice (Public Health Nursing, Health Visiting)

University of Bedfordshire B22

BA (Hons): 1 year full-time or 2 years part-time
HE credits: 60, RN, RM

Specialist Community Public Health Nursing (Health Visiting and School Nursing)

Manchester Metropolitan University M40

BSc (Hons): 3 years full-time
HE credits: 240, RN, RM

Specialist Nursing

Glasgow Caledonian University G42
BSc/BSc (Hons): 3 - 5 years part-time
RN, RM

Specialist Nursing Practice (Community Mental Health Nursing)

Staffordshire University S72
BSc (Hons): 1 year full-time or 2 years part-time
HE credits: 240, RN

Specialist Nursing Practice (Community Nursing)

Coventry University C85
BSc (Hons): 2 - 5 years part-time
RN, RM, HP
NMC

Specialist Nursing Practice (Community Nursing in the Home, District Nursing)

Staffordshire University S72
BSc (Hons): 1 year full-time or 2 years part-time
HE credits: 240, RN, RM

Specialist Nursing Practice (General Practice Nursing)

Staffordshire University S72
BSc (Hons): 1 year full-time or 2 years part-time
RN, RM

Specialist Nursing Practice (Oncology)

Coventry University C85
BSc (Hons): 2 years part-time
RN

Specialist Nursing Practice (Palliative Care)

Coventry University C85
BSc (Hons): 2 years part-time
RN

Specialist Nursing Practice (Public Health Nursing/Health Visiting)

Staffordshire University S72
BSc (Hons): 1 year full-time or 2 years part-time
RN, RM

Specialist Nursing Practice (School Nursing)

Staffordshire University S72
BSc (Hons): 1 year full-time or 2 years part-time
RN, RM

Specialist Practice in Public Health (Health Visiting/District Nursing)

City University C60
BSc: 1 year full-time or 2 years part-time
HE credits: 240, RN, RM

Specialist Practice (post-qualifying framework)

Bristol, University of the West of England B80
BSc (Hons): 1 year full-time or 4 years part-time – B990
RN, RM, HP

Supportive and Palliative Care

St Luke's Hospice (Education and Resource Centre)
BA (Hons): 2 - 5 years part-time day
RN, RM, HP

Supportive and Palliative Care (Specialist Practitioner, Adult)

Sheffield Hallam University S21
BA (Hons): 2 - 6 years part-time
HE credits: 240, RN
NMC

St Luke's Hospice (Education and Resource Centre)
BA (Hons): 2 - 5 years part-time day
RN

Surgical Care Practitioner

University of Teesside T20
BSc (Hons): 1 year full-time or 2 - 5 years part-time
HE credits: 120

Tissue Viability

University of Hertfordshire H36
BSc (Hons): 2 - 6 years part-time
HE credits: 120, RN

Optometry and Audiology

Including:
Ophthalmic Dispensing
Ophthalmology
Optometry
Audiology

What would you study?

Courses in this chapter will enable you to assist people with problems with vision and hearing. Some are three- or four-year degree courses while others are offered as Foundation degree courses over two years, the latter mainly aimed at the career of dispensing optician.

Optometry

The topics studied include anatomy, physiology and pharmacology. More specific to optometry are subjects such as:

- Binocular anomalies
- Law relating to optometrists
- Mathematics and geometric optics
- Optical dispensing
- Ocular examination techniques.

Audiology

There has been considerable expansion of higher education for audiologists in recent years. There are now nine degree courses in the UK and they take four years (including a year's practical experience in the third year).

The course content, as with most courses in the healthcare field, includes a range of science-based study. A typical course starts with two years at university gaining a theoretical background to the job. Subjects studied and skills tackled will include:

- Biology and psychology relevant to communication issues
- Deafness in the community
- Hearing aid fitting
- Hearing science
- Introduction to assessment techniques
- Supervised practical sessions
- Tinnitus.

The third year will normally be a practical year (usually paid) spent in a clinic experiencing the job first hand, before returning to university for the final year, which will still include a considerable amount of practical work and also a dissertation. There is often an opportunity to acquire signing skills, though some institutions like applicants to have had some experience of this from the start.

Getting in

Once again the emphasis is on science subjects and you might expect to be asked to show evidence of at least one subject from biology, chemistry, physics, mathematics or psychology. Admissions tutors will be looking for people who can communicate well. Professionals in this field have to be able to apply the theory they have learnt to the practicalities of each patient's circumstances, so a logical approach is also necessary.

Each university decides on its own entry requirements. You can see the range of UCAS points asked by each one by consulting the course listings on the following pages. However, many Foundation degree courses exercise a more flexible admissions procedure which enables them to take into account factors such as work experience in their entrance requirements and which cannot therefore be expressed as part of the UCAS tariff framework.

Graduate outlook

Qualifications in this area can lead to a variety of careers. The main ones are summarised in the paragraphs below.

Optometrist

Optometrists can deal with people of all ages but some decide to specialise in areas such as children's vision, low vision or contact lenses. There are around 7500 of them working in many different environments – hospitals, large national companies (such as Specsavers, Boots or Dollond & Aitchison), in business on their own or in partnerships. There are also opportunities for work as a locum – providing professional cover for any optician's business the area – and there is plenty of opportunity for part-time work.

Optometrists work with other medical professionals such as GPs or eye specialists in the sense that examination and testing of eyes can reveal other medical conditions of which the patient may not yet be aware. Thes could be specific to the eye, in which case there will be a referral to a hospital eye department. There the patient may be seen by an ophthalmi medical practitioner or an ophthalmologist – both fully qualified doctors who specialise in eye care. Other more general conditions, such as diabetes, could also be identified and would initially be referred to a GP. Optometry graduates have to undertake a pre-registration year before th can consider themselves to be professionally qualified.

Orthoptist

Orthoptists normally work in hospitals, in a team with ophthalmologists, assessing and treating conditions such as squints or double vision. Much of the work is with children – and keeping their parents involved and co-operative is an essential part of the job. See the chapter on **Therapies** fo more detail about this career.

Dispensing optician

Dispensing opticians are an integral part of the eyecare team, putting the finishing touches to the work of the others. They discuss with patients ho the prescription and recommendations from the optometrist might best b achieved in the light of their particular circumstances. They take into account patients' lifestyles, preferred fashion styles and preferences for frames and lenses or contact lenses. In effect, the dispensing optician helps patients by putting the required prescriptions into the most appropriate package for them. Following that, they are available for providing advice, adjustment and repairs.

Audiologist

Audiologists work mainly with children and the elderly as those groups a most likely to have hearing problems. Balance problems often have the same causes as hearing problems and are therefore an important part o their role. Audiologists work as part of a team with ear, nose and throat doctors, speech therapists and, often, teachers of the deaf and educatio audiologists. Most audiologists work in hospitals.

As a result of a recent modernisation programme, new digital devices and cochlear implants have made their way into the audiologists' armoury – much to the benefit of their patients. It is therefore a technical job in that audiologists must understand the technology behi the latest devices developed to assist those with hearing difficulties. However, technical prowess is not much use if it is not applied proper to the needs of each individual patient. Therefore the audiologist must have excellent communication skills to work with a group of people fo whom communication may not be easy. Counselling skills may also be required in order to help the patient come to terms with his or her problem, and motivational skills are important in order to keep the patient enthusiastic about following the treatment strategies which ha been prescribed.

In the NHS, careers may progress from junior audiologist all the way up consultant level. Other career opportunities occur in higher education teaching or working for local education authorities.

What would you earn?

Salary scales for audiologists and orthoptists employed in the NHS are a scale from approximately £19,000 to £31,000. Promotion could bring salaries up to £36,400 and very senior posts are paid up to £61,000.

These examples are based on April 2006 salary scales. At the time of writing this book the public sector unions had not accepted the pay increase of around 2.5%, which had been offered in April 2007.

Dispensing opticians earn around £15,000 to £30,000. Partners in practices can earn over £80,000. Optometrists can earn from £17,000 £36,000.

Case Study

Sarah Broderick

Sarah is in the Final Year of a BSc in Optometry at Aston University.

'When I started to look at degree courses I knew that I wanted to do something leading to a career in health care and also thought about pharmacy and radiography before deciding on optometry. Radiography would have given me the same mix of science and patient contact but there seemed to be too much physics in it, so I chose optometry – and I'm glad that I did. I'm thoroughly enjoying the course. It is a very good one for someone who likes patient contact and who likes fitting together what the patients says, their symptoms and scientific knowledge to solve a problem.

'I did the Irish Leaving Certificate and I didn't take physics to Higher Level. I wondered whether I might find that a problem but I haven't done so. There are students on my course who hadn't taken physics A level either and they find the same. We had a module on introductory physics in the first year – and we could always ask for help if we needed to.

'In the first year, the course was more about science than optometry. There was a lot of biology, with some modules in optics – and the one in physics. Teaching was done through lectures to the year group (of 120), some tutorials and laboratory practicals which we did in smaller groups. All our work is done in the School of Life Sciences building, and all as optometry students. We have no shared lectures with students from other courses.

'The second year was very much like the first year but with a bit more practical work. This year it has all come together and is really, really interesting. We have a smaller number of lectures – one every day from 9am–10am and one every Tuesday from 4pm–6pm. The remainder of the time is spent on clinical work and on our individual dissertations. The school has its own optometry clinic where paying members of the public come as patients. I do eye tests which last one hour then work out what type of glasses or contact lenses patients might need. This is a much longer time than a normal eye test would take but the patients know that we are students and are taking extra time. One of the staff always checks our work and they are the ones who explain the results and discuss them with patients. The clinic timetable changes regularly because every student has to see a specified number of patients in order to qualify and we also have to see all kinds of eye conditions. So our hours have to fit around the patients who come in.

'I have spent a lot of time this year on my dissertation – which I have just finished. We can choose between literature-based and practical-based titles. Mine is on "Does nutrition have an aetiological role in myopia onset and development?" Because it is literature-based I have not been conducting experiments or interviewing patients but researching in the library and on the internet. Not much has been written on this particular aspect of myopia so I have to search hard. There is a lot to find on nutrition however as knowledge on this is constantly being updated. I have collated all my findings and written up the results now. The final dissertation is about 8000 words in length.

'The relationship between staff and students is very good. We are asked to complete a questionnaire at the end of each year – and they do take note of the answers. We have benefited from some changes that the year group above us suggested – and the staff say that as a result of these changes our skills have improved.'

Advanced Ophthalmic Dispensing (top-up)

City University C60
BSc (Hons): 1 year full-time – B512
HND, Fd

Audiology

Aston University A80
BSc (Hons): 4 years sandwich – B610
A2: BBC

University of Bristol B78
BSc (Hons): 4 years sandwich – B610
A2: BBB - ABB BTEC: DDM SQA: BBBBB - AABBB
IB: 32 - 33

Castle College Nottingham [De Montfort University] ▲
BSc (Hons): 4 years full-time – B610 V
Tariff: 240 IB: 26

De Montfort University D26
BSc (Hons): 4 years sandwich – B610
Tariff: 180 - 240 IB: 26

University of Leeds L23
BSc (Hons): 4 years full-time – B611
A2: CCC BTEC: MMM

University of Manchester M20
BSc (Hons): 4 years full-time – B610
A2: BBB BTEC: DDM SQA: AABBB ILC: AABBB IB: 30

Queen Margaret University, Edinburgh Q25
BSc (Hons): 4 years full-time – B610
Tariff: 278 - 280

University of Southampton S27
BSc (Hons): 4 years full-time – B610
Tariff: 350 IB: 34 Interview

University of Wales, Swansea S93
BSc (Hons): 3 years full-time – B610
Tariff: 240

University College London, University of London U80
BSc (Hons): 4 years full-time – B610
A2: BBB IB: 32 Interview

Dispensing Optics

City University C60
FdA: 2 years full-time – B511
Tariff: 180

Ophthalmic Dispensing

Anglia Ruskin University A60
BSc (Hons): 3 years full-time – B590
Tariff: 140 - 200

Anglia Ruskin University A60
FdSc: 2 years full-time
A2: CC

City University C60
FdSc: 2 years full-time or 3 years part-time – B511
Tariff: 180

City and Islington College [City University] ▲
FdSc: 3 years part-time day-release
Tariff: 180

Glasgow Caledonian University G42
BSc: 3 years full-time – B502
Tariff: 120
ABDO, GOC

Ophthalmic Dispensing with Management

Bradford College [Leeds Metropolitan University] B60
BSc (Hons): 3 years full-time – B503
Tariff: 120 - 160
ABDO, GOC

Bradford College [Leeds Metropolitan University] B60
FdSc: 2 years full-time – B500
Tariff: 120

Ophthalmic Science and Technology

Castle College Nottingham [Nottingham Trent University] C21
FdSc: 2 years full-time – B500
Tariff: 120

Optometry

Anglia Ruskin University A60
BOptom (Hons): 3 years full-time – B513
A2: ABB ILC: AAAAB IB: 33

Aston University A80
BSc (Hons): 3 years full-time – B510
A2: AAB SQA: AAABB IB: 35 HP
GOC

University of Bradford B56
BSc (Hons): 3 years full-time – B510
Tariff: 320 IB: 33
GOC

Cardiff University C15
BSc (Hons): 3 years full-time – B510
Tariff: 340 IB: 34 - 36 Interview
BCO, GOC

City University C60
BSc (Hons): 3 years full-time – B510
A2: ABB SQA: AABBB IB: 33
GOC

Glasgow Caledonian University G42
BSc: 4 years full-time BSc (Hons): 4 years full-time – B510
A2: ABB SQA: BBBBB ILC: AAABBB HP
BCO, GOC

University of Manchester M20
BSc (Hons): 3 years full-time – B510
A2: ABB BTEC: DDM SQA: AAABB ILC: AABBB IB: 33
BCO, GOC

University of Manchester M20
MOptom (Hons): 4 years full-time – B511
A2: ABB BTEC: DDM SQA: AAABB ILC: AABBB IB: 33
BCO, GOC

University of Ulster U20
BSc (Hons): 3 years full-time – B510 C
Tariff: 340 IB: 37
GOC

Optometry (with a preliminary year

Cardiff University C15
BSc (Hons): 4 years full-time including foundation year – B511
Interview

Orthoptics

University of Liverpool L41
BSc (Hons): 3 years full-time – B520
A2: CCC SQA: BBBCC ILC: BBBCC IB: 26
HPC

University of Sheffield S18
BMedSci (Hons): 3 years full-time – B520
A2: BBB SQA: AABB ILC: ABBBB IB: 32
HPC

Pharmacology and Pharmacy

What would you study?

Pharmacology

Pharmacology is a research-orientated subject and studies the uses, effects and modes of action of drugs. It is a subject in its own right but also forms an essential part of other degrees such as Medicine, Dentistry, Veterinary Science and, of course, Pharmacy.

Pharmacy

Pharmacy is the science governing the dispensing and preparation of drugs. How is a drug used most effectively and with the least chance of unwanted side effects? What sort of carrying agent is best for any given condition – for example, is the 'active ingredient' best formulated as a cream, a spray, or delivered as an injection?

All Pharmacy courses are accredited by the Royal Pharmaceutical Society (www.rpsgb.org.uk) and are four years in duration, leading to a Master of Pharmacy (MPharm). Subjects included in the courses are:

- Microbiology
- Molecular biology
- Pharmaceutical and biological chemistry
- Pharmaceutics
- Pharmacy practice
- Physiology.

Getting in

Tariff point requirements vary across the many higher education establishments offering degree courses in this chapter. Institutions are most likely to ask for A levels (or equivalent) in chemistry and biology.

However, many Foundation degree courses exercise a more flexible admissions procedure which enables them to take into account factors such as work experience in their entrance requirements and which cannot therefore be expressed as part of the UCAS tariff framework.

Graduate outlook

Pharmacology

Pharmacologists are constantly searching for new drugs, identifying new medicines and assessing how they work in the body. As part of their work, they will develop biological tests in cell or tissue systems or whole animals. Pharmacologists may still rely upon tests involving animals but some universities have structured their courses to avoid this and the profession as a whole is making advances in the use of computer simulations both as a teaching and as an experimental tool.

Careers opportunities for pharmacologists tend to be in research and development for the pharmaceutical industry, or academic higher education research and teaching. As a profession it is regulated by the British Pharmacological Society (www.bps.ac.uk).

Pharmacy

All graduate pharmacists have to undertake a pre-registration year following their accredited degree course. They will be employed during this time. After the pre-registration year an exam must be taken to satisfy the standards of the Royal Pharmaceutical Society of Great Britain before their name is entered into the register of pharmaceutical chemists. There are around 35,000 practising pharmacists in the UK. There are three main branches of the pharmacist's profession:

Community pharmacy

This branch employs around two-thirds of qualified pharmacists. These are the people who work in your local chemist's store. Many of them run individual small businesses in which the chemist supplies customers with the drugs and medicines which have been prescribed by their doctors. They will also sell non-prescription medication and other goods. These pharmacists are effectively running their own businesses and employing their own staff so they have to be familiar with all the record keeping, accounti and property-management aspects of business life. There is now a trend away from the small business towards the high-street chain. Here, there a opportunities for pharmacists to work as staff in a store or as store managers. You could also find work in a pharmacy based in a health cent Wherever they are, pharmacists also have to take responsibility for the wc of those in their team such as dispensing technicians.

Not only do pharmacists prepare and dispense medicines, they frequently also act as informal sources of medical expertise, giving advice to the pub about treatment for minor ailments like giving up smoking, healthy eating and diet and family planning. Less well-known perhaps is the fact that the may offer advice to the prescribing doctor about the appropriate dosage le for any given situation. They may draw on a variety of continuing educatio courses to keep themselves abreast of new developments.

It is possible for undergraduates, often during their vacations, to obtain paid work experience with some of the large high street chains.

Hospital pharmacy

About 8000 hospital pharmacists work with the hospital team. They are daily contact with all the other healthcare professionals in the hospital a also with the patients themselves. They advise other staff on the correct dosage for any given clinical condition. Outpatients, nursing homes and patients of local healthcare centres might also look to a hospital pharmacist for advice.

Your early years in hospital pharmacy would probably be spent working alongside experienced pharmacists in a range of different ward types in or to gain wide experience before deciding on a specialism for your career.

Hospital pharmacies are heavily computerised. Most hospitals also have library of drug information. Prospects include promotion to pharmacy management and, indeed, many pharmacists use that as a springboard other management posts in the wider NHS.

Industrial pharmacy

Industrial pharmacists work for large pharmaceutical manufacturing companies carrying out a range of different types of work. For example they could work on the techniques for the actual manufacturing of any given drug, answering questions like 'in what form should an "active ingredient" be presented – pills, lozenges or creams …?' and 'how sho it be packaged?' Industrial pharmacists could be working alongside chemists, pharmacologists, toxicologists and the business and commer experts within the company. Quality control pharmacists would assist in determining the stability of the product and its shelf life. There is a dem for pharmacists in the manufacture of agricultural and veterinary produ

The skill and knowledge of pharmacists working in this sector provide t expertise needed to go for careers in sales and marketing, performing tasks like writing up literature on a drug, post-marketing surveillance a liaison with medical staff.

The publication *What do graduates do?* provides statistics for Pharmaco logy, Toxicology and Pharmacy graduates. It shows that of 1695 studen who responded to a survey in 2005 (the latest year for which figures ar available):

- 65.5 % were in employment in the UK
- 11.4% were doing full-time further study.
- 16.9% were working and studying
- 2.8% were unemployed

…. six months after graduation.

(The figures do not total 100% because some graduates answered th survey stating that they were not available for work.)

The majority of those in employment were using their degrees directly their careers, working as health professionals and associate health professionals (79%) while a further 3.8% were in scientific research a alysis. Around 2.7% were in commercial, industrial and public sector anagement. A number had used their degree as a level of qualification her than as a specific vocational training and had entered careers as ferent as business, finance, marketing, sales, advertising, IT work and ailing.

hat would you earn?

is varies considerably between the different branches of the profession. general, the industrial side pays the highest salaries. Pharmacologists can earn between £17,000 and £70,000, community pharmacists from £25,000 to £55,000 and industrial pharmacists £22,000 to £60,000. Salary scales for pharmacists working in the NHS are on a scale from approximately £19,000 to £31,000. Promotion could bring salaries up to £36,400 and very senior posts are paid over £73,000.

These examples are based on April 2006 salary scales. At the time of writing this book the public sector unions had not accepted the pay increase of around 2.5%, which had been offered in April 2007.

Case Study

Barry McCann

Barry is in the final year of an MPharm (Hons) course at the University of Manchester.

'My A level choices at school focused on chemistry – a subject I really enjoyed and wanted more of at university. Pharmacy allowed me to continue my interest in chemistry. I chose Manchester on the back of a good Quality Assurance Agency (QAA) report. I did voluntary work on a hospital ward and had work experience with mentally handicapped people. Before this, I was not sure how I would manage communicating with patients, but I gained confidence from befriending patients and shadowing a doctor.

'In the first year, surprisingly, much of what we had to study did not, at first sight, relate directly to pharmacy. People had come from different science backgrounds and we needed a common base. I needed more biology, others more physics or mathematics. The year was mainly lectures, tutorials and some practical work in labs. Each lecture threw up more reading and research. I will use these learning skills to keep up to date later in my career. We had exams to pass in order to continue.

'As I progressed through the second and third year, the exams we had began to count towards our ultimate degree grades. I found that the amount of self-directed work I put in to supplement lectures and practicals had a significant influence on my grades.

'By the third year we were spending more time in practical work experience situations in local Manchester hospitals. For example, "Disease Management" involved tutorials followed by work on the wards with experienced pharmacists and the rest of the ward medical team.

'The final year introduced problem-based learning. We split into small groups and took a case study on a particular disease. The idea is that you control your own learning by pooling what you already know as a group, then agree what else you need to know and do the necessary research.

'After my degree I will do the normal pre-registration year. We decide, by the third year, what branch of pharmacy we want to pursue as a career. The choice is:

- Retail work (in the chemists' shop)
- Hospital pharmacy
- Pharmaceutical manufacture (working for a drug research and manufacturing company).

Pre-registration job interviews took place at the beginning of the final year so we know in advance where we will be working after graduation.

'I have really enjoyed Manchester for the course and for the social life. I had time to take part-time jobs early on. In fact, the course handbook makes suggestions about how much time you could reasonably commit to earning money without compromising your learning. The final year, however, is too hectic to allow time for a job, so my coursework effort is up but my finances are down at the moment. I also found time during the course to be chairman of Manchester University Pharmaceutical Society – organising freshers' parties and a black tie ball.'

Applied Pharmacology

Queen Margaret University, Edinburgh Q25
BSc/BSc (Hons): 3 years full-time or 4 years full-time – B210
Tariff: 156 - 160 HND

Biochemistry (Pharmacology)

University of Surrey S85
BSc (Hons): 3 years full-time or 4 years sandwich – C7B2
Tariff: 260 - 300 IB: 30 - 32

Biomedical Sciences (Pharmacology)

University of Aberdeen A20
BSc (Hons): 4 years full-time – B9B2
A2: BCC - ABB SQA: ABBB ILC: ABBBB IB: 32

Cardiff University C15
BSc (Hons): 4 years sandwich – B212
Tariff: 300 - 320

Cardiff University C15
BSc (Hons): 3 years full-time – B211
Tariff: 300 - 320 IB: 32

Pharmaceutical Chemistry

University of Dundee D65
BSc (Hons): 5 years sandwich including foundation year – F154
Tariff: 240 IB: 26

University of Dundee D65
BSc (Hons): 4 years sandwich – F153
Tariff: 300 IB: 32 HND

Pharmacology

University of Aberdeen A20
BSc (Hons): 4 years full-time – B210
A2: CDD SQA: BBBB ILC: BCCCC - BBCC IB: 26

University of Bath B16
BSc (Hons): 3 years full-time – B210
A2: BBB - AAB IB: 34

University of Bath B16
MPharm (Hons): 4 years sandwich – B213
A2: BBB - AAB IB: 34

University of Bradford B56
BSc (Hons): 3 years full-time or 4 years sandwich – B210
Tariff: 260 IB: 24
HPC

University of Bradford B56
BSc (Hons): 3 years full-time or 4 years sandwich – B201
Tariff: 260

University of Bristol B78
BSc (Hons): 3 years full-time or 4 years sandwich – B210
A2: BBB BTEC: DMM - DDM SQA: BBBBB IB: 32

Chichester College [University of Portsmouth] ▲
BSc (Hons) (Foundation): 1 year full-time – B218 C
A2 Interview

University of Dundee D65
BSc (Hons): 4 years full-time – B210
Tariff: 240 IB: 26

University of Dundee D65
BSc (Hons): 3 years full-time – B211
Tariff: 300 IB: 32 HND

University of East London E28
BSc (Hons): 3 years full-time or 4 years sandwich – B210
A2: CC BTEC: MMM SQA: CCCC

University of East London E28
BSc (Hons): 5 years sandwich including foundation year – B218
Tariff: 60

University of Edinburgh E56
BSc (Hons): 4 years full-time – B210
A2: BBB SQA: BBBB IB: 30

University of Glasgow G28
MSci (Hons): 5 years sandwich – B211
A2: BCC SQA: BBBB ILC: BBBB IB: 28 HND

University of Glasgow G28
BSc: 3 years full-time BSc (Hons): 4 years full-time – B210
A2: BCC SQA: BBBB ILC: BBBB IB: 28 HND

Glasgow Caledonian University G42
BSc: 3 years full-time BSc (Hons): 4 years full-time – B110
A2: DDD SQA: BBC - BCCC HND

University of Hertfordshire H36
BSc/BSc (Hons): 3 years full-time or 4 years full-time including foundation year or 4 years sandwich or 5 years sandwich including foundation year – B210
Tariff: 200 IB: 24
IOB

King's College London (University of London) K60
BSc (Hons): 3 years full-time or 4 years sandwich – B210
A2: BBB SQA: ABBBB ILC: AABBBB IB: 32

Kingston University K84
BSc (Hons): 3 years full-time or 6 years part-time – B210
Tariff: 200 - 240

Kingston University K84
BSc (Hons): 4 years sandwich – B211
Tariff: 200 - 240

Kingston University K84
BSc (Hons): 4 years full-time including foundation year – B212
Tariff: 40 Interview

University of Leeds L23
BSc (Hons): 3 years full-time or 4 years full-time with time abroad or 4 years sandwich – B210
Tariff: 300 IB: 32

University of Liverpool L41
BSc (Hons): 3 years full-time – B210
A2: BBC - BBB BTEC: MMM - DMM SQA: ABBBC ILC: BBBBC IB: 26

London Metropolitan University L68
BSc (Hons): 3 years full-time – B210
Tariff: 160 IB: 28

University of Manchester M20
BSc (Hons): 3 years full-time – B210
A2: BBB - AAB BTEC: DDM - DDD SQA: AABBB - AAAA
ILC: AAABB IB: 32 - 35 Interview

Newcastle University N21
BSc (Hons): 3 years full-time – B210
A2: ABB BTEC ILC: ABBBB IB: 30 - 32

University of Portsmouth P80
BSc (Hons): 3 years full-time – B210
Tariff: 200 - 280

University of Southampton S27
BSc (Hons): 3 years full-time or 4 years sandwich – B21
A2: BCC BTEC: MMM SQA: BBCCC

University of Strathclyde S78
BSc (Hons): 4 years sandwich – B210
A2: BBC SQA: BBBB HND

University of Sunderland S84
BSc (Hons): 3 years full-time – B210
Tariff: 180

City of Sunderland College [University Sunderland] ▲
BSc (Hons) (Foundation): 1 year full-time – B218 K
Tariff: 80

University of Ulster U20
BSc (Hons): 3 years full-time – B210 C
Tariff: 300 IB: 33

University College London, University London U80
BSc (Hons): 3 years full-time – B210
A2: BBB BTEC: MDD SQA: AAABB IB: 32

University of Wolverhampton W75
BSc (Hons): 3 years full-time or 4 years sandwich or 4 years part-time – B210
Tariff: 160 - 200

Pharmacology and Anthropology

University of East London E28
BA (Hons)/BSc (Hons): 3 years full-time – BL26
Tariff: 160

Pharmacology and Biochemistry

University of Wolverhampton W75
BSc (Hons): 3 years full-time or 4 years sandwich – CB
Tariff: 240 - 300 IB: 30

Pharmacology with Biochemistry

University of East London E28
BSc (Hons): 3 years full-time – B2C7
Tariff: 160

Pharmacology and Biotechnology

University of Wolverhampton W75
BSc (Hons): 3 years full-time or 4 years sandwich – BJ
Tariff: 220 - 240

harmacology with Business

ngston University K84
: (Hons): 3 years full-time – B2N1
iff: 200 - 240

ngston University K84
: (Hons): 4 years sandwich – B2NC
iff: 200 - 240

harmacology with Criminology

iversity of East London E28
: (Hons): 3 years full-time – B2M9
iff: 160

harmacology with Health Services anagement

iversity of East London E28
: (Hons): 3 years full-time – B2N2
iff: 160

harmacology and Human Biology

iversity of Wolverhampton W75
(Hons): 3 years full-time or 4 years sandwich – BC21
f: 260 - 320

harmacology with Human Biology

iversity of East London E28
(Hons): 3 years full-time – B2B1
f: 160

harmacology and Human Physiology

iversity of Wolverhampton W75
(Hons): 3 years full-time or 4 years sandwich – B210
f: 160 - 200

armacology (with industrial or ofessional experience)

versity of Manchester M20
(Hons): 4 years sandwich – B211
BB - AAB BTEC: DDM - DDD SQA: AABBB - AAAAB
AABB IB: 32 - 35 Interview

armacology with Medical crobiology

versity of East London E28
(Hons): 3 years full-time – B2C5
: 160

armacology with a Modern nguage

versity of Manchester M20
Hons): 4 years full-time with time abroad – B212
BB - AAB BTEC: DDM - DDD SQA: AABBB - AAAAB
2 A2 A2 B2 B2 - A1 A1 A1 B1 B1 IB: 32 - 35
iew

Pharmacology and Molecular Genomics

King's College London (University of London) K60
BSc (Hons): 3 years full-time or 4 years sandwich – BC24
A2: BBB SQA: BBBBB ILC: AABBBB IB: 32

Pharmacology and Neuroscience

Nottingham Trent University N91
BSc (Hons): 3 years full-time – BB21
Tariff: 180

Pharmacology and Physiological Sciences

University of Dundee D65
BSc (Hons): 4 years full-time – BB21
Tariff: 240

University of Dundee D65
BSc (Hons): 3 years full-time – BB2C
Tariff: 300 IB: 32 HND

Pharmacology and Physiology

University of Leeds L23
BSc (Hons): 3 years full-time or 4 years full-time including foundation year – BB12
A2: CCC - BCC

University of Manchester M20
BSc (Hons): 3 years full-time – BB12
A2: BBB - AAB BTEC: DDM - DDD SQA: AABBB - AAAAB
ILC: AAABB IB: 32 - 35 Interview

University of Manchester M20
BSc (Hons): 4 years sandwich – BBC2
A2: BBB - AAB BTEC: DDM - DDD SQA: AABBB - AAAAB
ILC: AAABB IB: 32 - 35 Interview

Pharmacology and Third World Development

University of East London E28
BA (Hons)/BSc (Hons): 3 years full-time – BL29
Tariff: 160

Pharmacology with Toxicology

University of East London E28
BSc (Hons): 3 years full-time – B290
Tariff: 160

Pharmacology (with year in Europe)

University of Hertfordshire H36
BSc/BSc (Hons): 4 years full-time with time abroad or 5 years full-time with time abroad and foundation year – B211
Tariff: 200 IB: 24
IOB

Pharmacology (with year in North America)

University of Hertfordshire H36
BSc/BSc (Hons): 4 years full-time with time abroad or 5 years full-time with time abroad and foundation year – B212
Tariff: 200 IB: 24
IOB

Pharmacy

Aston University A80
MPharm (Hons): 4 years full-time – B230
A2: BBB - ABB SQA: AABBB IB: 32
RPSGB

University of Bath B16
MPharm (Hons): 4 years full-time or 4 years full-time with time abroad – B230
A2: BBB - AAB IB: 34
RPSGB

Birkbeck, University of London
Fd: 3 years part-time
HP

University of Bradford B56
MPharm (Hons): 4 years full-time – B230
Tariff: 280
RPSGB

University of Bradford B56
MPharm (Hons): 5 years sandwich – B231
Tariff: 280
RPSGB

University of Brighton B72
MPharm (Hons): 4 years full-time – B230
Tariff: 320 IB: 32
RPSGB

Cardiff University C15
MPharm (Hons): 4 years full-time – B230
Tariff: 320 IB: 32
RPSGB

De Montfort University D26
MPharm: 4 years full-time – B230 Y
A2: BCC - BBB BTEC: MMD ILC: BBBBBB
RPSGB

University of East Anglia E14
MPharm (Hons): 4 years full-time – B230
A2: BBB - ABB SQA: BBBBB - AABBB ILC: BBBBBB - AABBBB IB: 31 - 32

University of Hertfordshire H36
MPharm: 4 years full-time – B230
Tariff: 320

University of Hertfordshire H36
MPharm: 4 years full-time – BCF0
Tariff: 280

Keele University K12
MPharm: 4 years full-time – B230
A2: BBB IB: 32
RPSGB

University of Kent K24
MPharm (Hons): 4 years full-time – B230 K
Tariff: 300 IB: 32

King's College London (University of London) K60
MPharm (Hons): 4 years full-time – B230
A2: ABB SQA: AAABB ILC: AAAABB IB: 32
RPSGB

Kingston University K84
MPharm (Hons): 4 years full-time – B230
Tariff: 300

Kingston University K84
MPharm (Hons): 5 years full-time including foundation year – B231
Tariff: 40 Interview

Liverpool John Moores University L51
MPharm: 4 years full-time or 5 years sandwich – B201
A2: CCC - AAA Interview
RPSGB

University of Manchester M20
MPharm (Hons): 4 years full-time – B230
A2: ABB - AAB BTEC: DDM - DDD ILC: A1A1A1B1B1
IB: 33 - 35

University of Nottingham N84
MPharm: 4 years full-time – B230
A2: BBB IB: 32
RPSGB

University of Portsmouth P80
MPharm (Hons): 4 years full-time – B230
A2: BBB BTEC: DDD
RPSGB

Queen's University Belfast Q75
MPharm (Hons): 4 years full-time – B230
A2: ABB - AAB IB: 32
PSNI, RPSGB

University of Reading R12
MPharm: 4 years full-time – B230
Tariff: 320 IB: 33

Robert Gordon University R36
MPharm (Hons): 4 years full-time – B201
A2: BBB SQA: BBBCC - ABBB ILC: BBBBB
RPSGB

School of Pharmacy, University of London S12
MPharm (Hons): 4 years full-time – B230
A2: ABB SQA: AAABB ILC: AAAABB IB: 32
RPSGB, RSC

University of Strathclyde S78
MPharm: 4 years full-time – B230
A2: BBB SQA: BBBB ILC: AABBB IB: 7 6 6
RPSGB

University of Sunderland S84
MPharm: 4 years full-time – B230
Tariff: 280
RPSGB

University of Wolverhampton W75
MPharm: 4 years full-time – B231
Tariff: 300 - 360

Pharmacy (conversion entry programme)

King's College London (University of London) K60
MPharm (Hons): 5 years full-time including foundation year – B231
A2: BBB - ADD BTEC: MMM SQA: AABBBB ILC: AABBE
IB: 34

Pharmacy (with Health foundation year)

Keele University K12
MPharm: 5 years full-time including foundation year – B2
A2: BBB

Pharmacy Services

Merton College [Kingston University] ▲
FdSc: 2 years full-time – B232 M
HP

Preston College [University of Central Lancashire]
FdSc: 3 years part-time
Tariff: 40 - 80

Psychology

BSc courses only

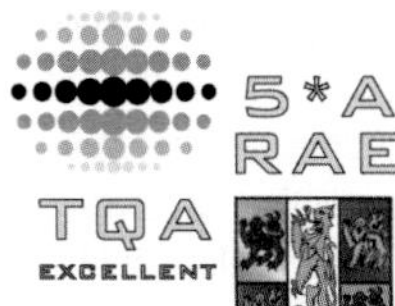

What would you study?

'Psychology is the study of people: How they think. How they act, react and interact. Psychology is concerned with all aspects of behaviour and the thoughts feelings and motivations underlying such behaviour.'

That is a definition taken from the British Psychological Society (BPS) website (www.bps.org.uk) which is well worth checking if you want to know more before deciding whether to take a psychology course. There are over 350 single-subject degree courses on offer in the UK. Psychology is both an art and a science and there are two separate types of course offered by higher education institutions: you can take the subject as a BA or as a BSc degree. The BSc courses only are covered in this guide. Both arts and science courses cover a similar range of topics. You can also study psychology in combination with many other subjects.

The first rule when choosing your course is to check that the degree for which you are applying meets the requirements of the Graduate Basis for Registration (GBR). The GBR is your guarantee that, by the end of your degree course, your studies will be the platform for professional qualification (if that is the way you want to go). GBR-accredited courses tend to cover the same broad range of topics in the first two years. Subjects will include:

- Abnormal psychology
- Cognition
- Health psychology
- Learning theory
- Neuropsychology
- Psychobiology
- Psychopathology.

With the core of psychology dealt with in years one and two, the third year tends to offer more freedom for students to specialise in aspects of the subject that interest them most.

Getting in

Statistics feature strongly, so confidence in mathematics is advisable (though you do not have to have the A level or equivalent). Above all, you need curiosity about people's behaviour, problems and attitudes. Each university decides on its own entry requirements. You can see the range of UCAS points asked by each one by consulting the course listings on the following pages. However, many Foundation degree courses exercise a more flexible admissions procedure which enables them to take into account factors such as work experience in their entrance requirements and which cannot therefore be expressed as part of the UCAS tariff framework.

Graduate outlook

After your degree, your route will vary according to the branch of psychology you have chosen. The pathway to professional qualification could take several years depending on the specialism you choose to take.

The case study overleaf shows one graduate's route to qualification as a clinical psychologist. Most branches of the profession will involve a similar pattern – a postgraduate qualification to at least Master's level. You will need to check the precise route towards the branch you want to specialise in during your first-degree course. In order to apply for the next stage, you need to show that you have practical experience that is relevant to your chosen field – the chances are, therefore, that after your first degree, you will have to find a job which offers this, so the good news is that you are not just a student throughout the process – you could be working and earning as well as studying.

Some of the psychology professions are outlined below:

- **Clinical Psychologists** work in hospitals, health centres, with social services or in the private sector. Their clients come from any age and background, and include those who have mental health problems, addictive behaviour, neurological problems, relationship problems, anxiety or depression.
- **Educational Psychologists** work mainly in schools for education authorities. They advise teachers about approaches to learning, both f individual pupils and for groups. They assess pupils with learning or behavioural difficulties, and engage with parents or guardians to enlis their support in tackling whatever problem their children are facing. They will often study for a teaching qualification as part of the qualification process.
- **Forensic Psychologists** deal with offending behaviour, both assisting its detection and generating strategies for its reduction. They are ofter called as expert witnesses in court, and they also work in the justice system with organisations such as the police, the courts or the probation service.
- **Counselling Psychologists** are found mainly in the NHS though they can work in education or with large employers, sometimes on a freelance basis. They help people manage traumatic experiences suc as bereavement or mental health issues.
- **Occupational Psychologists** are involved with issues connected wit work, training for work and how both organisations and the individua within them can become more effective and less stressed.

If you are thinking 'What about psychiatry?', you should be looking in the chapter dealing with **Medicine** courses. However, only around 15% of graduates in Psychology actually end up as professional psychologists. S what do the rest do? The fact is that a Psychology degree is a versatile qualification and helps students develop skills that can be applied in a variety of career areas, such as:

- **Human Resource management (HR):** your degree will have discuss behaviour in groups and how to influence it. Large employers use HR specialists to advise on how an organisation can change in order to allow staff to be as effective in their work as they possibly can be. Training techniques, skills analysis, staff appraisal and selection techniques all have roots in the study of psychology.
- **Guidance and counselling work** is available in various areas, including careers guidance, education and social care.
- **Advertising, market research and marketing** may not be purist psychology but statistical and analytical techniques gained from the courses in this guide can be adapted to the business of finding out h sections of the population think, and how to change group perceptio and behaviour.

The publication *What do graduates do?* provides statistics for Psycholog graduates. It shows that of 8560 students who responded to a survey in 2005 (the latest year for which figures are available):

- 59.4 % were in employment in the UK
- 14.3% were doing full-time further study.
- 9.8% were working and studying
- 6.0% were unemployed

.... six months after graduation.

(The figures do not total 100% because some graduates answered the survey stating that they were not available for work.)

The majority of those in employment were working as social and welfa professionals and associate professionals (16.8%) while a further 4% were in educational professions. Around 7.5% were in commercial, industrial and public sector management and 4.1% were in marketing sales and advertising. A number had used their degree as a level of qualification rather than as a specific vocational training and had ente careers as varied as finance (6.3%), retailing, IT and hospitality.

What would you earn?

With psychologists popping up in so many different places, it is difficult to make generalisations about earnings. However, according to the British Psychological Society educational psychologists might earn between £25,000 and £59,000, forensic psychologists from £20,000 to £60,000, counselling psychologists from £26,000 to £70,000 and occupational psychologists up to £70,000.

Salary scales for clinical psychologists in the NHS are on a scale from approximately £27,600 to £42,000. Very senior posts are paid up to £78,000. These examples are based on April 2006 salary scales. At the time of writing this book the public sector unions had not accepted the pay increase of around 2.5%, which had been offered in April 2007.

Ergonomics

Ergonomics is a subject that is often offered on degree courses in psychology, however it can sometimes be studied in a combined degree (possibly with psychology) or on its own. What is it?

According to the Ergonomics Society it is 'the application of scientific information concerning humans to the design of objects, systems and environment for human use. It comes into everything which involves people. Work systems, sports and leisure, health and safety should all embody ergonomics principles if well designed.'

So ergonomists scientifically study the relationship between people, equipment and environments. Those working professionally as ergonomists improve human interaction with processes and systems.

On an ergonomics course you would study modules such as:

- Introduction to ergonomics
- Anatomy and physiology
- Communication and study skills
- Ergonomics and design
- Ergonomics and manufacturing systems
- Ergonomics of disability and ageing
- Experiment, design and analysis
- Forensic ergonomics
- Human diversity
- Human factors and product design
- Human performance at environmental extremes
- Human response to noise and vibration
- Issues in occupational psychology
- Occupational safety and health
- Organisational behaviour
- Physiology of physical activity
- Qualitative methods for ergonomists.

As a graduate beginning a career in ergonomics you could expect to earn between £18,000 and £24,000. Senior ergonomists can earn over £55,000.

Case Study

Fran Garrard Cole – Currently Senior Tutor in Psychology Department.

'I am from St Albans and came through clearing to the University of Wales, Bangor in 1997 after speaking to a very friendly person who helped me along the way. When I arrived in Bangor I settled into my Student Halls and set about researching the important things in life (pub locations, late-licence bars...). Having been very worried about whether I would find friends or get on with anybody I soon found on my arrival day that I couldn't get rid of my mum quick enough! In between lectures in my first year I also spent a great deal of my time climbing and walking in the local area.

I was a relatively conscientious student, I attended most lectures and handed in most of my assignments on time! Before I began my course at Bangor I wasn't quite aware of the world-wide reputation of the Psychology degree course here, but the enthusiasm and support provided by the Staff was fantastic. For me, one of the best things about the course was the diversity of the subject - I had no idea how broad 'Psychology' was. The combination of lecture based material and small-group seminars made it really easy to interact with the tutors. A new experience for me came in the form of research articles. These were not something I had encountered at school and I found it really exciting that new research was coming out all the time and that topics of 'science' were not set in stone but instead were hotly debated and that I could participate in that debate. Towards the middle of my final year my thoughts turned to 'what next?'. I discovered that I had only just scratched the surface of Psychology. I was particularly interested in Cognitive Psychology and the idea that we can run experiments on student participants that might help us understand the workings of the human mind in both a 'normal' and 'clinical' population.

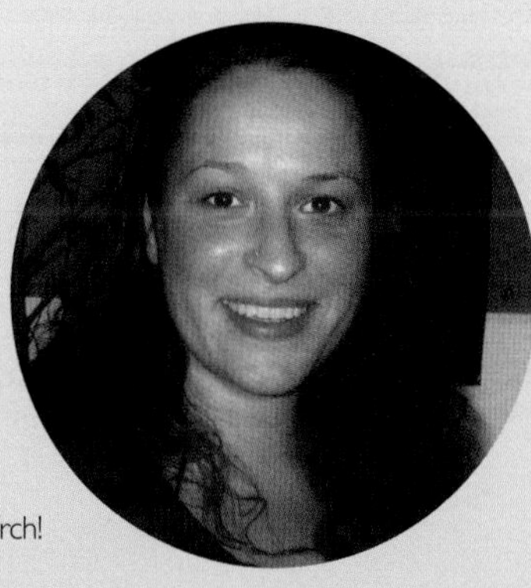

After getting a 2:1 degree I not only secured a place and funding here. During my PhD, I investigated developmental aspects of visual attention and even managed to incorporate playing video games into my research!

After I finished my PhD I worked as a Rehabilitation Support Worker in an Acquired Brain Injury unit but found I was missing Bangor. I was then lucky enough to get a job as a Research Assistant investing speech perception in infants. This was only a Part-time position so when the opportunity came up to also take a Teaching Associate job I did so. In September 2005 I became a full-time teaching Associate with a Year 3 module to teach, projects to supervise and personal tutees. I discovered that I really, really enjoyed teaching and seemed to be quite good at it. I had a job I loved in an area I loved and then in May 2006 I left!

My son was born in June at home in Bethesda and for 8 months I stayed at home with him. In February 2007 I came back to work 2 days a week, again as a Teaching Associate and I am now delighted that I have been offered the position of Senior Tutor from the beginning of August 2007. I love interacting with the students and always try to give as much support as I can. It is particularly satisfying being able to reassure students that all is not lost when they are in the depths of panic, I know because I have been there! '

Applied Psychology

University of Bedfordshire B22
BSc (Hons): 4 years sandwich – C810
Tariff: 160 - 200

Cardiff University C15
BSc (Hons): 4 years sandwich – C810
A2: AAA
BPS

University of Central Lancashire C30
BSc (Hons): 3 years full-time – C810
Tariff: 240
BPS

University of Cumbria C99
BSc (Hons): 3 years full-time – C810 C
Tariff: 200

University of Durham D86
BSc (Hons): 3 years full-time – C810 S
A2: BBC ILC: ABBBBB IB: 30
BPS

University of Durham D86
BSc (Hons): 4 years full-time including foundation year – C813 S
Interview

University of Glamorgan G14
BSc (Hons): 3 years full-time – C810
Tariff: 220 - 260

Heriot-Watt University H24
BSc: 3 years full-time BSc (Hons): 4 years full-time – C810
A2: DDD - CCC SQA: BBB

University of Kent K24
BSc (Hons): 4 years sandwich – C850
A2: BBB - ABC IB: 33
BPS

Liverpool John Moores University L51
BSc (Hons): 3 years full-time or 4 - 6 years part-time – C870
Tariff: 220 IB: 28
BPS

Applied Psychology with Clinical Psychology

University of Kent K24
BSc (Hons): 4 years sandwich – C823
A2: ABB IB: 35
BPS

Applied Psychology and Criminology

Liverpool John Moores University L51
BA (Hons)/BSc (Hons): 3 years full-time or 4 - 6 years part-time – MC28
Tariff: 160 - 260

Applied Psychology and Sociology

University of Surrey S85
BSc (Hons): 4 years sandwich – CL83
Tariff: 260 - 300 IB: 30 - 32
BPS

Behavioural Science

University of Abertay Dundee A30
BSc (Hons): 4 years full-time – C890
Tariff: 168 - 180
BPS

Behavioural Sciences

University of Huddersfield H60
BSc/BSc (Hons): 3 years full-time – C830
Tariff: 200
BPS

Clinical Psychology

University of East London E28
BSc (Hons): 3 years full-time – B120
Tariff: 160

Cognitive Neuroscience

University of Sussex S90
BSc (Hons): 3 years full-time – B141
A2: ABB IB: 34

Cognitive Science

University of Edinburgh E56
BSc (Hons): 4 years full-time – C850
A2: BBB SQA: BBBB

University of Hertfordshire H36
BSc (Hons): 3 years full-time – C801
Tariff: 220 IB: 30
BPS

University of Leeds L23
BSc (Hons): 3 years full-time – CG84
A2: ABB SQA: AAAAB IB: 33
BPS

University of Westminster W50
BSc (Hons): 3 years full-time – C850
Tariff: 160 IB: 26
BPS

Cognitive Science (with year in Europe)

University of Hertfordshire H36
BSc (Hons): 4 years full-time with time abroad – C803
Tariff: 220

Counselling Psychology

University of Wolverhampton W75
BSc (Hons): 3 years full-time or 5 - 6 years part-time – C813
Tariff: 240 - 300 IB: 24

Criminological Psychology

Buckinghamshire Chilterns University College B94
BSc (Hons): 3 years full-time – C890
A2: DD

Developmental Psychology

University of Glamorgan G14
BSc (Hons): 3 years full-time – C820
Tariff: 220 - 260

Ergonomics (Human Factors)

Loughborough University L79
BSc (Hons): 4 years sandwich – J961
Tariff: 260 - 280 IB: 28 - 30
ES

Loughborough University L79
BSc (Hons): 3 years full-time – J920
Tariff: 260 - 280 IB: 28 - 30
ES

Experimental Psychology

University of Oxford O33
BA (Hons): 3 years full-time – C830
A2: AAB - AAA SQA: AAAAB - AAAAA IB: 38
BPS

Forensic Psychology

University of Central Lancashire C30
BSc (Hons): 3 years full-time – C8B1
A2: BCC
BPS

Leeds, Trinity & All Saints [University of Leeds] L24
BSc (Hons): 3 years full-time – CF84
Tariff: 160 - 240

University of Portsmouth P80
BSc (Hons): 3 years full-time or 6 years part-time – C81
Tariff: 300

Staffordshire University S72
BSc (Hons): 3 years full-time – C890
Tariff: 240 IB: 28
BPS

University of Teesside T20
BSc (Hons): 3 years full-time – C890
Tariff: 240 IB: 26
BPS

Health Psychology

Anglia Ruskin University A60
BSc (Hons): 3 years full-time – C841
Tariff: 240 IB: 30

University of Bedfordshire B22
BSc (Hons): 3 years full-time – C841
Tariff: 160 - 200

Queen Margaret University, Edinburgh Q25
BSc: 3 years full-time BSc (Hons): 4 years full-time – C840
Tariff: 228 - 264 HND

University of Teesside T20
BSc (Hons): 3 years full-time – C841
Tariff: 180 - 220 IB: 26

uman Psychology

ston University A80
c (Hons): 3 years full-time – C880
, BBB SQA: ABBBB IB: 32
S

ston University A80
c (Hons): 4 years sandwich – C881
BBB SQA: ABBBB IB: 32
S

e Montfort University D26
c/BSc (Hons): 3 years full-time – C883 Y
iff: 240

uman Psychology and Public Policy nd Management

ton University A80
(Hons): 3 years full-time or 4 years sandwich – CL8F
ff: 300

uman Psychology and Sociology

ton University A80
(Hons): 3 years full-time or 4 years sandwich – CL83
ff: 300

ajor/Minor Honours (Psychology)

iversity of Glamorgan G14
(Hons)/BSc (Hons): 3 years full-time – Y002
f: 180 - 240

europsychology

iversity of Central Lancashire C30
(Hons): 3 years full-time – C860
CCC

europsychology (intercalated)

iversity of Wales, Bangor B06
1 year full-time
f: 260 - 300

ychological Studies

iversity Centre Barnsley [University of ddersfield] ▲
(Hons): 3 years full-time – C8L3 X
f: 160

ychology

iversity of Aberdeen A20
3 years full-time BSc (Hons): 4 years full-time –
0
CDD SQA: BBBB ILC: BCCCC - BBCC IB: 26

versity of Abertay Dundee A30
(Hons): 4 years full-time – C800
f: 180

Anglia Ruskin University A60
BSc (Hons): 3 years full-time – C800
Tariff: 240

University of Wales, Bangor B06
BSc (Hons): 3 years full-time – C800
Tariff: 260 - 300
BPS

University of Bath B16
BSc (Hons): 4 years sandwich – C800
A2: AAA IB: 36
BPS

Bath Spa University B20
BSc (Hons): 3 years full-time or 5 years part-time – C800
Tariff: 200 - 240

Bath Spa University B20
DipHE: 2 years full-time – C801
Tariff: 80 - 120

University of Bedfordshire B22
BSc (Hons): 4 years full-time including foundation year – C803
Interview

University of Bedfordshire B22
BSc (Hons): 3 years full-time – C800
Tariff: 160 - 200
BPS

Birkbeck, University of London
BSc (Hons): 4 years part-time evening
A2: C Interview
BPS

University of Birmingham B32
BSc (Hons): 3 years full-time – C800
Tariff: 320 IB: 34 - 36
BPS

University of Bolton B44
BSc (Hons): 3 years full-time or 5 years part-time – C801
Tariff: 180 IB: 24
BPS

University of Bradford B56
BSc (Hons): 3 years full-time – C801
Tariff: 240

University of Bristol B78
BSc (Hons): 3 years full-time – C801
A2: ABB - AAB BTEC: DDM SQA: AAAAB IB: 34 - 36
BPS

Bristol, University of the West of England B80
BSc (Hons): 3 years full-time or part-time day – C800
Tariff: 260 - 300
BPS

Brunel University B84
BSc (Hons): 3 years full-time – C801
Tariff: 300 IB: 32
BPS

University of Buckingham B90
BSc (Hons): 2 years full-time – C800
Tariff: 230 IB: 26

Buckinghamshire Chilterns University College B94
BSc (Hons): 3 years full time – C800
Tariff: 120 IB: 27
BPS

Canterbury Christ Church University C10
BSc (Hons): 3 years full-time or 5 - 6 years part-time – C800
A2: CC SQA: CCCC ILC: CCCCC IB: 24

Cardiff University C15
BSc (Hons): 3 years full-time – C800
Tariff: 360 IB: 33
BPS

University of Wales Institute, Cardiff C20
BSc (Hons): 3 years full-time or 6 years part-time day – C800
Tariff: 200
BPS

University of Central Lancashire C30
BSc (Hons): 3 years full-time or 4 - 6 years part-time – C801
A2: BCC
BPS

University of Chester C55
BSc (Hons): 3 years full-time – C800
Tariff: 260 IB: 30
BPS

City University C60
BSc (Hons): 3 years full-time or 4 years sandwich – C800
Tariff: 300 - 320 IB: 30
BPS

Coventry University C85
BSc (Hons): 3 years full-time or 5 years part-time – C800
Tariff: 280
BPS

University of Derby D39
BSc (Hons): 3 years full-time or 6 years part-time – C800
A2: CCC BTEC: DMM SQA: BBBCC IB: 30
BPS

University of Dundee D65
BSc (Hons): 4 years full-time – C800
Tariff: 240 IB: 26
BPS

University of Dundee D65
BSc (Hons): 3 years full-time – C803
Tariff: 300
BPS

University of Durham D86
BSc (Hons): 3 years full-time – C800
Tariff: 320 IB: 33
BPS

University of East London E28
BSc (Hons): 3 years full-time or 4 - 4.5 years part-time – C800
Tariff: 160 - 180 IB: 24
BPS

Edge Hill University E42
BSc (Hons): 3 years full-time – C800
Tariff: 180

University of Edinburgh E56
BSc (Hons): 4 years full-time – C800
A2: BBB SQA: BBBB IB: 34
BPS

University of Essex E70
BSc (Hons): 3 years full-time – C800
Tariff: 300 IB: 32
BPS

versity of Exeter E84
Hons): 3 years full-time – C802
340 - 360 IB: 35 - 36

versity of Glamorgan G14
Hons): 3 years full-time – C800
220

versity of Glasgow G28
Hons): 4 years full-time – C800
CC SQA: BBBB ILC: BBBB IB: 28 HND

sgow Caledonian University G42
3 years full-time BSc (Hons): 4 years full-time –

240 - 280

versity of Gloucestershire G50
Hons): 3 years full-time – C800
240

dsmiths, University of London G56
Hons): 3 years full-time – C800
BC BTEC: DMM SQA: BBBBC IB: 30

versity of Greenwich G70
Hons): 3 years full-time or 6 years part-time – C800
200

versity of Hertfordshire H36
Hons): 3 years full-time or 4 years sandwich – C802
180 - 280

versity of Hertfordshire H36
Hons): 3 years full-time – C800
280

versity of Huddersfield H60
3Sc (Hons): 3 years full-time – C800
240

versity of Hull H72
Hons): 3 years full-time – C800
280

le University K12
Hons): 4 years full-time including foundation year –

C

versity of Kent K24
Hons): 3 years full-time – C800
BB - ABC IB: 33

gston University K84
Hons): 3 years full-time or 6 years part-time day –

260

caster University L14
Hons): 3 years full-time – C800
320 IB: 34

University of Leeds L23
BSc (Hons): 3 years full-time – C800
A2: AAB IB: 33
BPS

Leeds, Trinity & All Saints [University of Leeds] L24
BSc (Hons): 3 years full-time or 6 years part-time – C800
Tariff: 160 - 240 IB: 24
BPS

University of Leicester L34
BSc (Hons): 3 years full-time – C800
Tariff: 320 - 340 IB: 30 - 33
BPS

University of Lincoln L39
BSc (Hons): 3 years full-time – C800 L
Tariff: 260 IB: 28
BPS

University of Liverpool L41
BSc (Hons): 3 years full-time – C800
A2: ABB SQA: AABBB ILC: ABBBB IB: 32
BPS

University of Liverpool L41
BSc (Hons): 4 years full-time including foundation year – C801
Interview
BPS

Liverpool Hope University L46
BSc (Hons): 3 years full-time – C800
Tariff: 180 - 240

London Metropolitan University L68
BSc (Hons): 3 years full-time or 4 - 6 years part-time day – C830
Tariff: 240 IB: 28
BPS

London South Bank University L75
BSc (Hons): 3 years full-time – C800
A2: CCC
BPS

Loughborough University L79
BSc (Hons): 3 years full-time – C800
A2: ABB - AAB BTEC: DDM IB: 32 - 34
BPS

Loughborough University L79
BSc (Hons): 4 years sandwich – C801
A2: ABB - AAB BTEC: DDM IB: 32 - 34
BPS

University of Manchester M20
BSc (Hons): 3 years full-time – C800
A2: AAB BTEC: DDD SQA: AAABB ILC: AAABB IB: 33 - 35
BPS

Manchester College of Arts and Technology [Manchester Metropolitan University] M10
BSc (Hons): 6 years part-time
Tariff: 240

Manchester Metropolitan University M40
BSc (Hons): 3 years full-time or 6 years part-time or 4 - 6 years mixed mode – C800
Tariff: 280
BPS

Manchester Metropolitan University M40
BSc (Hons): 4 years full-time including foundation year – C801
Tariff: 180

Middlesex University M80
BSc (Hons): 3 years full-time or 4 years sandwich – C800 E
Tariff: 160 - 240
BPS

Newcastle University N21
BSc (Hons): 3 years full-time – C800
A2: BBB - AAB ILC: ABBBB - AAABB IB: 34
BPS

Newman College of Higher Education [University of Leicester] N36
BSc (Hons): 3 years full-time – C800
Tariff: 160 IB: 24
BPS

University of Wales, Newport N37
BSc (Hons): 3 years full-time or 6 years part-time – C800
Tariff: 200

University of Northampton N38
BSc (Hons): 3 years full-time or part-time – C800
Tariff: 180 - 220 IB: 24
BPS

Northumbria University N77
BSc (Hons): 3 years full-time – C800
Tariff: 280
BPS

University of Nottingham N84
BSc (Hons): 3 years full-time – C800
A2: ABB ILC: AABBB IB: 31 - 34
BPS

Nottingham Trent University N91
BSc (Hons): 3 years full-time – C800
Tariff: 280
BPS

Oxford Brookes University O66
BSc (Hons): 3 years full-time – C800
A2: BBB IB: 30

University of Paisley P20
BSc: 3 years full-time BSc (Hons): 4 years full-time – C800
A2: DD SQA: BCCC - BBC

University of Plymouth P60
BSc (Hons): 3 years full-time or 4 years sandwich – C800
Tariff: 220 - 280 IB: 30
BPS

University of Portsmouth P80
BSc (Hons): 3 years full-time – C800
Tariff: 300
BPS

Queen Margaret University, Edinburgh Q25
BSc: 3 years full-time BSc (Hons): 4 years full-time – C800
Tariff: 228 - 264 HND
BPS

Queen's University Belfast Q75
BSc (Hons): 3 years full-time – C800
A2: BBB - ABB SQA: ABBB IB: 29
BPS

University of Reading R12
BSc (Hons): 3 years full-time – C800
A2: AAB IB: 34
BPS

Roehampton University R48
BSc (Hons): 3 years full-time or 4 - 7 years part-time – C800
A2: CCD BTEC: DDD SQA: BBC IB: 30
BPS

Royal Holloway, University of London R72
BSc (Hons): 3 years full-time – C800
Tariff: 320 - 340 IB: 34 - 36
BPS

University of St Andrews S36
BSc (Hons): 4 years full-time – C800
A2: AAB SQA: AABB IB: 36
BPS

University of Salford S03
BSc (Hons): 3 years full-time – C802
Tariff: 240 IB: 27

University of Sheffield S18
BSc (Hons): 3 years full-time – C800
A2: AAB SQA: AAAA ILC: AAABB IB: 35
BPS

Sheffield Hallam University S21
BSc (Hons): 3 years full-time or 6 years part-time – C800
Tariff: 300
BPS

University of Southampton S27
BSc (Hons): 3 years full-time – C800
A2: AAB BTEC: MMM SQA: AAABB IB: 33
BPS

Southampton Solent University S30
BSc (Hons): 3 years full-time – C800
Tariff: 220 Interview
BPS

Staffordshire University S72
BSc (Hons): 3 years full-time – C800
Tariff: 240 IB: 28
BPS

Staffordshire University Regional Federation S73
BSc (Hons): 4 years full-time including foundation year – C800 L
Tariff: 60 Interview

University of Stirling S75
BSc: 3 years full-time BSc (Hons): 4 years full-time – C800
A2: BCC BTEC: MMM SQA: BBBB IB: 30
BPS

University of Sunderland S84
BSc (Hons): 3 years full-time or 5 years part-time – C800
Tariff: 220
BPS

University of Surrey S85
BSc (Hons): 4 years sandwich – C800
A2: ABB BTEC: DDM IB: 34
BPS

University of Sussex S90
BSc (Hons): 3 years full-time – C800
A2: ABB - AAB IB: 34 - 36
BPS

University of Wales, Swansea S93
BSc (Hons): 3 years full-time – C800
A2: BCC - BBB BTEC: DMM SQA: AABBB ILC: AABBBB IB: 32
BPS

University of Teesside T20
BSc (Hons): 3 years full-time – C800
Tariff: 240 IB: 26
BPS

Thames Valley University T40
BSc (Hons): 3 years full-time or 5 - 7 years part-time – C800
Tariff: 240 IB: 36

University of Ulster U20
BSc (Hons): 3 years full-time or 6 years part-time – C815 M
Tariff: 280 IB: 32
BPS

University College London, University of London U80
BSc (Hons): 3 years full-time – C800
A2: AAB BTEC: MMM SQA IB: 36
BPS

University of Warwick W20
BSc (Hons): 3 years full-time – C800
A2: AAB ILC: AAABBB IB: 36 Interview
BPS

University of Westminster W50
BSc (Hons): 3 years full-time or 5 years part-time day – C801
A2: BBB IB: 28
BPS

University of Wolverhampton W75
BSc (Hons): 3 years full-time or 5 - 6 years part-time – C800
Tariff: 240 - 300 IB: 30
BPS

University of Worcester W80
BSc (Hons): 3 years full-time – C800
Tariff: 160 IB: 28
BPS

University of York Y50
BSc (Hons): 3 years full-time – C800
A2: ABB - AAB SQA: AAAABB ILC: AAAABB IB: 36
BPS

York St John University Y75
BSc (Hons): 3 years full-time – C800
Tariff: 200 IB: 24

Psychology with Accounting

University of Northampton N38
BA (Hons)/BSc (Hons): 3 years full-time or 4 - 6 years part-time – C8N4
Tariff: 180 - 220
BPS

Psychology with American Studies

Canterbury Christ Church University C10
BA (Hons)/BSc (Hons): 3 years full-time – C8T7
A2

University of Sunderland S84
BA (Hons)/BSc (Hons): 3 years full-time – C8T7
Tariff: 220 - 360

University of Sussex S90
BSc (Hons): 4 years full-time with time abroad – C8T7
A2: ABB - AAB IB: 34 - 36
BPS

Psychology with Animal Behaviour

University of Chester C55
BSc (Hons): 3 years full-time – C8D3
Tariff: 240 IB: 30

Psychology with Applied Criminolog

Canterbury Christ Church University C1
BA (Hons)/BSc (Hons): 3 years full-time – C8Mx
Tariff: 160 IB: 24

Psychology (Applied) and Health Studies

London Metropolitan University L68
BA (Hons)/BSc (Hons): 3 years full-time – CL84
Tariff: 160 - 200 IB: 28

Psychology with Art

Canterbury Christ Church University C
BA (Hons)/BSc (Hons): 3 years full-time – C8W1
A2: CC

Psychology with Artificial Intelligen (with year in Europe)

University of Hertfordshire H36
BSc (Hons): 4 years full-time with time abroad – CG87
Tariff: 220
BPS

Psychology and Astronomy

University of Hertfordshire H36
BSc (Hons): 3 years full-time – C8F5
Tariff: 180 - 280
BPS

Psychology with Biological Conservation

University of Northampton N38
BA (Hons)/BSc (Hons): 3 years full-time or 4 - 6 years time – C8C1
Tariff: 180 - 220
BPS

Psychology and Biology

Kingston University K84
BA (Hons)/BSc (Hons): 3 years full-time – CC81
Tariff: 220 - 320

verpool John Moores University L51
c (Hons): 3 years full-time or 4 years sandwich or 4 years
t-time – CC18
iff: 220 IB: 24
S

iversity of Reading R12
c (Hons): 3 years full-time – CC18
: AAB IB: 34

sychology with Biology

iversity of Chester C55
: (Hons): 3 years full-time – C8C1
iff: 240 IB: 30

iversity of East London E28
: (Hons): 3 years full-time – C8C1
iff: 180 IB: 24

iversity of Leicester L34
: (Hons): 3 years full-time – C8C1
ff: 300 - 320 IB: 30 - 33

sychology and Biology for sychologists

iversity of Worcester W80
'Hons)/BSc (Hons): 3 years full-time – CC81
f: 160 IB: 26

sychology with Biosciences

nterbury Christ Church University C10
Hons)/BSc (Hons): 3 years full-time or 5 - 6 years part-
– C8C1
CC BTEC: MM SQA: CCCC ILC: CCCCC IB: 24

ychology and Business

versity of Central Lancashire C30
(Hons): 3 years full-time – CN81
: 240

versity of Hertfordshire H36
(Hons): 3 years full-time – C8N1
: 220 - 260 IB: 26 - 28

ychology with Business

versity of Northampton N38
Hons)/BSc (Hons): 3 years full-time or 4 - 6 years part-
– C8N1
: 180 - 220

ychology with Business Computing

terbury Christ Church University C10
Hons)/BSc (Hons): 3 years full-time – C8G5
: 160 IB: 24

Psychology with Business Entrepreneurship

University of Northampton N38
BA (Hons)/BSc (Hons): 3 years full-time or 4 - 6 years part-time – C8NF
Tariff: 180 - 220
BPS

Psychology with Business Studies

University of Buckingham B90
BSc (Hons): 2 years full-time – C8N1
Tariff: 230 IB: 26

Canterbury Christ Church University C10
BA (Hons)/BSc (Hons): 3 years full-time – C8N1
A2: CC

University of Sunderland S84
BA (Hons)/BSc (Hons): 3 years full-time – C8N1
Tariff: 180 - 360

Psychology with Chemistry

University of Sunderland S84
BA (Hons)/BSc (Hons): 3 years full-time – C8F1
Tariff: 180 - 360 IB: 32

Psychology with Child Development

London South Bank University L75
BSc (Hons): 3 years full-time – C8X3
A2: CCC
BPS

Psychology with Child and Language Development

University of Wales, Bangor B06
BSc (Hons): 3 years full-time – C8X9
Tariff: 260 - 300 IB: 30

Psychology with Child and Youth Studies

University of Lincoln L39
BSc (Hons): 3 years full-time – C8L5 L
Tariff: 260 IB: 28

Psychology, Childhood and Ageing

University of Reading R12
BSc (Hons): 3 years full-time – C805
A2: AAB - AAA IB: 34

Psychology with Clinical and Health Psychology

University of Wales, Bangor B06
BSc (Hons): 3 years full-time – C880
Tariff: 260 - 300 IB: 30
BPS

Psychology (Clinical Psychology)

London South Bank University L75
BSc (Hons): 3 years full-time – C840
A2: CCC
BPS

Psychology with Clinical Psychology

University of Kent K24
BSc (Hons): 3 years full-time – C822
A2: ABB IB: 35
BPS

University of Lincoln L39
BSc (Hons): 3 years full-time – C840 L
Tariff: 260 IB: 28
BPS

Psychology and Cognitive Neuroscience

University of Nottingham N84
BSc (Hons): 3 years full-time – C850
A2: ABB ILC: AABBB IB: 35

Psychology with Cognitive Science

University of Sussex S90
BSc (Hons): 3 years full-time – CG87
A2: ABB - AAB IB: 34 - 36

Psychology with Communication Studies

Canterbury Christ Church University C10
BA (Hons)/BSc (Hons): 3 years full-time – C8P9
Tariff: 160 IB: 24

Psychology with Comparative Literature

University of Sunderland S84
BA (Hons)/BSc (Hons): 3 years full-time – C8Q2
Tariff: 180 - 360

Psychology and Computer Science

University of Wales, Swansea S93
BSc (Hons): 3 years full-time – CG84
A2: BBC BTEC: DDM SQA: ABBBB ILC: ABBBBB IB: 30
BPS

Psychology with Computer Science

University of Chester C55
BSc (Hons): 3 years full-time – C8G4
Tariff: 240 IB: 30

Psychology with Computer Studies

University of Sunderland S84
BA (Hons)/BSc (Hons): 3 years full-time – C8G4
Tariff: 220 - 360 IB: 32

Psychology and Computing

Bournemouth University B50
BSc (Hons): 3 years full-time – CG84
Tariff: 180 - 280

University of Hertfordshire H36
BSc (Hons): 3 years full-time – C8G4
Tariff: 220 - 260 IB: 26 - 28
BPS

Psychology with Computing

Canterbury Christ Church University C10
BA (Hons)/BSc (Hons): 3 years full-time – C8GK
A2: CC

University of Northampton N38
BA (Hons)/BSc (Hons): 3 years full-time or 4 - 6 years part-time – C8G4
Tariff: 180 - 220
BPS

Psychology and Counselling

University of Wales, Newport N37
BSc (Hons): 3 years full-time or 6 years part-time – C8B9
Tariff: 200

Roehampton University R48
BSc (Hons): 3 years full-time – C845
A2: CCD BTEC: DDD SQA: BBC IB: 30
BPS

University of Teesside T20
BSc (Hons): 3 years full-time – L550
Tariff: 240 IB: 26
BPS

Psychology with Counselling

University of Huddersfield H60
BSc (Hons): 3 years full-time – C8B9
Tariff: 260 Interview

University of Hull H72
BSc (Hons): 3 years full-time – C822
Tariff: 280
BPS

Psychology with Counselling Skills

Middlesex University M80
BSc (Hons): 3 years full-time – C8B9 E
Tariff: 160 - 240

Psychology and Counselling Studies

University of Derby D39
BSc (Hons): 3 years full-time or 6 years part-time – CL85
Tariff: 160

Psychology with Counselling Theory

Thames Valley University T40
BSc (Hons): 3 years full-time or 3 - 7 years part-time – C8B9
Tariff: 240

Psychology and Crime

Bedford College [University of Bedfordshire]
Fd: 2 years part-time
A2: E - EE BTEC: PP - PPP

University of Bradford B56
BSc (Hons): 3 years full-time – CL83
Tariff: 180 - 220

Psychology and Criminal Behaviour

University of Bedfordshire B22
FdSc: 2 years full-time – C880
Tariff: 80 - 120

University of Bedfordshire B22
BSc (Hons): 3 years full-time – CL83

Milton Keynes College [University of Bedfordshire] ▲
FdSc: 2 years full-time – C880 M
Tariff: 80

Psychology and Criminal Justice

University of Wolverhampton W75
BA (Hons)/BSc (Hons): 3 years full-time or 4 years sandwich – CM8X
Tariff: 200 - 260

Psychology with Criminal Justice Studies

University of Plymouth P60
BA (Hons)/BSc (Hons): 3 years full-time – C8M9
Tariff: 220 - 280 IB: 30
BPS

Psychology and Criminology

Anglia Ruskin University A60
BSc (Hons): 3 years full-time – C8MX
Tariff: 220 - 260

University of Bedfordshire B22
BSc (Hons): 3 years full-time – CM89
Tariff: 160 - 200

Buckinghamshire Chilterns University College B94
BSc (Hons): 3 years full-time – CM89
Tariff: 120

Cardiff University C15
BSc (Hons): 3 years full-time – CM89
Tariff: 360 IB: 33

University of Central Lancashire C30
BSc (Hons): 3 years full-time – CMV9
A2: CCC

Coventry University C85
BSc (Hons): 3 years full-time or 5 years part-time – CM82
Tariff: 260
BPS

University of Lincoln L39
BA (Hons)/BSc (Hons): 3 years full-time – CM89 L
Tariff: 260
BPS

Staffordshire University S72
BSc (Hons): 3 years full-time – CMV1
Tariff: 240 IB: 28
BPS

University Campus Suffolk [University of East Anglia, University of Essex] S82
BSc (Hons): 3 years full-time or 5 - 9 years part-time – CL8H I
Tariff: 120 - 180

University of Teesside T20
BSc (Hons): 3 years full-time – CM89
Tariff: 240 IB: 26
BPS

Psychology with Criminology

Buckinghamshire Chilterns University College B94
BSc (Hons): 3 years full-time – C8M9
Tariff: 120

University of Chester C55
BSc (Hons): 3 years full-time – C8M9
Tariff: 240 IB: 30

University of East London E28
BSc (Hons): 3 years full-time – C8M9
Tariff: 180 IB: 24

University of Huddersfield H60
BSc (Hons): 3 years full-time – C8M2
Tariff: 240

University of Hull H72
BSc (Hons): 3 years full-time – C8M9
Tariff: 280
BPS

Middlesex University M80
BSc (Hons): 3 years full-time – CM89 E
Tariff: 160 - 240

University of Northampton N38
BA (Hons)/BSc (Hons): 3 years full-time or 4 - 6 years [part-]time – C8M9
Tariff: 180 - 220
BPS

Nottingham Trent University N91
BSc (Hons): 3 years full-time – C800
Tariff: 280 IB: 24

University of Portsmouth P80
BSc (Hons): 3 years full-time – C8M9
Tariff: 300
BPS

University of Sunderland S84
BA (Hons)/BSc (Hons): 3 years full-time – C8M9
Tariff: 180 - 360 IB: 32

sychology with Criminology and riminal Justice

iversity of Glamorgan G14
c (Hons): 3 years full-time – C8M9
iff: 220 IB: 24

sychology with Cultural Studies

Mary's University College, ickenham S64
(Hons)/BSc (Hons): 3 years full-time – C8V9
ff: 160

sychology with Dance

iversity of Northampton N38
(Hons)/BSc (Hons): 3 years full-time or 4 - 6 years part- – C8W5
f: 180 - 220

iversity of Sunderland S84
Hons)/BSc (Hons): 3 years full-time – C8W5
f: 160 - 360 IB: 31

sychology and Deaf Studies

iversity of Wolverhampton W75
Hons)/BSc (Hons): 3 years full-time or 4 years wich – CB85
f: 200 - 260

sychology (with Diploma in dustrial Studies/Diploma in Area udies)

iversity of Ulster U20
(Hons): 3 years full-time or 4 years sandwich – C
f: 280 IB: 32

ychology with Drama

versity of Northampton N38
Hons)/BSc (Hons): 3 years full-time or 4 - 6 years part- – C8W4
: 180 - 220

ychology and Early Childhood udies

versity Campus Suffolk [University of t Anglia, University of Essex] S82
Hons): 3 years full-time or 5 - 9 years part-time – I
. 120 - 180

ychology with Early Childhood udies

terbury Christ Church University C10
ons)/BSc (Hons): 3 years full-time – C8X3
C

University of East London E28
BA (Hons)/BSc (Hons): 3 years full-time – C8X3
Tariff: 160

Psychology and Economics

University of Hertfordshire H36
BSc (Hons): 3 years full-time – C8L1
Tariff: 220 - 260 IB: 26 - 28
BPS

Psychology and Education

University of Central Lancashire C30
BSc (Hons): 3 years full-time – CX83
Tariff: 240

University of Exeter E84
BSc (Hons): 3 years full-time – CX83
A2: AAB - AAA

University of Sunderland S84
BA (Hons)/BSc (Hons): 3 years full-time – CX83
Tariff: 180 - 360

Psychology with Education

University of Sunderland S84
BA (Hons)/BSc (Hons): 3 years full-time – C8X3
Tariff: 180 - 360 IB: 32

Psychology with Education and Employment

St Mary's University College, Twickenham S64
BA (Hons)/BSc (Hons): 3 years full-time – C8X3
Tariff: 160

Psychology and Education Studies

University of Teesside T20
BSc (Hons): 3 years full-time – CX83
Tariff: 240

Psychology with Education Studies

University of Northampton N38
BA (Hons)/BSc (Hons): 3 years full-time or 4 - 6 years part-time – C8X3
Tariff: 180 - 220
BPS

Psychology and English

University of Glamorgan G14
BSc (Hons): 3 years full-time – CQ83
Tariff: 220 - 260

University of Lincoln L39
BA (Hons)/BSc (Hons): 3 years full-time – CQ83 L
Tariff: 260
BPS

Psychology with English

Canterbury Christ Church University C10
BA (Hons)/BSc (Hons): 3 years full-time – C8Q3
A2: CC

University of Northampton N38
BA (Hons)/BSc (Hons): 3 years full-time or 4 - 6 years part-time – C8Q3
Tariff: 180 - 220
BPS

St Mary's University College, Twickenham S64
BA (Hons)/BSc (Hons): 3 years full-time – C8Q3
Tariff: 160

Psychology and English Language and Communications

University of Hertfordshire H36
BSc (Hons): 3 years full-time – C8Q1
Tariff: 220 - 260 IB: 26 - 28
BPS

Psychology with English Language Studies (EFL)

University of Buckingham B90
BSc (Hons): 2 years full-time – C8Q3
Tariff: 230 IB: 26

Psychology with English Literature

University of Buckingham B90
BSc (Hons): 2 years full-time – C8Q2
Tariff: 230 IB: 26

Psychology with English Studies

University of Sunderland S84
BA (Hons)/BSc (Hons): 3 years full-time – C8Q3
Tariff: 180 - 360 IB: 32

Psychology and Environmental Studies

University of Hertfordshire H36
BSc (Hons): 3 years full-time – C8F9
Tariff: 220 - 260 IB: 26 - 28
BPS

Psychology with Ergonomics

Loughborough University L79
BSc (Hons): 3 years full-time – C8J9
A2: ABB BTEC: DDM IB: 32 - 34
BPS, ES

Loughborough University L79
BSc (Hons): 4 years sandwich – C8JX
A2: ABB BTEC: DDM IB: 32 - 34
BPS, ES

Psychology with European Studies

University of Sunderland S84
BA (Hons)/BSc (Hons): 3 years full-time – C8R9
Tariff: 180 - 360 IB: 32

Psychology and Film, Radio and Television Studies

Canterbury Christ Church University C10
BA (Hons)/BSc (Hons): 3 years full-time – CW86
A2: CC

Psychology with Film, Radio and Television Studies

Canterbury Christ Church University C10
BA (Hons)/BSc (Hons): 3 years full-time or 5 - 6 years part-time – C8W6
A2: CC

Psychology and Film and Screen Studies

Bath Spa University B20
BA (Hons)/BSc (Hons): 3 years full-time or 4 years sandwich – WC68
Tariff: 200 - 260

Psychology with Fine Art Painting and Drawing

University of Northampton N38
BA (Hons)/BSc (Hons): 3 years full-time or 4 - 6 years part-time – C8W1
Tariff: 180 - 220
BPS

Psychology with Forensic Biology

University of Chester C55
BSc (Hons): 3 years full-time – C8F4
Tariff: 240 IB: 30

Leeds Metropolitan University L27
BSc (Hons): 3 years full-time or 5 years part-time – C8F4
Tariff: 180 - 240 IB: 24

Liverpool Hope University L46
BA (Hons)/BSc (Hons): 3 years full-time – C8FK
Tariff: 180 - 240
BPS

Psychology with Forensic Computing

University of Chester C55
BSc (Hons): 3 years full-time – C8FK
Tariff: 240 IB: 30

Psychology and Forensic Science

Bristol, University of the West of England B80
BSc (Hons): 3 years full-time – CF84
Tariff: 220

University of Central Lancashire C30
BSc (Hons): 3 years full-time – CFV4
Tariff: 240

Psychology with French

University of Aberdeen A20
BSc (Hons): 4 years full-time – C8R1
A2: CDD SQA: BBBB ILC: BCCCC - BBCC IB: 26
BPS

University of Buckingham B90
BSc (Hons): 2 years full-time – C8R1
Tariff: 230 IB: 26

University of Northampton N38
BA (Hons)/BSc (Hons): 3 years full-time or 4 - 6 years part-time – C8R1
Tariff: 180 - 220
BPS

University of St Andrews S36
BSc (Hons): 4 years full-time – C8R1
A2: AAB SQA: AABB IB: 36

University of St Andrews S36
BSc (Hons): 5 years full-time with time abroad – C8RC
A2: AAB SQA: AABB IB: 36

Psychology with Gaelic

University of Aberdeen A20
BSc (Hons): 4 years full-time – C8QN
A2: CDD SQA: BBBB ILC: BCCCC - BBCC IB: 26
BPS

Psychology with Gender Studies

University of Sunderland S84
BA (Hons)/BSc (Hons): 3 years full-time – C8LH
Tariff: 180 - 360 IB: 32

Psychology and Geographic Information Systems

Bath Spa University B20
DipHE: 2 years full-time – FC68
Tariff: 80 - 120 Interview, Portfolio

Psychology with Geography

University of Chester C55
BSc (Hons): 3 years full-time – C8F8
Tariff: 240 IB: 30

Newman College of Higher Education [University of Leicester] N36
BSc (Hons): 3 years full-time – C8F8
Tariff: 160 - 240

University of Sunderland S84
BA (Hons)/BSc (Hons): 3 years full-time – C8L7
Tariff: 180 - 360 IB: 32

Psychology with German

University of Aberdeen A20
BSc (Hons): 4 years full-time – C8R2
A2: CDD SQA: BBBB ILC: BCCCC - BBCC IB: 26
BPS

University of Chester C55
BSc (Hons): 3 years full-time – C8R2
Tariff: 240 IB: 30

Psychology and Health

Roehampton University R48
BSc (Hons): 3 years full-time or 4 - 7 years part-time – C841
Tariff: 160

Psychology with Health

Thames Valley University T40
BSc (Hons): 3 years full-time or 5 years part-time – CB8
Tariff: 240

Psychology with Health and Exercis

St Mary's University College, Twickenham S64
BA (Hons)/BSc (Hons): 3 years full-time – C8BY
Tariff: 140 - 160

Psychology and Health Studies

University of Central Lancashire C30
BSc (Hons): 3 years full-time – CL85
Tariff: 240

Psychology with Health Studies

University of East London E28
BSc (Hons): 3 years full-time – C8B9
Tariff: 180 IB: 24

University of Northampton N38
BA (Hons)/BSc (Hons): 3 years full-time or 4 - 6 years time – C8L4
Tariff: 180 - 220
BPS

University of Sunderland S84
BA (Hons)/BSc (Hons): 3 years full-time – C8B9
Tariff: 180 - 360 IB: 32

Psychology and History

University of Glamorgan G14
BSc (Hons): 3 years full-time – CV81
Tariff: 220

Psychology with History

Canterbury Christ Church University C
BA (Hons)/BSc (Hons): 3 years full-time – C8V1
A2: CC

iversity of Northampton N38
(Hons)/BSc (Hons): 3 years full-time or 4 - 6 years part-
e – C8V1
iff: 180 - 220
S

Mary's University College,
vickenham S64
(Hons)/BSc (Hons): 3 years full-time – C8V1
iff: 140 - 160

iversity of Sunderland S84
(Hons)/BSc (Hons): 3 years full-time – C8V1
iff: 180 - 360 IB: 32

sychology with History of Art and esign

iversity of Northampton N38
(Hons)/BSc (Hons): 3 years full-time or 4 - 6 years part-
– C8V3
ff: 180 - 220

sychology and Human Biology

versity of Wales Institute, Cardiff C20
: 3 years full-time – CB81
ff: 120

iversity of Hertfordshire H36
(Hons): 3 years full-time – C8B1
f: 220 - 260

ychology with Human Biology

iversity of Northampton N38
Hons)/BSc (Hons): 3 years full-time or 4 - 6 years part-
– C8B1
: 180 - 220

versity of Plymouth P60
Hons)/BSc (Hons): 3 years full-time – C8C1
: 220 - 280 IB: 30

Mary's University College,
ckenham S64
Hons)/BSc (Hons): 3 years full-time – C8C1
: 140 - 160

ychology and Human Geography

versity of Hertfordshire H36
Hons): 3 years full-time – C8L7
: 220 - 260

ychology with Human Geography

versity of Northampton N38
ons)/BSc (Hons): 3 years full-time or 4 - 6 years part-
– C8L7
180 - 220

Psychology and Human Resource Management

University of Wolverhampton W75
BA (Hons)/BSc (Hons): 3 - 4 years full-time – CN86
Tariff: 200 - 260

Psychology with Human Resource Management

University of East London E28
BA (Hons)/BSc (Hons): 3 years full-time – C8N6
Tariff: 160

Middlesex University M80
BSc (Hons): 3 years full-time – CN86 E
Tariff: 160 - 240

University of Northampton N38
BA (Hons)/BSc (Hons): 3 years full-time or 4 - 6 years part-time – C8N6
Tariff: 180 - 220
BPS

Psychology with Human Rights

Kingston University K84
BA (Hons)/BSc (Hons): 3 years full-time or 6 years part-time – C8LF
Tariff: 220 - 320

Psychology in Education

Lancaster University L14
BSc (Hons): 3 years full-time – C812
Tariff: 320 IB: 34

Psychology in Society

City College Norwich [University of East Anglia] N82
BSc (Hons): 3 years full-time – C880
Tariff: 160

Psychology (including foundation studies)

University of Bolton B44
BSc (Hons): 4 years full-time – C802
Tariff: 80

Psychology and Information Systems

Keele University K12
BSc (Hons): 3 years full-time – CG8L
Tariff: 260

Psychology with Information Systems

University of Buckingham B90
BSc (Hons): 2 years full-time – C8G5
Tariff: 230 IB: 26

Psychology with Information Technology

Newman College of Higher Education [University of Leicester] N36
BSc (Hons): 3 years full-time – C8G5
Tariff: 160 - 240

University of Sunderland S84
BA (Hons)/BSc (Hons): 3 years full-time – C8GM
Tariff: 180 - 360 IB: 32

Psychology and International Development Studies

University of Chester C55
BSc (Hons): 3 years full-time – CL89
Tariff: 240 IB: 30

Psychology with International Development Studies

University of Chester C55
BSc (Hons): 3 years full-time – C8L9
Tariff: 240 IB: 30

Psychology with Internet Computing

Canterbury Christ Church University C10
BA (Hons)/BSc (Hons): 3 years full-time – C8GL
Tariff: 160 IB: 24

Psychology with Internet Technologies

University of Chester C55
BSc (Hons): 3 years full-time – C8H6
Tariff: 240 IB: 30

Psychology with Journalism

University of Sunderland S84
BA (Hons)/BSc (Hons): 3 years full-time – C8P5
Tariff: 180 - 360

Psychology and Law

Anglia Ruskin University A60
BSc (Hons): 3 years full-time – C8M1
Tariff: 220 - 260

University of Central Lancashire C30
BSc (Hons): 3 years full-time – CM81
Tariff: 240

University of Kent K24
BSc (Hons): 4 years full-time – CM81
Tariff: 320 IB: 33

Sheffield Hallam University S21
BA (Hons): 4 years sandwich – MC18
Tariff: 260
BC, BPS

University of Wales, Swansea S93
BSc (Hons): 3 years full-time – CM8C
A2: BBC BTEC: DDM SQA: ABBBB ILC: ABBBBB IB: 30
BPS, LS

University of Wolverhampton W75
BA (Hons)/BSc (Hons): 3 years full-time or 4 years sandwich – CM81
Tariff: 200 - 260

Psychology with Law

University of Northampton N38
BA (Hons)/BSc (Hons): 3 years full-time or 4 - 6 years part-time – C8M1
Tariff: 180 - 220
BPS

University of Plymouth P60
BA (Hons)/BSc (Hons): 3 years full-time – C8M2
Tariff: 220 - 280
BPS

Psychology with Linguistics

University of St Andrews S36
BSc (Hons): 4 years full-time – C8QC
A2: AAB SQA: AABB IB: 36

Psychology with Management

University of Northampton N38
BA (Hons)/BSc (Hons): 3 years full-time or 4 - 6 years part-time – C8N2
Tariff: 180 - 220
BPS

University of Sunderland S84
BA (Hons)/BSc (Hons): 3 years full-time – C8N2
Tariff: 180 - 360

Psychology and Management Science

University of Hertfordshire H36
BSc (Hons): 3 years full-time – C8G2
Tariff: 220 - 260
BPS

Psychology with Management Studies

St Mary's University College, Twickenham S64
BA (Hons)/BSc (Hons): 3 years full-time – C8N2
Tariff: 160 - 200

Psychology with Marketing

University of Buckingham B90
BSc (Hons): 2 years full-time – C8N5
Tariff: 230 IB: 26

Canterbury Christ Church University C10
BA (Hons)/BSc (Hons): 3 years full-time – C8N5
A2: CC

Middlesex University M80
BSc (Hons): 3 years full-time – C8N5 E
Tariff: 160 - 240

University of Northampton N38
BA (Hons)/BSc (Hons): 3 years full-time or 4 - 6 years part-time – C8N5
Tariff: 180 - 220
BPS

University of Sunderland S84
BA (Hons)/BSc (Hons): 3 years full-time – C8N5
Tariff: 180 - 360

Psychology with Mathematics

University of Chester C55
BSc (Hons): 3 years full-time – C8G1
Tariff: 240 IB: 30

University of Northampton N38
BA (Hons)/BSc (Hons): 3 years full-time or 4 - 6 years part-time – C8G1
Tariff: 180 - 220
BPS

Psychology with Media Communications

University of Buckingham B90
BSc (Hons): 2 years full-time – C8P3
Tariff: 230 IB: 26

Psychology with Media and Cultural Studies

Canterbury Christ Church University C10
BA (Hons)/BSc (Hons): 3 years full-time – C8P3
A2: CC

Psychology and Media Production

University of Glamorgan G14
BSc (Hons): 3 years full-time – PCH8
Tariff: 220

Psychology with Media Studies

University of Sunderland S84
BA (Hons)/BSc (Hons): 3 years full-time – C8P3
Tariff: 180 - 360 IB: 32

Psychology, Mental and Physical Health

University of Reading R12
BSc (Hons): 3 years full-time – C806
A2: AAB - AAA IB: 34

Psychology and Multimedia Communication

University of Hertfordshire H36
BSc (Hons): 3 years full-time – C8H6
Tariff: 160 - 220
BPS

Psychology with Multimedia Technologies

University of Chester C55
BSc (Hons): 3 years full-time – C8PJ
Tariff: 240 IB: 30

Psychology and Music

Anglia Ruskin University A60
BSc (Hons): 3 years full-time – C8W3
Tariff: 220

Psychology with Music

Canterbury Christ Church University C1
BA (Hons)/BSc (Hons): 3 years full-time – C8W3
A2: CC

University of Sunderland S84
BA (Hons)/BSc (Hons): 3 years full-time – C8W3
Tariff: 180 - 360 IB: 31

Psychology with Natural Hazard Management

University of Chester C55
BSc (Hons): 3 years full-time – C8WP
Tariff: 240 IB: 30

University of Chester C55
BSc (Hons): 3 years full-time – C8FV
Tariff: 240 IB: 30

Psychology with Neuropsychology

University of Wales, Bangor B06
BSc (Hons): 3 years full-time – C801
Tariff: 260 - 300 IB: 30

Psychology and Neuroscience

University of Manchester M20
BSc (Hons): 3 years full-time – BC18
A2: ABB - AAB SQA: AAABB - AAAAB ILC: AAABBB - AAAAAB IB: 33 - 35

University of Manchester M20
BSc (Hons): 4 years full-time – BCC8
A2: ABB - AAB SQA: AAABB - AAAAB ILC: AAABBB - AAAAAB IB: 33 - 35

Psychology with Neuroscience

University of Leicester L34
BSc (Hons): 3 years full-time – C8B1
Tariff: 300 - 320 IB: 30 - 33
BPS

University of Sussex S90
BSc (Hons): 3 years full-time – CB81
A2: ABB - AAB IB: 34 - 36

University of Westminster W50
BSc (Hons): 3 years full-time or 5 years part-time – C8
A2: CC BTEC: MMP IB: 26

iversity of Westminster W50

: (Hons): 4 years full-time – C8BC
CC BTEC: MMP IB: 26

sychology with Nutrition

iversity of Chester C55

: (Hons): 3 years full-time – C8B4
ff: 240 IB: 30

erpool Hope University L46

Hons)/BSc (Hons): 3 years full-time – C8B4
ff: 180 - 240

Mary's University College, ickenham S64

Hons)/BSc (Hons): 3 years full-time – C8BK
f: 140 - 160

sychology with Nutrition and Health

eds, Trinity & All Saints [University of eds] L24

(Hons): 3 years full-time – C8B4
f: 160 - 240

sychology of Nutrition and nsumer Choice

iversity of Wales Institute, Cardiff C20

3 years full-time or 4 years sandwich – C890
: 200

ychology of Sport and Exercise

nchester Metropolitan University M40

(Hons): 3 years full-time – C841
: 200

ychology and Outdoor Recreation

versity of Derby D39

Hons): 3 years full-time – CNV2
: 140 - 160

ychology with Performance

versity of Northampton N38

Hons)/BSc (Hons): 3 years full-time or 4 - 6 years part- – C8WK
: 180 - 220

ychology and Philosophy

versity of Hertfordshire H36

Hons): 3 years full-time – C8V5
220 - 260

versity of Nottingham N84

Hons): 3 years full-time – CV85
BB IB: 35

University of Wolverhampton W75

BA (Hons)/BSc (Hons): 3 years full-time or 4 years sandwich – CV85
Tariff: 160 - 220

Psychology with Philosophy

University of Glamorgan G14

BSc (Hons): 3 years full-time – C8V5
Tariff: 220 - 260 IB: 24

University of Hull H72

BSc (Hons): 3 years full-time – C8V5
Tariff: 280
BPS

University of Northampton N38

BA (Hons)/BSc (Hons): 3 years full-time or 4 - 6 years part-time – C8V5
Tariff: 180 - 220
BPS

St Mary's University College, Twickenham S64

BA (Hons)/BSc (Hons): 3 years full-time – C8V5
Tariff: 160 - 200

Psychology with Photography

University of Sunderland S84

BA (Hons)/BSc (Hons): 3 years full-time – C8W6
Tariff: 180 - 360 IB: 32

Psychology with Physiology

University of Sunderland S84

BA (Hons)/BSc (Hons): 3 years full-time – C8B1
Tariff: 180 - 360 IB: 32

Psychology with Politics

Canterbury Christ Church University C10

BA (Hons)/BSc (Hons): 3 years full-time – C8LG
A2: CC

University of Sunderland S84

BA (Hons)/BSc (Hons): 3 years full-time – C8L2
Tariff: 180 - 360 IB: 32

Psychology and Popular Music Production

University of Derby D39

BSc (Hons): 3 years full-time or 4 - 6 years part-time – CW83
Tariff: 140 - 160 IB: 26

Psychology with Professional and Creative Writing

St Mary's University College, Twickenham S64

BA (Hons)/BSc (Hons): 3 years full-time – C8W8
Tariff: 160 - 200

Psychology and Religion, Philosophy and Ethics

University of Gloucestershire G50

BA (Hons)/BSc (Hons): 3 years full-time – CVM6
Tariff: 200 - 260 IB: 26 - 30
BPS

Psychology and Religious Studies

Canterbury Christ Church University C10

BA (Hons)/BSc (Hons): 3 years full-time – CV86
A2: CC

Psychology with Religious Studies

Canterbury Christ Church University C10

BA (Hons)/BSc (Hons): 3 years full-time – C8V6
A2: CC

Psychology and Robotics

Bristol, University of the West of England B80

BA (Hons)/BSc (Hons): 3 years full-time – CH86
Tariff: 240 - 300 IB: 24 - 28
BPS

Psychology and Science of Sport and Exercise

Roehampton University R48

BA (Hons)/BSc (Hons): 3 years full-time – CCP8
Tariff: 160
BPS

Psychology with Science of the Environment

Canterbury Christ Church University C10

BA (Hons)/BSc (Hons): 3 years full-time – C8F8
A2: CC

Psychology with Sexuality

London South Bank University L75

BSc (Hons): 3 years full-time – C8L3
A2: CCC BTEC

Psychology and Social Anthropology

Brunel University B84

BSc (Hons): 3 years full-time – CL8P
Tariff: 300 IB: 30
BPS

University of Kent K24

BSc (Hons): 3 years full-time – CL86
A2: BBB - ABC IB: 33

Roehampton University R48

BA (Hons)/BSc (Hons): 3 years full-time – CL8Q
Tariff: 160 - 200
BPS

Psychology and Social Anthropology (thin sandwich)

Brunel University B84
BSc (Hons): 4 years sandwich – CL86
Tariff: 300 IB: 32
BPS

Psychology and Social Care Studies

University of Winchester W76
DipHE: 2 years full-time – LC3W
Tariff: 80

Psychology and Social History

Manchester Metropolitan University M40
BSc (Hons): 3 years full-time – CV83
Tariff: 160 - 240
BPS

Psychology and Social Justice

Manchester Metropolitan University M40
BA (Hons)/BSc (Hons): 3 years full-time – MC28
Tariff: 200

Psychology and Social Policy

University of Lincoln L39
BA (Hons)/BSc (Hons): 3 years full-time – CL84 L
Tariff: 260
BPS

London South Bank University L75
BA (Hons)/BSc (Hons): 3 years full-time – CLV4
A2: CCC
BPS

Psychology and Social Policy and Administration

Roehampton University R48
BA (Hons)/BSc (Hons): 3 years full-time – CL84
Tariff: 160 - 200
BPS

Psychology and Social Science

Canterbury Christ Church University C10
BA (Hons)/BSc (Hons): 3 years full-time – LC38
A2: CC

Psychology with Social Science

Canterbury Christ Church University C10
BA (Hons)/BSc (Hons): 3 years full-time – C8L3
A2: CC

Psychology and Social Science of Sport

Roehampton University R48
BA (Hons)/BSc (Hons): 3 years full-time – LCH8
Tariff: 160 - 200
BPS

Psychology and Social Welfare

University of Worcester W80
BA (Hons)/BSc (Hons): 3 years full-time – CL85
Tariff: 160 IB: 26
BPS

Psychology with Social Welfare

University of Northampton N38
BA (Hons)/BSc (Hons): 3 years full-time or 4 - 6 years part-time – C8L5
Tariff: 180 - 220
BPS

Psychology with Socio-Legal Studies

University of Buckingham B90
BSc (Hons): 2 years full-time – C8M1
Tariff: 230 IB: 26

Psychology and Sociology

Anglia Ruskin University A60
BSc (Hons): 3 years full-time – C813
Tariff: 220 - 260 HND

Bath Spa University B20
DipHE: 2 years full-time – LC38
Tariff: 80 - 120

Bath Spa University B20
BA (Hons)/BSc (Hons): 3 years full-time – CL83
Tariff: 200 - 240

Bridgwater College [Bath Spa University] ▲
BA (Hons)/BSc (Hons): 3 years full-time – CL83 F
Tariff: 200 - 240

Bristol, University of the West of England B80
BA (Hons)/BSc (Hons): 3 years full-time – CL83
Tariff: 200 - 280 IB: 24 - 28
BPS

Brunel University B84
BSc (Hons): 3 years full-time – CL8H
Tariff: 300 IB: 32
BPS

Buckinghamshire Chilterns University College B94
BSc (Hons): 3 years full-time – CL83
Tariff: 120 - 240

University of Chester C55
BSc (Hons): 3 years full-time – LC38
Tariff: 240 IB: 30

Coventry University C85
BSc (Hons): 3 years full-time or 5 years part-time – CL83
Tariff: 260
BPS

University of Derby D39
BA (Hons): 3 years full-time or 4 - 6 years part-time – CL8H
Tariff: 140 - 160 IB: 26

University of Glamorgan G14
BSc (Hons): 3 years full-time – LC38
Tariff: 220 IB: 24

University of Gloucestershire G50
BA (Hons)/BSc (Hons): 3 years full-time – LC38
Tariff: 200 - 280 IB: 26 - 30
BPS

Keele University K12
BA (Hons)/BSc (Hons): 3 years full-time – CL83
Tariff: 300 - 320

University of Kent K24
BSc (Hons): 3 years full-time – CL83
A2: BBB - ABC IB: 33

University of Leeds L23
BSc (Hons): 3 years full-time – LC38
A2: BCC - ABB

Liverpool Hope University L46
BA (Hons): 3 years full-time – CL83
Tariff: 240
BPS

London South Bank University L75
BA (Hons)/BSc (Hons): 3 years full-time – CL83
A2: CCC
BPS

Manchester Metropolitan University M
BA (Hons)/BSc (Hons): 3 years full-time – CLV3
Tariff: 200

Manchester Metropolitan University M
BSc (Hons): 3 years full-time – CL83
Tariff: 280 IB: 30
BPS

Oxford Brookes University O66
BA (Hons)/BSc (Hons): 3 years full-time or 4 years sandwich – CL83
A2: ABB
BPS

Queen Margaret University, Edinburgh Q25
BSc: 3 years full-time BSc (Hons): 4 years full-time – C
Tariff: 180 - 220 HND

Roehampton University R48
BA (Hons)/BSc (Hons): 3 years full-time – CL83
Tariff: 160 - 200
BPS

St Mary's University College, Twickenham S64
BA (Hons)/BSc (Hons): 3 years full-time – CL83
Tariff: 160

Staffordshire University S72
BA (Hons)/BSc (Hons): 3 years full-time – LC38
Tariff: 240

University Campus Suffolk [University East Anglia, University of Essex] S82
BSc (Hons): 3 years full-time or 5 - 9 years part-time – LC38 I
Tariff: 120 - 180

University of Sunderland S84
BA (Hons)/BSc (Hons): 3 years full-time – CL83
Tariff: 180 - 360 IB: 32

University of Worcester W80
BA (Hons)/BSc (Hons): 3 years full-time – CL83
Tariff: 160 IB: 26
BPS

sychology with Sociology

uckinghamshire Chilterns University ollege B94
c (Hons): 3 years full-time – C8L3
iff: 120

iversity of Chester C55
c (Hons): 3 years full-time – C8L3
iff: 240 IB: 30

iversity of East London E28
c (Hons): 3 years full-time – C8L3
iff: 160

iversity of Glamorgan G14
c (Hons): 3 years full-time – C8L3
iff: 220 IB: 24

iversity of Hull H72
c (Hons): 3 years full-time – C8L3
iff: 280
S

iversity of Leicester L34
c (Hons): 3 years full-time – C8L3
ff: 300 - 320 IB: 30 - 33
S

rth Devon College [University of ymouth] ▲
c: 2 years full-time – C8LH
ff: 80

iversity of Northampton N38
(Hons)/BSc (Hons): 3 years full-time or 4 - 6 years part- – C8L3
ff: 180 - 220

ttingham Trent University N91
(Hons): 3 years full-time – C8LH
f: 240 IB: 24

iversity of Plymouth P60
Hons)/BSc (Hons): 3 years full-time – C8L3
f: 220 - 280 IB: 30

Mary's University College, ickenham S64
Hons)/BSc (Hons): 3 years full-time – C8L3
f: 140 - 160

iversity of Sunderland S84
Hons)/BSc (Hons): 3 years full-time – C8L3
f: 180 - 360 IB: 32

iversity of Sussex S90
(Hons): 3 years full-time – C8L3
ABB - AAB IB: 34 - 36

ychology and Sociology (Applied)

ndon Metropolitan University L68
Hons)/BSc (Hons): 3 years full-time – CL83
: 160 - 200 IB: 28

Psychology and Sociology (thin sandwich)

Brunel University B84
BSc (Hons): 4 years sandwich – CL83
Tariff: 300 IB: 32
BPS

Psychology and Spanish

University of Hertfordshire H36
BSc (Hons): 3 years full-time – C8R4
Tariff: 220 - 260 IB: 26 - 28
BPS

Roehampton University R48
BA (Hons)/BSc (Hons): 3 years full-time – CR84
Tariff: 160 IB: 28
BPS

Psychology with Spanish

University of Buckingham B90
BSc (Hons): 2 years full-time – C8R4
Tariff: 230 IB: 26

University of Chester C55
BSc (Hons): 3 years full-time – C8R4
Tariff: 240 IB: 30

University of St Andrews S36
BSc (Hons): 4 years full-time – C8R4
A2: AAB SQA: AABB IB: 36

University of St Andrews S36
BSc (Hons): 5 years full-time with time abroad – C8RK
A2: AAB SQA: AABB IB: 36

Psychology and Spanish (4 years)

University of Wales, Swansea S93
BA (Hons): 4 years full-time with time abroad – CR84
A2: BCC - BBC
BPS

Psychology with Special Educational Needs

University of East London E28
BA (Hons)/BSc (Hons): 3 years full-time – C8X1
Tariff: 160

Psychology and Special Effects Technology

Manchester Metropolitan University M40
BSc (Hons): 3 years full-time – CWV6
Tariff: 160 - 240
BPS

Psychology and Special Needs

Liverpool Hope University L46
BA (Hons)/BSc (Hons): 3 years full-time – XC18
Tariff: 180 - 240 IB: 25
BPS

Psychology and Speech Pathology

Manchester Metropolitan University M40
BSc (Hons): 4 years full-time – BC68
Tariff: 300
BPS, RCSLT

Psychology and Sport

Manchester Metropolitan University M40
BA (Hons)/BSc (Hons): 3 years full-time – CC68
Tariff: 200 IB: 28

Psychology with Sport and Exercise

Leeds, Trinity & All Saints [University of Leeds] L24
BSc (Hons): 3 years full-time – C8C6
Tariff: 160 - 240

Psychology, Sport and Exercise

Staffordshire University S72
BSc (Hons): 3 years full-time – CC86
Tariff: 240 IB: 28
BPS

Psychology and Sport and Exercise Science

Canterbury Christ Church University C10
BA (Hons)/BSc (Hons): 3 years full-time – CC86
A2: CC BTEC: MM SQA: CCCC ILC: CCCCC IB: 24

Psychology with Sport and Exercise Science

University of Exeter E84
BSc (Hons): 3 years full-time – C8C6
A2: AAB - AAA

University of Huddersfield H60
BSc (Hons): 3 years full-time – C8C6
Tariff: 240

Psychology and Sport and Exercise Sciences

University of Gloucestershire G50
BA (Hons)/BSc (Hons): 3 years full-time – CC68
Tariff: 200 - 260 IB: 26 - 30
BPS

Psychology with Sport and Exercise Sciences

University of Chester C55
BSc (Hons): 3 years full-time – C8C6
Tariff: 240 IB: 30

Psychology and Sport Psychology

Canterbury Christ Church University C10
BA (Hons)/BSc (Hons): 3 years full-time or 5 - 6 years part-time – C893
A2: CC

Psychology and Sport Science

University of Gloucestershire G50
BA (Hons)/BSc (Hons): 3 years full-time – CC8Q
Tariff: 200 - 260 IB: 26 - 30
BPS

St Mary's University College, Twickenham S64
BA (Hons)/BSc (Hons): 3 years full-time – CC86
Tariff: 160

Psychology with Sport Science

Canterbury Christ Church University C10
BA (Hons)/BSc (Hons): 3 years full-time – C8C6
A2: CC

Northumbria University N77
BSc (Hons): 3 years full-time – C8C6
Tariff: 280 IB: 26
BPS

Nottingham Trent University N91
BSc (Hons): 3 years full-time – C8C6
Tariff: 240 IB: 24
BPS

St Mary's University College, Twickenham S64
BA (Hons)/BSc (Hons): 3 years full-time – C8C6
Tariff: 140 - 160

Psychology and Sport Studies

Liverpool Hope University L46
BA (Hons)/BSc (Hons): 3 years full-time – CC86
Tariff: 180 - 240
BPS

Psychology with Sport Studies

University of Northampton N38
BA (Hons)/BSc (Hons): 3 years full-time or 4 - 6 years part-time – C8C6
Tariff: 180 - 220
BPS

Psychology and Sports Biology

Bristol, University of the West of England B80
BSc (Hons): 3 years full-time – CC68
Tariff: 180 - 220 IB: 24 - 26

Psychology and Sports and Coaching Studies

Oxford Brookes University O66
BA (Hons)/BSc (Hons): 3 years full-time or 4 years sandwich – CC68
A2: ABB IB: 34
BPS

Psychology and Sports Development

University of Gloucestershire G50
BA (Hons)/BSc (Hons): 3 years full-time – CL8J
Tariff: 200 - 260 IB: 26 - 30
BPS

Liverpool Hope University L46
BA (Hons)/BSc (Hons): 3 years full-time – CC68
Tariff: 180 - 240
BPS

University of Winchester W76
DipHE: 2 years full-time – CNV2
Tariff: 80

Psychology and Sports Education

University of Gloucestershire G50
BA (Hons)/BSc (Hons): 3 years full-time – CX8J
Tariff: 200 - 260 IB: 26 - 30
BPS

Psychology with Sports Science

University of Hull H72
BSc (Hons): 3 years full-time – C8C6
Tariff: 280
BPS

Psychology and Sports Studies

University of Hertfordshire H36
BSc (Hons): 3 years full-time – C8C6
Tariff: 180 - 280
BPS

University of Winchester W76
DipHE: 2 years full-time – CL8J
Tariff: 80

Psychology with Sports Studies

Newman College of Higher Education [University of Leicester] N36
BSc (Hons): 3 years full-time – C8C6
Tariff: 160 - 240

Psychology and Statistics

University of Hertfordshire H36
BSc (Hons): 3 years full-time – C8G3
Tariff: 180 - 280
BPS

Lancaster University L14
BSc (Hons): 3 years full-time – CG83
Tariff: 300 IB: 33

Newcastle University N21
BSc (Hons): 3 years full-time or 4 years full-time including foundation year – CG83
A2: ABB SQA: AABBB

Oxford Brookes University O66
BA (Hons)/BSc (Hons): 3 years full-time or 4 years sandwich – CG83
A2: ABB IB: 34
BPS

University of Reading R12
BSc (Hons): 3 years full-time – CG83
A2: AAB

Psychology Studies and Counselling Studies

University of Salford S03
BSc (Hons): 3 years full-time or 6 years part-time – CL85
Tariff: 260 IB: 27

Psychology Studies and Health Sciences

University of Salford S03
BSc (Hons): 3 years full-time or 6 years part-time – BC98
Tariff: 280 IB: 27

Psychology with Studies in English Language/Linguistics

University of Sunderland S84
BA (Hons)/BSc (Hons): 3 years full-time – C8Q1
Tariff: 180 - 360 IB: 32

Psychology (with studies in Europe)

University of Kent K24
BSc (Hons): 4 years full-time with time abroad – C881
A2: BBB - ABC IB: 34
BPS

Psychology and Study of Religions

Bath Spa University B20
BA (Hons)/BSc (Hons): 3 years full-time – CV86
Tariff: 220 - 260

Bath Spa University B20
DipHE: 2 years full-time – VC68
Tariff: 80 - 120

Psychology and Teaching English a a Foreign Language

Manchester Metropolitan University M
BSc (Hons): 3 years full-time – CX81
Tariff: 160 - 240
BPS

Psychology and Theatre Studies

University of Glasgow G28
MA (Hons): 4 years full-time – CW84
A2: ABB SQA: ABBB ILC: ABBB IB: 30

Psychology with Theology

Canterbury Christ Church University C
BA (Hons)/BSc (Hons): 3 years full-time – C8VP
A2: CC

Psychology and Theology and Religious Studies

University of Glasgow G28
MA (Hons): 4 years full-time – CV86
A2: ABB SQA: ABBB ILC: ABBB IB: 30

verpool Hope University L46

, (Hons)/BSc (Hons): 3 years full-time – CV86
iff: 180 - 240
S

: Mary's University College, vickenham S64

(Hons)/BSc (Hons): 3 years full-time – CV86
iff: 160

niversity of Winchester W76

HE: 2 years full-time – LV76
iff: 80

sychology with Theology and eligious Studies

Mary's University College, vickenham S64

(Hons)/BSc (Hons): 3 years full-time – C8V6
iff: 140 - 160

sychology (thin sandwich)

unel University B84

: (Hons): 4 years sandwich – C800
iff: 300 IB: 32

sychology with Third World evelopment

iversity of Northampton N38

(Hons)/BSc (Hons): 3 years full-time or 4 - 6 years part-
– C8LX
ff: 180 - 220

sychology and Time-Based Digital edia

iversity of Worcester W80

(Hons)/BSc (Hons): 3 years full-time – CG84
ff: 160 IB: 26

sychology and Tourism

stol, University of the West of England
0

(Hons)/BSc (Hons): 3 years full-time – CN88
f: 200 - 280 IB: 24 - 28

erpool Hope University L46

Hons)/BSc (Hons): 3 years full-time – CN88
f: 180 - 240

ndon South Bank University L75

Hons)/BSc (Hons): 3 years full-time – CN88
CCC

Mary's University College, ckenham S64

Hons)/BSc (Hons): 3 years full-time – CN88
: 160

Psychology with Tourism

University of Northampton N38

BA (Hons)/BSc (Hons): 3 years full-time or 4 - 6 years part-time – C8N8
Tariff: 180 - 220
BPS

St Mary's University College, Twickenham S64

BA (Hons)/BSc (Hons): 3 years full-time – C8N8
Tariff: 140 - 160

Psychology and Tourism and Heritage Management

University of Winchester W76

DipHE: 2 years full-time – NC8W
Tariff: 80

Psychology and Tourism and Leisure Studies

Canterbury Christ Church University C10

BA (Hons)/BSc (Hons): 3 years full-time – CN28
A2: CC

Psychology with Tourism and Leisure Studies

Canterbury Christ Church University C10

BA (Hons)/BSc (Hons): 3 years full-time – C8N8
A2: CC

Psychology and Urban Studies

Manchester Metropolitan University M40

BSc (Hons): 3 years full-time – CK84
Tariff: 160 - 240
BPS

Psychology and Visual Arts

Manchester Metropolitan University M40

BA (Hons)/BSc (Hons): 3 years full-time – WC18

University of Worcester W80

BA (Hons)/BSc (Hons): 3 years full-time – CW82
Tariff: 160 IB: 26
BPS

Psychology with Working with Children Young People and Families

Newman College of Higher Education [University of Leicester] N36

BA (Hons)/BSc (Hons): 3 years full-time – C8L5
Tariff: 160 - 240 IB: 24

Psychology and Writing

Manchester Metropolitan University M40

BA (Hons)/BSc (Hons): 3 years full-time – WC88
Tariff: 200 IB: 28

Psychology and Youth Studies

University Campus Suffolk [University of East Anglia, University of Essex] S82

BSc (Hons): 3 years full-time or 5 - 9 years part-time – CL85 I
Tariff: 120 - 180

Psychology and Zoology

University of Bristol B78

BSc (Hons): 3 years full-time – CC83
A2: BBB - AAB BTEC: DDM SQA: AAABB IB: 32 - 36
BPS

Sport and Exercise Psychology

University of Bolton B44

BSc (Hons): 3 years full-time or 5 years part-time – C800
Tariff: 180
BPS

Canterbury Christ Church University C10

BSc (Hons): 3 years full-time or 5 - 6 years part-time – C813
Tariff: 160

University of East London E28

BSc (Hons): 3 years full-time – C890
Tariff: 160

University of Teesside T20

BSc (Hons): 3 years full-time – C820
Tariff: 240 IB: 26

Sport Psychology

University of Central Lancashire C30

BSc (Hons): 3 years full-time – C8C6
A2: BCC
BPS

Liverpool Hope University L46

BSc (Hons): 3 years full-time – C891
Tariff: 180 - 240

Sport Psychology and American Studies

Canterbury Christ Church University C10

BA (Hons)/BSc (Hons): 3 years full-time or 5 - 6 years part-time – TC78
A2: CC

Sport Psychology with American Studies

Canterbury Christ Church University C10

BA (Hons)/BSc (Hons): 3 years full-time or 5 - 6 years part-time – C8TR
A2: CC

Sport Psychology with Applied Criminology

Canterbury Christ Church University C10

BA (Hons)/BSc (Hons): 3 years full-time or 5 - 6 years part-time – C8M9
A2: CC

Sport Psychology and Art

Canterbury Christ Church University C10

BA (Hons)/BSc (Hons): 3 years full-time or 5 - 6 years part-time – WC18
A2: CC

Sport Psychology with Art

Canterbury Christ Church University C10

BA (Hons)/BSc (Hons): 3 years full-time or 5 - 6 years part-time – C8WC
A2: CC

Sport Psychology and Biosciences

Canterbury Christ Church University C10

BA (Hons)/BSc (Hons): 3 years full-time or 5 - 6 years part-time – CC78
A2: CC

Sport Psychology with Biosciences

Canterbury Christ Church University C10

BA (Hons)/BSc (Hons): 3 years full-time or 5 - 6 years part-time – C8C7
A2: CC

Sport Psychology and Business Studies

Canterbury Christ Church University C10

BA (Hons)/BSc (Hons): 3 years full-time or 5 - 6 years part-time – CN81
A2: CC

Sport Psychology with Business Studies

Canterbury Christ Church University C10

BA (Hons)/BSc (Hons): 3 years full-time or 5 - 6 years part-time – C8NC
A2: CC

Sport Psychology with Computing

Canterbury Christ Church University C10

BA (Hons)/BSc (Hons): 3 years full-time or 5 - 6 years part-time – C8GL
A2: CC

Sport Psychology and Digital Culture, Arts and Media

Canterbury Christ Church University C10

BA (Hons)/BSc (Hons): 3 years full-time or 5 - 6 years part-time – CGW4
A2: CC

Sport Psychology with Digital Culture, Arts and Media

Canterbury Christ Church University C10

BA (Hons)/BSc (Hons): 3 years full-time or 5 - 6 years part-time – C8G9
A2: CC

Sport Psychology and Early Childhood Studies

Canterbury Christ Church University C10

BA (Hons)/BSc (Hons): 3 years full-time or 5 - 6 years part-time – CX83
A2: CC

Sport Psychology with Early Childhood Studies

Canterbury Christ Church University C10

BA (Hons)/BSc (Hons): 3 years full-time or 5 - 6 years part-time – C8XH
A2: CC

Sport Psychology with English

Canterbury Christ Church University C10

BA (Hons)/BSc (Hons): 3 years full-time or 5 - 6 years part-time – C8QH
A2: CC

Sport Psychology with French

Canterbury Christ Church University C10

BA (Hons)/BSc (Hons): 3 years full-time or 5 - 6 years part-time – C8RC
A2: CC

Sport Psychology with Geography

Canterbury Christ Church University C10

BA (Hons)/BSc (Hons): 3 years full-time or 5 - 6 years part-time – C8FX
A2: CC

Sport Psychology with History

Canterbury Christ Church University C10

BA (Hons)/BSc (Hons): 3 years full-time or 5 - 6 years part-time – C8VC
A2: CC

Sport Psychology and Marketing

Canterbury Christ Church University C10

BA (Hons)/BSc (Hons): 3 years full-time or 5 - 6 years part-time – CN85
A2: CC

Sport Psychology with Marketing

Canterbury Christ Church University C10

BA (Hons)/BSc (Hons): 3 years full-time or 5 - 6 years part-time – C8NM
A2: CC

Sport Psychology and Media and Cultural Studies

Canterbury Christ Church University C10

BA (Hons)/BSc (Hons): 3 years full-time or 5 - 6 years part-time – CPW3
A2: CC

Sport Psychology with Media and Cultural Studies

Canterbury Christ Church University C1

BA (Hons)/BSc (Hons): 3 years full-time or 5 - 6 years pa
time – C8PJ
A2: CC

Sport Psychology with Music

Canterbury Christ Church University C1

BA (Hons)/BSc (Hons): 3 years full-time or 5 - 6 years pa
time – C8WH
A2: CC

Sport Psychology and Religious Studies

Canterbury Christ Church University C1

BA (Hons)/BSc (Hons): 3 years full-time or 5 - 6 years pa
time – CV66
A2: CC

Sport Psychology with Religious Studies

Canterbury Christ Church University C1

BA (Hons)/BSc (Hons): 3 years full-time or 5 - 6 years pa
time – C8VQ
A2: CC

Sport Psychology with Social Scien

Canterbury Christ Church University C

BA (Hons)/BSc (Hons): 3 years full-time or 5 - 6 years p
time – C8LH
A2: CC

Sport Psychology and Sociology

Canterbury Christ Church University C

BA (Hons)/BSc (Hons): 3 years full-time or 5 - 6 years p
time – CL83
A2: CC

Sport Psychology and Theology

Canterbury Christ Church University C

BA (Hons)/BSc (Hons): 3 years full-time or 5 - 6 years p
time – CVW6
A2: CC

Sport Psychology with Theology

Canterbury Christ Church University C

BA (Hons)/BSc (Hons): 3 years full-time or 5 - 6 years p
time – C8V9
A2: CC

Sport Psychology and Tourism and Leisure Studies

Canterbury Christ Church University C

BA (Hons)/BSc (Hons): 3 years full-time or 5 - 6 years p
time – CN88
A2: CC

port Psychology with Tourism and eisure Studies

anterbury Christ Church University C10

(Hons)/BSc (Hons): 3 years full-time or 5 - 6 years part-
e – C8NV
CC

ports and Exercise Psychology

iversity of Huddersfield H60

: (Hons): 3 years full-time – C841
ff: 240

Sports Psychology

Anglia Ruskin University A60

BSc (Hons): 3 years full-time – C890
Tariff: 240 IB: 30

Buckinghamshire Chilterns University College B94

BSc (Hons): 3 years full-time – C601
Tariff: 180 - 240

University of Glamorgan G14

BSc (Hons): 3 years full-time – C601
Tariff: 200 - 220

Sports Psychology and Coaching Sciences

Bournemouth University B50

BSc (Hons): 4 years sandwich – CX81
Tariff: 260

Sports Psychology and Performance

London Metropolitan University L68

BSc (Hons): 3 years full-time – CC68
Tariff: 160 IB: 28

Therapies

Including:
Occupational Therapy
Orthoptics
Physiotherapy
Podiatry
Prosthetics (Orthotics)
Radiography (Therapeutic)
Speech Therapy

Overview

The 'mainstream'

The professions in this chapter are considered to be 'mainstream' healthcare and are well-recognised by the traditional medical professionals and within the NHS. Most of them qualify for the NHS bursary (a means of financial assistance) to encourage more students to apply. The course fees charged are the normal state-recognised rates for higher education. (This is in contrast to those careers featured in the chapter on **Complementary Medicine**.) Many of the courses in this chapter are widely available throughout the UK higher education system.

But even allowing for these distinctions, there is now the beginning of a blurring in the boundaries between the so-called complementary therapies and those in this chapter – see especially the physiotherapy paragraph below.

Validation and qualification

Most of the careers covered below are validated by the Health Professions Council (HPC), sometimes in conjunction with the professional body for the specific career. Course content is regulated to ensure that all courses offer the approved theoretical and clinical background.

In contrast to most of the courses in the chapters on **Anatomy and Physiology, Biomedical Sciences** and **Health Studies**, these subjects take you closer to qualification in particular professions or to postgraduate training – so it is a good idea to select a course from this chapter (rather than a more general healthcare course) if you have a clear idea of the profession in which you want to qualify. For example, Claire Collinge of Eaton Bank High School, Congleton says: 'It's good that my best subjects in the sixth form turned out to be science-based. I want a degree course that will get me as close as possible to my chosen career. I know I want to be a physiotherapist so that is the degree I am applying for.'

The courses

Some of these courses are offered in combination with a wide range of other courses. Where professional qualification is the aim you need to check that the course is accredited by the appropriate professional body. Where the subject is offered as one part of a joint honours course, there is less chance of covering all the ground required by professional bodies. All these courses include time 'in the field' for practical experience.

Each university decides on its own entry requirements. You can see the range of UCAS points asked by each one by consulting the course listings on the following pages. However, many Foundation degree courses exercise a more flexible admissions procedure which enables them to take into account factors such as work experience in their entrance requirements and which cannot therefore be expressed as part of the UCAS tariff framework.

Because the therapies included in this chapter are so diverse, they have each been treated separately in the paragraphs below.

Occupational therapy

Occupational therapy is a fast-growing profession. Therapists work with patients with physical, psychiatric and/or social problems, helping them to come to terms with developments in their lives, such as partial recovery from illness or accident. Following assessment of their patients' situations, lifestyle and domestic/work circumstances, they design a programme of exercise and activity to help them manage their lives in the best possible way. They work in conjunction with allied professionals including doctors, nurses, teachers and social workers.

Degree courses in Occupational Therapy usually take three years (or four in Scotland) but there are fast-track postgraduate courses for students from other disciplines and for mature applicants with relevant backgrounds. Both the College of Occupational Therapists (COT) and the HPC are involved in the accreditation process for this profession – further information is available from www.cot.co.uk.

Orthoptics

Orthoptists deal with eye disorders such as squints, lazy eye and double vision. They work with ophthalmic surgeons and ophthalmologists (see th chapter on **Optometry and Audiology**). Much of their work is with children. Degree courses usually take three years and registration, after you have graduated, is through the HPC. Further information is available from www.orthoptics.org.uk.

Physiotherapy

The Chartered Society of Physiotherapists (CSP) defines physiotherapy as 'a science-based healthcare profession, which views human movement a central to the health and well being of individuals:

- 'Physiotherapists identify and maximise movement potential through health promotion, preventive healthcare, treatment and rehabilitation. Th core skills used by chartered physiotherapists include manual therapy, therapeutic exercise and the application of electrophysical modalities
- 'Fundamental to the physiotherapist's approach, however, is an appreciation of the psychological, cultural and social factors which influence their clients and the patient's own active role in helping themselves maximise independence and function
- 'It uses physical approaches to promote, maintain and restore physica psychological and social well-being, taking account of variations in health status
- 'It is science-based, committed to extending, applying, evaluating and reviewing the evidence that underpins and informs its practice and delivery
- 'The exercise of clinical judgement and informed interpretation is at it core.'

Source: www.csp.org

Physiotherapists increasingly recognise the value of some of the alterna therapies and some have trained to offer treatments such as acupunctu or Pilates as extensions of their professional skills.

Courses in Physiotherapy take three or four years and are approved by t CSP and the HPC – essential for state registration to practise. Entry is qu competitive – applicants will usually be asked for grades equivalent to between 260 and 320 UCAS tariff points, with sciences featuring strong

Podiatry

This career is also known as **chiropody**. Podiatrists deal with the struct and function of the foot, the diagnosis of foot abnormalities and the administration of appropriate treatment. Practical elements in the trainin include examination, diagnosis and the making and fitting of remedial appliances. Many podiatrists work privately and are self-employed or w in small businesses. As with most careers in this chapter, registration is through the HPC. Further information is available from www.feetforlife.o

Prosthetics and Orthotics

Places on the four-year degree courses for these professions are limited Once again, the professions are regulated by the HPC. **Prosthetics** is th design and fitting of artificial replacements for upper and lower limbs a helping patients come to terms with using them. **Orthotics** is the desig and fitting of appliances such as braces, splints and special footwear to mobility and increase comfort.

Further information is available from www.bapo.com.

Radiography (therapeutic) and Radiotherapy

Therapeutic radiography deals with the use of ionising radiation in the treatment of tissue in the cure or alleviation of cancer and some non-malignant diseases. Therapeutic radiographers are responsible for the accurate delivery of radiation to the affected site and for calculating the precise dosage appropriate for each case. This is different from the rol the *diagnostic* radiographer described the chapter on **Medical Technology**.

eck the degree course carefully to make sure you are applying for one at takes you in the direction you want to go. Again, registration for the ofession is through the HPC after taking the approved degree course. ther information is available from www.sor.org.

eech therapy

eech therapists work mainly, though not exclusively, with children. They al with communication difficulties and sometimes also problems with ing and swallowing. In addition to the usual topics within degree urses related to medicine (anatomy, physiology and so on), Speech erapy courses will include:

- Acoustics
- Audiology
- Ear, nose and throat disorders
- Orthodontics
- Phonetics and linguistics
- Psychology.

e courses last for three or four years and you should apply for one that ccredited by the Royal College of Speech and Language Therapists. Registration to practise (through the HPC) is usually after one year of supervised experience.

Speech therapy opportunities are by no means confined to the NHS or private hospitals. They can be based in special schools or across a local education authority area. Speech therapists may well travel around an area dealing with patients in their own homes or schools. Further information is available from www.rcslt.org.

Salary scales for professionals in this chapter working in the NHS are on a scale from approximately £19,000 to £31,000. Promotion could bring salaries up to £36,400 and very senior posts are paid up to £61,000. (A head of psychology services would be on a salary scale rising to £88,000.)

These examples are based on April 2006 salary scales. At the time of writing this book the public sector unions had not accepted the pay increase of around 2.5%, which had been offered in April 2007.

Many chiropodists work in the private sector and are self-employed. Their earnings vary considerably and depend on the number of hours worked and practice expenses but according to the Society of Chiropodists and Podiatrists earnings are around £40 per hour.

Case Studies

To give you a broad range of opinion about the University of Plymouth, here are comments from a few of our students currently studying our Occupational Therapy, Physiotherapy and Podiatry courses.

Jason – 1st year student, BSc (Hons) in Occupational Therapy

'I'm finding this a highly enjoyable course. There is a lot of hands on practical experience through a range of classroom based workshops to develop our confidence for our practice placements, which are based across the South West. These practice placements have provided me with a range of opportunities and experience across different locations, which I may not have gained if I'd stayed in just one base. My range of experience so far and what is to come in my next two years with Plymouth is reinforcing my decision to study this profession.

'The creative skills development is great and the lecturers are very experienced and approachable. I'd recommend this course to anyone considering a career in Occupational Therapy.'

Jude – 2nd year student, BSc (Hons) in Physiotherapy

'I have had excellent clinical placements throughout Devon and Cornwall. There is also good access to facilities such as clinical skills labs, computing, a four storey new library and electronic journals, and all the staff are very approachable.

'One of the best features of my course is the problem-based learning approach which enables us to learn directly through our placements and individual cases. The interprofessional teaching elements also give us a good range of knowledge in learning alongside other professions.

'Plymouth is a vibrant city; compact and easy to get around on foot. There is a varied social life all around the university with pubs, theatres and cafes, also being close to watersports facilities, country walking and a dry ski slope. It's a lovely base for your studies.'

Chris – 2nd year student, BSc (Hons) in Podiatry

'The best aspect of the course is the amount of hands on experience; it's a great opportunity to put into practice the theory elements of study. The clinical skills facilities are excellent and new, there is also a specialist NHS shared Podiatry clinic where we get to work on real patients and good equipment and materials are at our disposal, leaving me feeling very confident as a trainee professional.

'Considering Plymouth? I would say go for it! Facilities, staff and opportunities are spot on, creating the ideal learning environment; coupled with living in Plymouth as a city makes it the ideal choice!'

Assisting Professional Practice (Occupational and Physiotherapy pathway)

Edge Hill University E42
FdSc: 2 years full-time – B900
Tariff: 40

Clinical Language Sciences (Speech and Language Therapy)

Leeds Metropolitan University L27
BSc (Hons): 3 years full-time – B630
A2: CCC IB: 28 Interview
RCSLT

Creative Expressive Therapies

University of Derby D39
BA (Hons): 3 years full-time – B360
A2: CDD BTEC: DMM SQA: CCCC IB: 26

Healing Arts and Heritage Conservation

University of Derby D39
BA (Hons): 3 years full-time or 4 - 6 years part-time – BD34
Tariff: 160

Healing Arts and History

University of Derby D39
BA (Hons): 3 years full-time or 4 - 6 years part-time – BV31
Tariff: 160

Healing Arts and Law

University of Derby D39
BA (Hons): 3 years full-time or 4 - 6 years part-time – MW19
Tariff: 160

Healing Arts and Marketing

University of Derby D39
BA (Hons): 3 years full-time or 4 - 6 years part-time – BN35
Tariff: 160

Healing Arts and Mathematics

University of Derby D39
BA (Hons): 3 years full-time or 4 - 6 years part-time – BG31
Tariff: 160

Healing Arts and Media Writing

University of Derby D39
BA (Hons): 3 years full-time or 4 - 6 years part-time – BW38
Tariff: 160

Healing Arts and Psychology

University of Derby D39
BA (Hons): 3 years full-time or 4 - 6 years part-time – BC38
Tariff: 160

Healing Arts and Sociology

University of Derby D39
BA (Hons): 3 years full-time or 4 - 6 years part-time – LW39
Tariff: 160

Healing Arts and Theatre Studies

University of Derby D39
BA (Hons): 3 years full-time or 4 - 6 years part-time – WW4X
Tariff: 160

Human Communication (Speech and Language Therapy)

De Montfort University D26
BSc (Hons): 3 years full-time – B620 Y
Tariff: 280

Integrated Therapy in Practice (top-up)

University of Salford S03
BSc (Hons): 1 year full-time or 2 - 3 years part-time – B931
HND, Fd, HE credits: 240, RN, RM, HP

Occupational Therapy

Bournemouth University B50
BSc (Hons): 3 years full-time – B930
Tariff: 180

University of Bradford B56
BSc (Hons): 3 years full-time – B930
Tariff: 240

Bristol, University of the West of England B80
BSc (Hons): 3 years full-time – B920
Tariff: 280 - 320 IB: 28 - 32
COT, HPC

Brunel University B84
BSc (Hons): 3 years full-time or 4 - 6 years part-time – B920
Tariff: 240 IB: 24
COT, HPC

Canterbury Christ Church University C10
BSc (Hons): 3 years full-time – B920
Tariff: 160 IB: 24
HPC

Cardiff University C15
BSc (Hons): 3 years full-time or 4 years part-time – B920
Tariff: 240 IB: 28
COT, HPC

Coventry University C85
BSc (Hons): 3 years full-time or 4 - 6 years part-time
B920
Tariff: 240
COT, HPC

University of Cumbria C99
BSc (Hons): 3 years full-time or 4 years part-time – B
Tariff: 300 IB: 28 Interview

University of Cumbria C99
BSc (Hons): 3 years full-time or 4 years part-time – B
Tariff: 300 IB: 28 Interview
HPC

University of Derby D39
BSc (Hons): 3 years full-time or 5 years part-time – B
A2: CCC BTEC: DDD SQA: BBCCC ILC: AABBCC IB:
COT, HPC

University of East Anglia E14
BSc (Hons): 3 years full-time – B920
A2: CCC SQA: BBBBB ILC: BBBBB IB: 32
COT, HPC

Glasgow Caledonian University G42
BSc (Hons): 4 years full-time – B920
Tariff: 216 Interview
COT, HPC, WFOT

University of Huddersfield H60
BSc (Hons): 3 years full-time – B930
A2: CCC
HPC

University of Liverpool L41
BSc (Hons): 3 years full-time – B920
A2: CCC SQA: BBBCC ILC: BBBCC IB: 26
COT, HPC, WFOT

London South Bank University L75
BSc/BSc (Hons): 4 years part-time
A2: CC
COT, HPC

North East Wales Institute of Higher Education [University of Wales] N56
BSc (Hons): 4 years part-time
A2 HP

University of Northampton N38
BSc (Hons): 3 years full-time or 4 years part-time – B
Tariff: 240
COT, HPC

Northumbria University N77
BSc (Hons): 3 years full-time – B920
Tariff: 240 IB: 26
HPC

Oxford Brookes University O66
BSc (Hons): 3 years full-time or 5 years part-time day
B920
A2: CCC
COT, HPC

University of Plymouth P60
BSc (Hons): 3 years full-time – B920
Tariff: 180 - 220

Queen Margaret University, Edinburg Q25
BSc: 3 years full-time BSc (Hons): 4 years full-time – B920
Tariff: 240 Interview
COT, HPC

bert Gordon University R36
 (Hons): 4 years full-time – B920
BCC SQA: BBCC ILC: BBBC
, HPC, WFOT

iversity of Salford S03
 (Hons): 3 years full-time – B920
ff: 240 IB: 28 Interview
, HPC

effield Hallam University S21
 (Hons): 3 years full-time or 5 years part-time – B920
ff: 240
, HPC

iversity of Southampton S27
(Hons): 3 years full-time – B920
f: 300 IB: 28
T, HPC

iversity of Teesside T20
(Hons): 3 years full-time – B920
f: 240 Interview
HPC

iversity of Ulster U20
(Hons): 3 years full-time – B930 J
AA BTEC: DDD SQA: AAAAA ILC: AAAA IB: 39
HPC, WFOT

k St John University Y75
 (Hons): 3 years full-time or 4 years part-time – B930
: 160 IB: 24 Interview
HPC

cupational Therapy (in-service te)

ventry University C85
(Hons): 3 years full-time or 4 - 6 years part-time
: 240
HPC

ysiotherapy

rnemouth University B50
Hons): 3 years full-time – B160
: 240

versity of Bradford B56
Hons): 3 years full-time – B160
: 300 IB: 32
HPC

versity of Brighton B72
Hons): 3 years full-time – B160
320 IB: 32
HPC

tol, University of the West of England
Hons): 3 years full-time – B160
280 - 340 IB: 32 - 34
HPC

nel University B84
Hons): 3 years full-time or 4 years part-time – B160
300 IB: 30
HPC

iff University C15
Hons): 3 years full-time – B160
340 IB: 30

University of Central Lancashire C30
BSc (Hons): 3 years full-time – B160
Tariff: 300

Colchester Institute [University of Essex] C75
BSc (Hons): 5 years part-time
A2: CC BTEC: PPP
CSP, HPC

Coventry University C85
BSc (Hons): 3 years full-time – B160
Tariff: 300
CSP, HPC

University of Cumbria C99
BSc (Hons): 3 years full-time – B160 C
Tariff: 360 IB: 36 Interview

University of East Anglia E14
BSc (Hons): 3 years full-time – B160
A2: BBB SQA: AABBB ILC: AABBB IB: 34
CSP, HPC

University of East London E28
BSc (Hons): 3 years full-time – B160
Tariff: 280 IB: 28
CSP, HPC

Glasgow Caledonian University G42
BSc (Hons): 4 years full-time – B160
A2: BBC SQA: BBBBB
CSP, HPC

University of Hertfordshire H36
BSc (Hons): 3 years full-time – B160
Tariff: 300 - 320 IB: 30
CSP, HPC

University of Huddersfield H60
BSc (Hons): 3 years full-time – B160
A2: BCC SQA: BBBB IB: 30
CSP, HPC

Keele University K12
BSc (Hons): 3 years full-time – B160
A2: BBB SQA: BBBB - ABBB ILC: BBBBB IB: 32
CSP, HPC

Keele University K12
BSc (Hons): 4 years full-time including foundation year – B1B9
A2: CCC

King's College London (University of London) K60
BSc (Hons): 3 years full-time – B962
A2: BBB SQA: AAABB ILC: AABBBB IB: 32
CSP, HPC

Leeds Metropolitan University L27
BSc (Hons): 3 years full-time – B160
Tariff: 200 - 280 IB: 30
CSP, HPC

University of Liverpool L41
BSc (Hons): 3 years full-time – B160
A2: BBB BTEC: DDM SQA: BBBBB ILC: BBBBB IB: 32
CSP, HPC

Manchester Metropolitan University M40
BSc (Hons): 3 years full-time – B160
Tariff: 300
CSP

Northumbria University N77
BSc (Hons): 3 years full-time – B160
Tariff: 300 IB: 32
CSP, HPC

University of Nottingham N84
BSc (Hons): 3 years full-time – B160
A2: BBB SQA: AABBB ILC: AABBBB IB: 32
CSP, HPC

Oxford Brookes University O66
BSc (Hons): 3 years full-time – B160
A2: BBB ILC: BBBBB IB: 32
CSP, HPC

University of Plymouth P60
BSc (Hons): 3 years full-time – B160
Tariff: 300

Queen Margaret University, Edinburgh Q25
BSc (Hons): 4 years full-time – B160
Tariff: 320 - 336 Interview
CSP, HPC

Robert Gordon University R36
BSc (Hons): 4 years full-time – B160
A2: BBB SQA: BBBB ILC: AABBBB
CSP, HPC

St George's, University of London S49
BSc (Hons): 3 years full-time – B160
Tariff: 240 Interview
HPC

University of Salford S03
BSc (Hons): 3 years full-time or 4 years part-time day – B160
Tariff: 300 IB: 32
CSP, HPC

Sheffield Hallam University S21
BSc (Hons): 3 years full-time – B160
Tariff: 300
CSP, HPC

University of Southampton S27
BSc (Hons): 3 years full-time – B160
Tariff: 370 IB: 33
CSP, HPC

University of Teesside T20
BSc (Hons): 3 years full-time – B160
Tariff: 300 Interview
CSP, HPC

University of Ulster U20
BSc (Hons): 3 years full-time – B160 J
A2: AAA BTEC: DDD SQA: AAAAA ILC: AAAA IB: 39
CSP, HPC

York St John University Y75
BHSc (Hons): 3 years full-time or 4 years part-time – B160
Tariff: 300 IB: 30 Interview

Physiotherapy (including state registration)

University of Birmingham B32
BSc (Hons): 3 - 6 years full-time or 4 - 6 years part-time – B160
Tariff: 320 IB: 33
CSP, HPC

Podiatric Medicine

University of East London E28
BSc (Hons): 3 years full-time or part-time – B330
Tariff: 180
HPC, SCP

Podiatry

University of Brighton B72
BSc (Hons): 3 years full-time – B985
Tariff: 200 IB: 28
HPC, SCP

University of Wales Institute, Cardiff C20
BSc (Hons): 3 years full-time – B985
Tariff: 160
SCP

Glasgow Caledonian University G42
BSc (Hons): 4 years full-time – B985
A2: CD SQA: BBCC
SCP

University of Huddersfield H60
BSc (Hons): 3 years full-time or 5 years part-time – B985
Tariff: 220 Interview
HPC, SCP

Matthew Boulton College of Further and Higher Education [Aston University] M60
BSc (Hons): 3 years full-time – B985
Tariff: 160
SCP

University of Plymouth P60
BSc (Hons): 3 years full-time – B985
Tariff: 160 - 180

Queen Margaret University, Edinburgh Q25
BSc: 3 years full-time BSc (Hons): 4 years full-time – B985
Tariff: 160 - 168 Interview
SCP

University of Salford S03
BSc (Hons): 3 years full-time – B985
Tariff: 240 Interview
SCP

University of Southampton S27
BSc (Hons): 3 years full-time – B985
Tariff: 300 IB: 28
SCP

University of Sunderland S84
BSc (Hons): 4 years full-time including foundation year – B988
Interview

University of Ulster U20
BSc (Hons): 3 years full-time – B985 J
A2: BCC SQA: AABB ILC: BBCCC IB: 30
HPC, SCP

Podiatry (Chiropody)

University of Northampton N38
BSc (Hons): 3 years full-time – B985
Tariff: 160 - 200
HPC, SCP

Podiatry (with foundation year and state registration)

New College Durham [University of Sunderland] N28
BSc (Hons): 4 years full-time including foundation year – B988
Interview
SCP

Podiatry Studies

University of Brighton B72
BSc (Hons): 15 months part-time
HP
HPC, SCP

Prosthetics and Orthotics

University of Salford S03
BSc (Hons): 4 years full-time – B984
Tariff: 240 IB: 28 Interview
BAPO, HPC

University of Strathclyde S78
BSc (Hons): 4 years full-time – B984
A2: CCC SQA: BBBB
BAPO

Radiation Oncology Science

Glasgow Caledonian University G42
BSc (Hons): 4 years full-time – B822
A2: CCD SQA: BBCC ILC: BBBB
HPC, SOR

Radiography (Radiotherapy and Oncology Practice)

Anglia Ruskin University A60
FdSc: 2 years full-time – B890
Interview

Radiography (Therapeutic)

Anglia Ruskin University A60
BSc (Hons): part-time
Interview

City University C60
BSc (Hons): 3 years full-time – B822
A2: CC

University of Portsmouth P80
BSc (Hons): 3 years full-time – B822
Tariff: 280 - 300 Interview
HPC, SOR

Radiography (Therapeutic, extended)

University of Portsmouth P80
BSc (Hons): 4 years full-time including foundation year – B828
Tariff: 260 Interview
HPC

Radiotherapy

Bristol, University of the West of Englan B80
BSc (Hons): 3 years full-time – B822
Tariff: 180 - 220 IB: 24
HPC, SOR

University of Liverpool L41
BSc (Hons): 3 years full-time – B822
A2: CCC BTEC: MMD SQA: BBBCC ILC: BBBCC IB: 26
HPC, SOR

UCE Birmingham C25
BSc (Hons): 3 years full-time or 6 years part-time – B82
Tariff: 220
HPC, SOR

Radiotherapy and Oncology

Cardiff University C15
BSc (Hons): 3 years full-time – B822
Tariff: 260

University of Hertfordshire H36
BSc (Hons): 3 years full-time or 5 years part-time – B82
Tariff: 240

Sheffield Hallam University S21
BSc (Hons): 3 years full-time – B822
Tariff: 160 Interview
HPC, SOR

Radiotherapy and Oncology in Practice

Sheffield Hallam University S21
DipHE: 2 years distance learning
A2: C
HPC, SOR

Rehabilitation

Oxford Brookes University O66
BA (Hons): 2 years full-time or 4 - 6 years part-time – B743
HP
NMC

York St John University Y75
FdA: 2 years full-time or 3 - 4 years part-time – L510
A2: CC Interview

Rehabilitation Studies

University of Wolverhampton W75
BSc (Hons): 3 years full-time or 4 - 6 years part-time – B930
HP

Rehabilitation Studies (top-up)

University of Central Lancashire C30
BSc (Hons): 1 year full-time – B930
Fd, HE credits: 240, HP

ehabilitation Work (Visual npairment)

CE Birmingham C25
HE: 2 years distance learning
: CC

ehabilitative Care

iversity of Glamorgan G14
: (Hons): 2 - 4 years part-time
credits: 120, HP

peech and Language Pathology

iversity of Strathclyde S78
: (Hons): 4 years full-time – B630
BBB SQA: BBBBBB - AABB ILC: BBBBB
LT

peech and Language Science

wcastle University N21
(Hons): 4 years full-time – B620
ABB ILC: AABBB IB: 35
LT

peech and Language Therapy

iversity of Wales Institute, Cardiff C20
(Hons): 4 years full-time – B620
BBB
LT

y University C60
(Hons): 4 years full-time – B620
BBB SQA: AABBB IB: 30
T

iversity of East Anglia E14
(Hons): 3 years full-time – B620
BBB SQA: AABBB IB: 34 Interview

versity of Manchester M20
(Hons): 4 years full-time – B620
ABB BTEC: DDM SQA: AABBB ILC: AAABBB IB: 33
T

Queen Margaret University, Edinburgh Q25
BSc (Hons): 4 years full-time – B630
Tariff: 320 - 324 Interview
HPC, RCSLT

University of Reading R12
BSc (Hons): 4 years full-time – B690
Tariff: 320 IB: 32
RCSLT

College of St Mark & St John [University of Exeter] M50
BSc (Hons): 3 years full-time – B620
Tariff: 240 - 280
RCSLT

UCE Birmingham C25
BSc (Hons): 3 - 6 years full-time or 6 years part-time – B620
Tariff: 260 HP
HPC, RCSLT

University of Ulster U20
BSc (Hons): 3 years full-time – B632 J
A2: AAA BTEC: DDD SQA: AAAAA ILC: AAAA IB: 39
HPC, RCSLT

Speech Pathology and Therapy

Manchester Metropolitan University M40
BSc (Hons): 3 years full-time – B630
Tariff: 300 IB: 32
RCSLT

Speech Science

University of Sheffield S18
BMedSci (Hons): 4 years full-time – B620
A2: ABB SQA: AAAB ILC: AABBB IB: 33
RCSLT

Speech Sciences

University College London, University of London U80
BSc (Hons): 4 years full-time – B620
A2: BBB - ABB BTEC: DDM IB: 32 - 34
RCSLT

Sport Rehabilitation

St Mary's University College, Twickenham S64
BSc (Hons): 3 years full-time – C602
Tariff: 160

Sport Rehabilitation and Injury Prevention

Middlesex University M80
BSc (Hons): 4 years sandwich – C610 E
Tariff: 160 - 220

Sports Rehabilitation

University of Hull H72
BSc (Hons): 3 years full-time – C602
Tariff: 280 IB: 28

University of Salford S03
BSc (Hons): 3 years full-time or 4 years distance learning – BC96
Tariff: 300 IB: 29

Therapeutic Radiography

Queen Margaret University, Edinburgh Q25
BSc (Hons): 4 years full-time – B822
Tariff: 180 Interview
SOR

Therapeutic Radiotherapy

St George's, University of London S49
BSc (Hons): 3 years full-time – B822
A2: CCD BTEC: DDM

Veterinary Science

Including:
Animal Behaviour
Animal Health
Animal Husbandry
Animal Nursing
Animal Science
Animal Welfare
Equine Studies
Veterinary Biochemistry/Veterinary Microbiology
Veterinary Medicine
Veterinary Physiology

What would you study?

Veterinary medicine/science

Courses are of a similar length to medicine degrees with the same opportunity to take an intercalated degree at the end of the pre-clinical phase. The course at Cambridge takes six years, and the remainder take five. The actual degrees offered by veterinary schools are Bachelor of Veterinary Science (BVetSci) or similar. At the end of your course you will gain registration with the Royal College of Veterinary Surgeons (RCVS).

The biology- and chemistry-based studies which feature (to a greater or lesser extent) in most of the courses listed in this directory are strongly represented in Veterinary Medicine/Science courses. Like medical degrees, veterinary degrees are divided into the pre-clinical and clinical phases. As mentioned above, the pre-clinical, theoretical phase can be extended by one year to allow you to turn it into an intercalated degree, probably BSc in Physiology or similar.

Other courses in this chapter

The courses divide into two main groups – those more focused on animal care and those focusing on the underlying science. The first group includes equine studies and animal behaviour/science/welfare and are available at degree and Foundation degree level. They still include some science, but look more at:

- Animal needs (in terms of space, bedding, ventilation and so on)
- Issues connected with prevention of infection
- Nutrition
- Spotting signs of health problems
- Training.

Courses falling into the second group – veterinary biochemistry/microbiology/physiology – are mainly offered at degree level and focus on the sciences connected with animal care. They look at subjects like:

- Animal disease
- Causes of disease
- Issues around prevention.

Getting in

Veterinary medicine/science

There are six veterinary schools in the UK. Competition for places is tough. With this in mind it is well worth re-reading the advice from Geraldine Giannopoulos of Edinburgh University quoted in the **Introduction** to this guide, particularly with regard to work experience. Each university decides on its own entry requirements. You can see the range of UCAS points asked by each one by consulting the course listings on the following pages.

Veterinary Medicine/Science applications may make up only four of your allowance of six UCAS course choices. If your UCAS choices include this subject, you must register your completed UCAS application by 15 October of the calendar year before you wish to start your course.

Admissions tests

For entry to some courses you will be required to take an entry test in addition to examination grades. This has been designed to help admissions staff by measuring general and personal skills and abilities not directly assessed in academic examinations. Institutions state clearly in their prospectuses whether or not applicants must take a test, which is known as the **BioMedical Admissions Test (BMAT)**. This is a 2 hour paper test consisting of multiple choice and essay questions. It costs £26 and takes place at the beginning of November. You have to register by 29 September. For more information, see www.bmat.org.uk

It is possible to access Veterinary Medicine/Science courses if you have a degree in a related subject such as physiology, anatomy or one of the veterinary variations on these listed in this chapter. However, this is by no means a guaranteed way in to the veterinary science courses and, at the best of times, chances of success are far lower than if you apply directly from school. Another issue on this point is that you will be able to access the normal student financial support package for your first degree, but you will need to check the support which is available to help you through wh would become your second degree.

Other courses in this chapter

Entry requirements for Foundation courses in equine studies and animal behaviour/science/welfare tend to be in the region of 40–100 UCAS tariff points. However, many Foundation courses exercise a more flexible admissions procedure which enables them to take into account factors such as work experience in their entrance requirements and which cann therefore be expressed as part of the UCAS tariff framework. Requireme for veterinary biochemistry/microbiology/physiology can be higher.

Graduate outlook

Veterinary medicine/science

Well, you could read the James Herriot books and yes, they will give you an idea of the range of animals that vets have to deal with – from budgerigars to bulls. They also tell you quite accurately how the animals owners are often key to the cure of any problems being experienced by animals themselves. Communication skills are a core requirement for a – especially if the animal involved is a terminally ill, much-loved pet and euthanasia is the likely outcome.

What the Herriot books don't cover is the increasingly sophisticated and technical range of treatments that vets have in their armoury these days reinforcing the need for a scientific background. They may also glamoris the vet's role somewhat. For example, it is a professional requirement th every vet is obliged to deal with any emergency for any animal at any time. It is a 24/7 job that can at times be demanding – even with the support of professional colleagues in a practice. For example, when Nick Barradale was interviewed for the case study at the end of this section, was unable to make the Sunday morning interview time that had been arranged. He then got caught up in a series of call-outs which kept him working all through the night and it was a few days before the interview actually happened.

Opportunities exist for vets to focus their careers on work with small animals, food-producing animals or horses. Large practices allow vets to continue working across the full range if they prefer. There are some opportunities for vets to work with the more exotic animals in zoos or wildlife parks, possibly as an employee of the zoo or as a vet in a practi that has such an organisation as a client.

Vets do not always work in professional practices. There are opportuniti for work:

- In the public sector (for organisations such as the Food Standards Agency, the Department for Environment, Food and Rural Affairs (DEFRA) and the Veterinary Medicines Directorate). The main aim of work here is to protect public health
- In universities, both in teaching and in research
- In other research organisations, whether publicly or privately funded sometimes involved with research into animal/human cross-over iss in diseases
- With pharmaceutical companies, either in developing animal medicir or on the marketing side
- With other organisations such as the RSPCA, PDSA or overseas organisations.

The profession is regulated by the Royal College of Veterinary Surgeons (www.rcvs.org.uk), which is responsible for ensuring the appropriate standards and content of Veterinary Science degree courses, as well as offering further postgraduate courses and training to help practising ve keep up to date or develop their career in a specialist direction.

ther courses in this chapter

e other courses in this section could lead to jobs like:

Animal inspector – carries out animal rescues, takes cases to court, checks conditions within animal establishments (like auctions and kennels) and administers first aid.

Animal technician – responsible for the welfare of animals used in universities and research establishments for biomedical research.

Equine/horse work – for example *race horse trainer* for which you will need to build experience, then gain a licence from the Jockey Club, or *farrier* for which you will need to complete a four-year apprenticeship period, gaining registration with the Farriers' Registration Council and passing the diploma of the Worshipful Company of Farriers.

Veterinary nurse – assists vets in their work by helping them to treat animals. To do this job you will need to complete a two-year Veterinary Nursing training scheme recognised by the Royal College of Veterinary Surgeons.

- **Zoo keeper** – working in safari, wildlife or birdlife parks, caring for or treating animals and talking to visitors about them.

The more scientific courses like veterinary biochemistry/microbiology/ physiology could lead to:

- Fast-track veterinary medicine/science degrees
- Research posts
- Work with veterinary product/pharmaceuticals companies and some government agencies.

What would you earn?

It's difficult to generalise as there are so many different types of careers involved and so many different sizes of veterinary practices. As a guide, however, you could expect around £20,000 in your first year as a practising veterinary surgeon. Some experienced vets earn over £65,000. Vets working in research could earn between £20,000 and £70,000. A veterinary nurse might earn between £15,000 and £22,000 depending on experience, and an animal inspector between £16,000 and £30,000.

Case Study

Nick Barradale

Nick graduated in 2005 with a degree in Veterinary Science from Liverpool University.

'I applied, in my sixth form, for my quota of vet schools. I remember my first interview vividly even though it was over six years ago now. They asked a load of questions about professional ethics. I was totally unprepared for it and, unsurprisingly, did not get an offer – but it meant that I was better-prepared by the time I got to the interview at Liverpool. They were keen to know about the work experience I had managed to undertake during the sixth form.

'I recommend reading articles from veterinary magazines and taking notes about what happened on work experience so it is all fresh in your mind at interview. I took A levels in chemistry, biology and mathematics and knew that I would have to get the best grades – that meant some extra tuition and revision for the exams. It paid off and I got the grades I needed.

'The science was certainly useful when I started at Liverpool. The first three years included subjects like anatomy, veterinary biology, biochemistry, metabolism and zoology. On the more practical side, we covered topics such as animal husbandry – looking at the requirements of cattle stock – space, ventilation, bedding and so on. The second year continued the first-year topics and introduced pharmacology where we had to learn all the drug names. The third year was tough. We got into pathology and looked at every organ and the diseases that can affect it. Parasitology was also a third-year subject.

'That completed the theoretical pre-clinical stage. We had exams throughout the course. The whole course was laced with work experience, even to the extent of cutting down our vacations to around four weeks per year. That meant there was no time for the traditional student vacation job and people's debts were soaring.

'Years four and five put all the theory into context for us. Liverpool University has a large animal field station out on the Wirral so we got to work in the countryside with the sort of animals that I wanted to specialise in. We rotated around three different activities – equine, large animals and small animals. This whole experience really brought the theory to life and made it seem much clearer. The practical approach continued through the fifth and final year and we also had clinical tutorials. I took 'elective' specialisms dealing with issues such as bovine reproduction and cattle herd health. By way of a change there were times when we had actors in to help us with developing communication skills – with the animal owners, that is!

'The vets were a really tight and supportive group, both academically and socially. Partying could be hectic at times. The course was thoroughly enjoyable and my choice of large animal specialisms paid off with a job in a practice looking after large animals in Cheshire.'

Animal Behaviour

Anglia Ruskin University A60
BSc (Hons): 3 years full-time or 6 years part-time – C120 C
Tariff: 220 IB: 24

University of Chester C55
BSc (Hons): 3 years full-time – D326
Tariff: 240 IB: 30

University of Exeter E84
BSc (Hons): 3 years full-time – D390
A2: BCC - BBB

Liverpool John Moores University L51
BSc (Hons): 3 years full-time or 4 years sandwich or 4 years part-time – C301
Tariff: 220

Manchester Metropolitan University M40
BSc (Hons): 3 years full-time

University of Sheffield S18
BSc (Hons): 3 years full-time – C120
A2: ABB SQA: AAAB ILC: AABBB IB: 33

University of Sheffield S18
MBioSci: 4 years full-time – C129
A2: ABB SQA: AAAB ILC: AABBB IB: 33

Animal Behaviour and Animal Welfare

Anglia Ruskin University A60
BSc (Hons): 3 years full-time or 6 years part-time – D390 C
Tariff: 220 IB: 24

Animal Behaviour and Applied Social Science

University of Chester C55
BSc (Hons): 3 years full-time – DL33
Tariff: 240 IB: 26

Animal Behaviour with Applied Social Science

University of Chester C55
BSc (Hons): 3 years full-time – D3L3
Tariff: 240 IB: 26

Animal Behaviour and Biology

University of Chester C55
BSc (Hons): 3 years full-time – DC31
Tariff: 240 IB: 26

Animal Behaviour with Biology

University of Chester C55
BSc (Hons): 3 years full-time – D3C1
Tariff: 240 IB: 26

Animal Behaviour and Communication Studies

University of Chester C55
BA (Hons): 3 years full-time – DP33
Tariff: 240 IB: 26

Animal Behaviour with Communication Studies

University of Chester C55
BA (Hons): 3 years full-time – D3P3
Tariff: 240 IB: 26

Animal Behaviour and Computer Science

University of Chester C55
BSc (Hons): 3 years full-time – DG34
Tariff: 240 IB: 26

Animal Behaviour with Computer Science

University of Chester C55
BSc (Hons): 3 years full-time – D3G4
Tariff: 240 IB: 26

Animal Behaviour and Ecology and Conservation

Anglia Ruskin University A60
BSc (Hons): 3 years full-time or 6 years part-time – DD34 C
Tariff: 200 IB: 24

Animal Behaviour and International Development Studies

University of Chester C55
BSc (Hons): 3 years full-time – DL39
Tariff: 240 IB: 26

Animal Behaviour with International Development Studies

University of Chester C55
BSc (Hons): 3 years full-time – D3L9
Tariff: 240 IB: 26

Animal Behaviour with Marketing

University of Chester C55
BA (Hons): 3 years full-time – D3N5
Tariff: 240 IB: 26

Animal Behaviour and Mathematics

University of Chester C55
BSc (Hons): 3 years full-time – DG31
Tariff: 240 IB: 26

Animal Behaviour with Mathematics

University of Chester C55
BSc (Hons): 3 years full-time – D3G1
Tariff: 240 IB: 26

Animal Behaviour and Psychology

Anglia Ruskin University A60
BSc (Hons): 3 years full-time – C1C8 C
Tariff: 220 IB: 26

University of Chester C55
BSc (Hons): 3 years full-time – DC38
Tariff: 240 IB: 26

Animal Behaviour with Psychology

University of Chester C55
BSc (Hons): 3 years full-time – D3C8
Tariff: 240 IB: 26

Animal Behaviour Science

University of Lincoln L39
BSc (Hons): 3 years full-time – D321 L
Tariff: 240 IB: 26

Animal Behaviour with Theology an[d] Religious Studies

University of Chester C55
BA (Hons): 3 years full-time – D3V6
Tariff: 240 IB: 26

Animal Behaviour with Tourism

University of Chester C55
BA (Hons): 3 years full-time – D3N8
Tariff: 240 IB: 26

Animal Behaviour and Welfare

Bournemouth University B50
FdSc: 2 years full-time – D328
Tariff: 80

University of Chester C55
BSc (Hons): 3 years full-time – D325
Tariff: 240 IB: 30

Guildford College of Further and High[er] Education G90
FdA: 2 years full-time or 2 - 3 years part-time – CD33
Tariff: 100

Harper Adams University College H12
BSc (Hons): 3 years full-time or 4 years sandwich – D3[…]
Tariff: 160 - 240

Hartpury College [Bristol, University of the West of England] ▲
BSc (Hons): 3 years full-time – D329 A
Tariff: 160 IB: 28

artpury College [Bristol, University of e West of England] ▲

Sc: 2 years full-time – D328 A
iff: 80 IB: 24

ngston Maurward College ournemouth University] ▲

Sc: 2 years full-time or up to 6 years part-time – D390 K
iff: 80

yerscough College [University of entral Lancashire] M99

c (Hons): 3 years full-time – D320
EE BTEC: MMM ILC: CCC IB: 26

nimal Behaviour and Wildlife iology

glia Ruskin University A60

(Hons): 3 years full-time or 6 years part-time – 33 C
ff: 200 IB: 24

nimal Behavioural Management op-up)

rkshire College of Agriculture uckinghamshire Chilterns University llege] ▲

(Hons): 1 year full-time or 2 years part-time – 20 C
), Fd

nimal Behavioural Science and elfare

dlow College [University of eenwich] ▲

c: 2 years full-time or 4 years part-time – D322 H
f: 60

nimal Biology and Art and Design

iversity of Worcester W80

Hons)/BSc (Hons): 3 years full-time – CW32
f: 160

nimal Biology and Business anagement

iversity of Worcester W80

Hons)/BSc (Hons): 3 years full-time – CN22
f: 160

nimal Biology and Computing

versity of Worcester W80

(Hons): 3 years full-time – CG25
: 160

imal Biology and Creative Digital edia

versity of Worcester W80

Hons)/BSc (Hons): 3 years full-time – CWH2
: 160

Animal Biology and Design Communication

University of Worcester W80

BA (Hons)/BSc (Hons): 3 years full-time – DW32
Tariff: 160 Interview

Animal Biology and Drama and Performance Studies

University of Worcester W80

BA (Hons)/BSc (Hons): 3 years full-time – CW24
Tariff: 160

Animal Biology and Ecology

University of Worcester W80

BSc (Hons): 3 years full-time – CC31
Tariff: 120

Animal Biology and Education Studies

University of Worcester W80

BA (Hons)/BSc (Hons): 3 years full-time – CX23
Tariff: 120

Animal Biology and Environmental Management

University of Worcester W80

BSc (Hons): 3 years full-time – CN29
Tariff: 120

Animal Biology and Geography

University of Worcester W80

BSc (Hons): 3 years full-time – CF28
Tariff: 140

Animal Biology and Health Studies

University of Worcester W80

BSc (Hons): 3 years full-time – CL25
Tariff: 120

Animal Biology and History

University of Worcester W80

BA (Hons)/BSc (Hons): 3 years full-time – CV21
Tariff: 140

Animal Biology and Human Biology

University of Worcester W80

BSc (Hons): 3 years full-time – CC3C
Tariff: 140

Animal Biology and Human Geography

University of Worcester W80

BA (Hons)/BSc (Hons): 3 years full-time – CL37
Tariff: 140

Animal Biology and Interactive Digital Media

University of Worcester W80

BA (Hons)/BSc (Hons): 3 years full-time – DG34
Tariff: 160

Animal Biology and Media and Cultural Studies

University of Worcester W80

BA (Hons)/BSc (Hons): 3 years full-time – CP23
Tariff: 160

Animal Biology and Physical Education

University of Worcester W80

BSc (Hons): 3 years full-time – DX33
Tariff: 200

Animal Biology and Physical Geography

University of Worcester W80

BSc (Hons): 3 years full-time – FC83
Tariff: 140

Animal Biology and Plant Science

University of Worcester W80

BSc (Hons): 3 years full-time – CC32
Tariff: 120

Animal Biology and Psychology

University of Worcester W80

BSc (Hons): 3 years full-time – CC28
Tariff: 160
BPS

Animal Biology and Sociology

University of Worcester W80

BA (Hons)/BSc (Hons): 3 years full-time – CL23
Tariff: 160

Animal Biology and Sports Coaching Science

University of Worcester W80

BSc (Hons): 3 years full-time – DC36
Tariff: 240

Animal Biology and Sports Studies

University of Worcester W80

BSc (Hons): 3 years full-time – CC26
Tariff: 200

Animal Biology and Time-Based Digital Media

University of Worcester W80
BA (Hons)/BSc (Hons): 3 years full-time – DGH4
Tariff: 160

Animal Biology and Visual Arts

University of Worcester W80
BA (Hons)/BSc (Hons): 3 years full-time – DW3F
Tariff: 160

Animal Care and Management

University of Wolverhampton W75
BSc (Hons): 3 years full-time or 4 years sandwich or 5 - 6 years part-time – D328
Tariff: 160 - 220 IB: 24

Animal Care Science (top-up)

Pershore Group of Colleges [University of Worcester] ▲
BSc: 1 year full-time – D329 P
HND

University of Worcester W80
BSc (Hons): 1 year full-time – D329
HND

Animal Conservation and Biodiversity

Hadlow College [University of Greenwich] ▲
FdSc: 2 years full-time or 4 years part-time – D390 H
Tariff: 60

Animal Conservation Science

University of Central Lancashire C30
BSc (Hons): 3 years full-time – D327 P
Tariff: 240

Animal Health and Welfare

NESCOT [Open University] N49
FdSc: 2 years full-time or 3 years part-time day and block-release – D330
A2: EE

Park Lane College [Leeds Metropolitan University] L21
FdSc: 2 years full-time – D320
A2: E IB: 20 Interview

Animal Industry Management (top-up)

Berkshire College of Agriculture [Buckinghamshire Chilterns University College] ▲
BA (Hons): 1 year full-time – D421 C
HND, Fd

Animal Management

Askham Bryan College [University of Leeds] A70
FdSc: 2 years full-time – D301
Tariff: 140

University of Greenwich G70
BSc (Hons): 3 years full-time – D300
Tariff: 180

Guildford College of Further and Higher Education G90
FdA: 2 years full-time – D328 M
Tariff: 100

Hadlow College [University of Greenwich] ▲
BSc (Hons): 3 years full-time or 4 years part-time – D300 H
Tariff: 160

Kingston Maurward College [Bournemouth University] ▲
FdSc: 2 years full-time – D328 K
Tariff: 80

Shuttleworth College [University of Essex]
FdSc: 2 years full-time
A2: C BTEC: MMM

Sparsholt College, Hampshire [University of Portsmouth] S34
FdSc: 2 years full-time – D329
Tariff: 40

Sparsholt College, Hampshire [University of Portsmouth] S34
BSc (Hons): 3 years full-time – D320
Tariff: 120

University Campus Suffolk [University of East Anglia, University of Essex] S82
FdSc: 2 years full-time or 3 - 4 years part-time – D420 O
Tariff: 60 - 120

Weston College [Bristol, University of the West of England] ▲
FdSc: 2 years full-time – D302 E
Tariff: 60 - 120

Writtle College [University of Essex] W85
FdSc: 2 years full-time – D391
Tariff: 60 IB: 24 Interview

Writtle College [University of Essex] W85
BSc (Hons): 3 years full-time – D291
Tariff: 160 IB: 24 Interview

Animal Management and Behaviour

Bishop Burton College [University of Lincoln] B37
FdSc: 2 years full-time – DC33
Tariff: 80

Animal Management, Health and Welfare (top-up)

Harper Adams University College H12
BSc/BSc (Hons): 2 years full-time – D740
HND

Animal Management and Science

Askham Bryan College [University of Leeds] A70
BSc (Hons): 3 years full-time – D302
Tariff: 220

Animal Management (top-up)

Askham Bryan College [University of Leeds] A70
BSc (Hons): 1 year full-time – D300
HND, Fd

Guildford College of Further and Higher Education G90
BSc (Hons): 1 year full-time or 1 - 2 years part-time – D3N2 M
HND, Fd

Writtle College [University of Essex] W8
BSc: 1 year full-time – D302
HND, Fd

Animal Management and Welfare

Brooksby Melton College [University of Lincoln] ▲
FdSc: 2 years full-time – D329 M
Tariff: 60

University of Lincoln L39
BSc (Hons): 3 years full-time – D426 L
Tariff: 180 IB: 24

Animal Science

University of Wales, Aberystwyth A40
BSc (Hons): 3 years full-time – D306
Tariff: 240

Bournemouth University B50
BSc (Hons): 3 years full-time – D305
Tariff: 80

Bournemouth University B50
FdSc: 2 years full-time – DN00
Tariff: 80

Bridgwater College [Bournemouth University] ▲
FdSc: 2 years full-time – D300 G
Tariff: 80

Bridgwater College [Bournemouth University] ▲
BSc (Hons): 3 years full-time – D305 G
Tariff: 80

Harper Adams University College H12
BSc (Hons): 3 years full-time or 4 years sandwich – D3
Tariff: 220 - 280

Hartpury College [Bristol, University of the West of England] ▲
BSc (Hons): 3 years full-time or 4 years sandwich – D320 A
Tariff: 160 IB: 28

artpury College [Bristol, University of e West of England] ▲

Sc: 2 years full-time – D321 A
iff: 80 IB: 24

niversity of Nottingham N84

c (Hons): 3 years full-time – D320
: CCC - BCC ILC: CCCCD IB: 24 - 30

ottingham Trent University N91

c (Hons): 3 years full-time or 4 years sandwich – D320
iff: 180

umpton College [University of ighton] ▲

Sc: 2 years full-time or 3 years part-time – D300 P
iff: 80 IB: 24

iversity of Plymouth P60

c (Hons): 3 years full-time or 4 years sandwich – D300
ff: 200 IB: 24

iversity of Reading R12

c (Hons): 3 years full-time – D320
ff: 280 IB: 30

ottish Agricultural College, Edinburgh niversity of Edinburgh] S01

: 3 years full-time BSc (Hons): 4 years full-time –
0 Z
CCD SQA: BBBC

ittle College [University of Essex] W85

c: 2 years full-time – D300
f: 60

ittle College [University of Essex] W85

(Hons): 3 years full-time – D321
f: 160 IB: 24

imal Science (Animal Husbandry)

chy College [University of Plymouth]
5

: 2 years full-time
: 80

imal Science (Behaviour)

chy College [University of Plymouth]
5

: 2 years full-time – D322
: 80

imal Science (Behaviour and elfare)

versity of Plymouth P60

(Hons): 3 years full-time or 4 years sandwich – D328
: 200

imal Science (Bird Biology)

chy College [University of Plymouth]
5

: 2 years full-time – D390
: 80

Animal Science, Care and Management

Canterbury Christ Church University C10

BSc (Hons): 3 years full-time or 6 years part-time – D300
A2: CC BTEC: MM SQA: CCCC ILC: CCCCC IB: 24

Animal Science (Companion Animal Studies)

Newcastle University N21

BSc (Hons): 3 years full-time – D300
A2: BBC - BBB BTEC: DMM - DDM ILC: BBBBB IB: 30 - 32

Animal Science (Deferred Choice)

Newcastle University N21

BSc (Hons): 3 years full-time – C305
A2: BBC - BBB BTEC: DMM - DDM ILC: BBBBB IB: 30 - 32

Animal Science (Equine) (top-up)

University of Plymouth P60

BSc (Hons): 2 years full-time – D301
HND, Fd

Animal Science with European Studies (Biosciences)

University of Nottingham N84

BSc (Hons): 4 years full-time with time abroad – D4RY
A2: CCC - BCC ILC: CCCCD IB: 24 - 30

Animal Science (Exotic)

Nottingham Trent University N91

BSc: 3 years full-time or 4 years sandwich – D300
Tariff: 180

Animal Science (Livestock Technology)

Newcastle University N21

BSc (Hons): 3 years full-time – D320
A2: BBC - BBB BTEC: DMM - DDM ILC: BBBBB IB: 30 - 32

Animal Science and Management

Wiltshire College [Royal Agricultural College] W74

FdSc: 2 years full-time – D300 L
Tariff: 80

Animal Science and Management (top-up)

Wiltshire College [Royal Agricultural College] ▲

BSc (Hons): 1 year full-time – D426 B
HND, Interview

Animal Science (top-up)

Writtle College [University of Essex] W85

BSc: 1 year full-time – D390
HND, Fd

Animal Science (Veterinary Nursing)

Duchy College [University of Plymouth] D55

FdSc: 2 years full-time – D311
Tariff: 80

Animal Science and Welfare

Easton College [University of East Anglia] ▲

FdSc: 2 years part-time – D300
Tariff: 80 IB: 24

Animal Studies

Nottingham Trent University N91

FdSc: 2 years full-time or 3 years sandwich – D325
Tariff: 120

Animal Studies with Management

Berkshire College of Agriculture [Buckinghamshire Chilterns University College] ▲

FdA: 2 years full-time – D3N2 C
A2: E

Animal Welfare

Anglia Ruskin University A60

BSc (Hons): 3 years full-time or 6 years part-time – D328 C
Tariff: 220 IB: 24

Warwickshire College, Royal Leamington Spa, Rugby and Moreton Morell [Coventry University] W25

BSc (Hons): 3 years full-time or 4 years sandwich – D329
Tariff: 160

Animal Welfare and Behaviour

University of Bristol B78

BSc (Hons): 3 years full-time – D390
A2: BBB - ABB BTEC: DDM SQA: AAAAB IB: 33

Animal Welfare (Management)

Warwickshire College, Royal Leamington Spa, Rugby and Moreton Morell [Coventry University] W25

Fd: 2 years full-time or 3 years sandwich – D390
Tariff: 80

Animal Welfare and Management

Harper Adams University College H12

FdSc: 2 years full-time – D320
Tariff: 40 - 100

Animal Welfare and Psychology

Anglia Ruskin University A60
BSc (Hons): 3 years full-time – D3C8 C
Tariff: 220 IB: 26

Animal Welfare (Science and Health)

Warwickshire College, Royal Leamington Spa, Rugby and Moreton Morell [Coventry University] W25
FdSc: 2 years full-time or 3 years part-time – D328
Tariff: 80

Animal Welfare (top-up)

Moulton College [University of Northampton] ▲
BSc (Hons): 1 year full-time – D321 M
HND

Applied Animal Behaviour and Training

Bishop Burton College [University of Lincoln] B37
BSc (Hons): 3 years full-time or part-time – C125
Tariff: 140

Applied Animal Science

Bishop Burton College [University of Lincoln] B37
BSc (Hons): 3 years full-time or part-time – D422
Tariff: 140

Scottish Agricultural College, Ayr S01
BSc (Hons): 3 years full-time – D300 Y
A2: CC SQA: BCC

Applied Animal Studies

University of Northampton N38
FdSc: 2 years full-time – D302
Tariff: 40

University of Northampton N38
BSc (Hons): 3 years full-time or 6 years part-time – D300
Tariff: 180 - 220

Applied Animal Studies (top-up)

University of Northampton N38
BSc (Hons): 1 year full-time or 2 years part-time – D301
HND

Applied Bioscience (Animal Science)

Scottish Agricultural College, Ayr [University of Glasgow] S01
BSc: 3 years full-time BSc (Hons): 4 years full-time – C300 Y
A2: CC SQA: BCC HND

Scottish Agricultural College, Edinburgh [University of Glasgow] S01
BSc: 3 years full-time BSc (Hons): 4 years full-time – C300 Z
A2: CC SQA: BCC HND

Bioveterinary Science

Harper Adams University College H12
BSc (Hons): 4 years sandwich – D300
Tariff: 220 - 240

Hartpury College [Bristol, University of the West of England] ▲
BSc (Hons): 3 years full-time – D390 A
Tariff: 200 IB: 30

Hartpury College [Bristol, University of the West of England] ▲
FdSc: 2 years full-time or 3 years part-time – CD93 A
Tariff: 100 IB: 24

University of Liverpool L41
BSc (Hons): 3 years full-time – D900
A2: BBB ILC: BBBBB IB: 32

Clinical Veterinary Nursing

Myerscough College [University of Central Lancashire] M99
BSc (Hons): 3 years part-time
HE credits: 120, HP

Equine Behaviour and Training

Duchy College [University of Plymouth] D55
FdSc: 2 years full-time or 5 years part-time – D426
Tariff: 100 - 120

Equine Behaviour and Welfare

Bournemouth University B50
FdSc: 2 years full-time
Tariff: 80

Equine Breeding and Stud Management

Writtle College [University of Essex] W85
FdSc: 2 years full-time – DN4F
Tariff: 40

Writtle College [University of Essex] W85
BSc (Hons): 3 years full-time – D426
Tariff: 160 IB: 24 Interview

Equine Breeding and Stud Management (top-up)

Writtle College [University of Essex] W85
BSc: 1 year full-time – DNKG
HND, Fd

Equine Dental Science

Hartpury College [Bristol, University of the West of England] ▲
BSc (Hons): 3 years full-time – D220 A
Tariff: 200 IB: 30

Equine Management

Askham Bryan College [University of Leeds] A70
FdSc: 2 years full-time – D422
Tariff: 140

College of Agriculture, Food and Rural Enterprise [University of Ulster] A45
BSc (Hons): 3 years full-time – D322
Tariff: 240 IB: 28

College of Agriculture, Food and Rural Enterprise [University of Ulster] A45
FdSc: 2 years full-time – 422D
Tariff: 40

University of Derby Buxton D39
FdA: 2 years full-time – D422 U
A2 BTEC SQA ILC

Easton College [University of East Anglia] ▲
FdSc: 2 years full-time or 3 years part-time – D426
Tariff: 80 IB: 24

Hadlow College [University of Greenwich] ▲
FdSc: 2 years full-time or 3 years part-time – NDF4 H
Tariff: 80

Hadlow College [University of Greenwich] ▲
BSc (Hons): 3 years full-time or 4 years sandwich – D422 H
Tariff: 180 Interview

Moulton College [University of Northampton] ▲
FdSc: 2 years full-time – D422 M
Tariff: 60 - 80

University of Northampton N38
FdSc: 2 years full-time – D422
Tariff: 40

University of Northampton N38
BSc (Hons): 3 years full-time or 6 years part-time – D4
Tariff: 180 - 220

Equine Management (Business)

Royal Agricultural College R54
BSc (Hons): 3 years full-time – D490
Tariff: 200

Equine Management Business and Equitation

Bishop Burton College [University of Lincoln] B37
FdA: 2 years full-time – ND24
Tariff: 80

quine Management with Equitation

skham Bryan College [University of eeds] A70
Sc: 2 years full-time – D426
iff: 60

quine Management (Science)

oyal Agricultural College R54
: (Hons): 3 years full-time – D491
iff: 200

quine Management (top-up)

skham Bryan College [University of eeds] A70
: (Hons): 1 year full-time – D425
D

uildford College of Further and Higher lucation G90
(Hons): 1 year full-time or 2 years part-time – D4N2
ff: 100

iversity of Northampton N38
: (Hons): 1 year full-time – D427
D

quine Performance

rtpury College [Bristol, University of West of England] ▲
: 2 years full-time – D427 A
f: 100

iversity Campus Suffolk [University of st Anglia, University of Essex] S82
: 2 years full-time – E422 0
f: 160 IB: 24

quine Science

iversity of Wales, Aberystwyth A40
(Hons): 3 years full-time – D322
f: 240

ingdon and Witney College [Oxford okes University] ▲
(Hons): 3 years full-time – D322
f: 220

glia Ruskin University A60
(Hons): 3 years full-time – D422
f: 200 IB: 24

hop Burton College [University of coln] B37
(Hons): 3 years full-time – D428
: 140 HND

dlow College [University of eenwich] ▲
: 2 years full-time or 3 years part-time – D426 H
: 80

tpury College [Bristol, University of West of England] ▲
: 2 years full-time – D426 A
: 100 IB: 24

Hartpury College [Bristol, University of the West of England] ▲
BSc (Hons): 3 years full-time or 4 years sandwich – D334 A
Tariff: 200 IB: 30

University of Lincoln L39
BSc (Hons): 3 years full-time – D320 L
Tariff: 240 IB: 26

Myerscough College [University of Central Lancashire] M99
FdSc: 2 years full-time or 3 years part-time – D422
Tariff: 80

Warwickshire College, Royal Leamington Spa, Rugby and Moreton Morell [Coventry University] W25
Fd: 2 years full-time or 3 years sandwich – D422
Tariff: 80

Warwickshire College, Royal Leamington Spa, Rugby and Moreton Morell [Coventry University] W25
BSc (Hons): 3 years full-time or 4 years sandwich – D323
Tariff: 160

Writtle College [University of Essex] W85
FdSc: 2 years full-time or 3 years sandwich – D428
Tariff: 60 IB: 24

Writtle College [University of Essex] W85
BSc (Hons): 3 years full-time – D322
Tariff: 160 IB: 24 - 28

Equine Science (International Thoroughbred Management)

Abingdon and Witney College [Oxford Brookes University] ▲
BSc (Hons): 4 years sandwich – D422
Tariff: 220

Equine Science and Management (Behaviour and Welfare)

Myerscough College [University of Central Lancashire] M99
BSc (Hons): 3 years full-time – DD34
Tariff: 120 IB: 26

Equine Science and Management (Physiology)

Myerscough College [University of Central Lancashire] M99
BSc (Hons): 3 years full-time – DDH4
Tariff: 120

Equine Science and Management (top-up)

Myerscough College [University of Central Lancashire] M99
BSc (Hons): 1 year full-time – DDJ4
HND, Fd

Equine Science (top-up)

Writtle College [University of Essex] W85
BSc: 1 year full-time – D427
HND, Fd

Equine Sport Performance and Coaching

Duchy College [University of Plymouth] D55
FdSc: 2 years full-time or 3 - 5 years part-time – DX41 S
Tariff: 80

Equine Sport Science

University of Wolverhampton W75
BSc (Hons): 3 years full-time or 4 years sandwich or 5 - 6 years part-time day/evening – DC46
Tariff: 140 - 200 IB: 24

Equine Sports Performance

Plumpton College [University of Brighton] ▲
BSc (Hons): 3 years full-time or 4 years sandwich or 5 years part-time – DC46 P
Tariff: 220 IB: 28 Interview

Equine Sports Performance (top-up)

Berkshire College of Agriculture [Buckinghamshire Chilterns University College] ▲
BA (Hons): 1 year full-time – D432 C
HND

Equine Sports Science

University of Lincoln L39
BSc (Hons): 3 years full-time – CD63 L
Tariff: 200 IB: 26

Nottingham Trent University N91
BSc (Hons): 3 years full-time or 4 years part-time – DC36
Tariff: 220

Equine Sports Science (Equine Psychology)

Nottingham Trent University N91
BSc (Hons): 3 years full-time or 4 years sandwich – D422
Tariff: 220

Equine Studies

University of Wales, Aberystwyth A40
Fd: 3 years sandwich – D324
Tariff: 80

Bicton College [University of Plymouth] ▲
FdSc: 2 years full-time – D422
Tariff: 60 - 80

Harper Adams University College H12
FdSc: 2 years full-time – D422
Tariff: 60 - 120

Otley College [University of East Anglia]
FdSc: 2 years full-time or 4 years part-time
Tariff: 60 - 120

Plumpton College [University of Brighton] ▲
FdSc: 2 years full-time or 3 years part-time – D422 P
Tariff: 80 IB: 24 Interview

Reaseheath College [Harper Adams University College] ▲
FdSc: 2 years full-time or 3 years sandwich – DN3F R
Tariff: 60 - 120

Sparsholt College, Hampshire [University of Portsmouth] S34
FdSc: 2 years full-time – D422
Tariff: 40

Sparsholt College, Hampshire [University of Portsmouth] S34
BSc (Hons): 3 years full-time – D322
Tariff: 120

Warwickshire College, Royal Leamington Spa, Rugby and Moreton Morell [Coventry University] W25
FdSc: 2 years full-time or 3 years sandwich or 4 years distance learning – D426
Tariff: 80

Warwickshire College, Royal Leamington Spa, Rugby and Moreton Morell [Coventry University] W25
BA (Hons): 3 years full-time or 4 years sandwich – D322
Tariff: 160

Writtle College [University of Essex] W85
BSc (Hons): 3 years full-time – D334
Tariff: 160 IB: 24 - 28

Writtle College [University of Essex] W85
FdSc: 2 years full-time or 2 - 4 years part-time – D429
Tariff: 60

Equine Studies and Business Management

Writtle College [University of Essex] W85
FdSc: 2 years full-time or 2 - 4 years part-time – DN4G
Tariff: 40

Writtle College [University of Essex] W85
BSc (Hons): 3 years full-time or 4 years sandwich – D323
Tariff: 160 IB: 24 - 28

Equine Studies with Business Management (top-up)

Writtle College [University of Essex] W85
BSc: 1 year full-time – DNLF
HND, Fd

Equine Studies with Management

Berkshire College of Agriculture [Buckinghamshire Chilterns University College] ▲
FdA: 2 years full-time – D4N2 C
A2

Equine Studies (The Performance Horse)

Kingston Maurward College [Bournemouth University] ▲
FdSc: 2 years full-time or up to 5 years part-time – D422 K
Tariff: 80

Equine Studies (top-up)

University of Wales, Aberystwyth A40
BSc (Hons): 1 year full-time – D325
HND

Rodbaston College [University of Wolverhampton] ▲
BSc (Hons): 1 year full-time – D322 R
HND, Fd

Writtle College [University of Essex] W85
BSc: 1 year full-time – D422
HND, Fd

Sports Horse Management and Training

Nottingham Trent University N91
FdSc: 2 years full-time or part-time – D323
Tariff: 120

Sports Science (Equitation Coaching)

Warwickshire College, Royal Leamington Spa, Rugby and Moreton Morell [Coventry University] W25
Fd: 2 years full-time or 3 years sandwich – DC46
Tariff: 80

Warwickshire College, Royal Leamington Spa, Rugby and Moreton Morell [Coventry University] W25
BSc (Hons): 3 years full-time or 4 years sandwich – DX41
Tariff: 180

Veterinary Health Studies

Sparsholt College, Hampshire [University of Portsmouth] S34
FdSc: 2 - 3 years part-time
Tariff: 40

Veterinary Medicine

University of Cambridge C05
VetMB: 6 years full-time – D100
Tariff: 360 IB: 36 - 40
RCVS

University of Edinburgh E56
BVM&S: 5 years full-time – D100
A2: AAB SQA: AAABB IB: 36 Interview
RCVS

University of Glasgow G28
BVMS: 5 years full-time – D100
A2: AAB SQA: AAABB Interview
RCVS

Royal Veterinary College, University of London R84
BVetMed: 5 years full-time – D100
A2: ABB - AAA SQA: AAAAA IB: 7 6 6 - 7 7 6 Interview
RCVS

Royal Veterinary College, University of London R84
BSc (Hons): 1 year full-time BVetMed: 6 years full-time - D101
A2: AAB - AAA SQA: AAAAA IB: 7 6 6 - 7 7 6 Interview
RCVS

Veterinary Medicine and Surgery

University of Nottingham N84
BVM BVS: 5 years full-time – D100
A2: AAB ILC: AAAAAB IB: 38

Veterinary Medicine and Surgery (with integrated Veterinary Medical Sciences)

University of Nottingham N84
BVM BVS: 6 years full-time – D104
A2: AAB

Veterinary Nursing

Askham Bryan College [University of Leeds] A70
FdSc: 2 years full-time – D310
Tariff: 140

Harper Adams University College H12
FdSc: 3 years sandwich – D311
Tariff: 140 - 180 Interview

Kingston Maurward College [Bournemouth University]
FdSc: 2 years part-time
HP

Middlesex University M80
BSc (Hons): 4 years full-time – D1B7 E
Tariff: 200 - 220

Myerscough College [University of Central Lancashire] M99
BSc (Hons): 3 years full-time – D310
Tariff: 220 Interview

Myerscough College [University of Central Lancashire] M99
FdSc: 2 years full-time – D313
Tariff: 100 - 180 Interview

Napier University N07
BSc (Hons): 4 years full-time – D310
A2: BCD SQA: BBBC

ottingham Trent University N91
Sc: 2 years full-time – D310
iff: 160

umpton College
2 years full-time – D310
iff: 80

oyal Veterinary College, University of
ndon R84
Sc: 2 years full-time – D310
E

iversity of Wolverhampton W75
Sc: 3 - 4 years part-time
ff: 60 - 120

eterinary Nursing with Business anagement

arwickshire College, Royal Leamington
a, Rugby and Moreton Morell
oventry University] W25
(Hons): 3 years full-time or 4 years sandwich – D3N2
ff: 160
'S

eterinary Nursing January entry op-up)

ddlesex University M80
(Hons): 1 year full-time or 3 years part-time – D311 E

eterinary Nursing and Practice dministration

iversity of Bristol B78
(Hons): 4 years full-time including foundation year –
2
CC BTEC: DDM SQA: CCCC IB: 26
S

terinary Nursing and Practice anagement

rper Adams University College H12
(Hons): 3 years full-time or 4 years sandwich – D310
: 220 - 280

Veterinary Nursing with Practice Management

Warwickshire College, Royal Leamington Spa, Rugby and Moreton Morell [Coventry University] W25
FdSc: 3 years full-time – D3D9
Tariff: 80
RCVS

Veterinary Nursing Science

Hartpury College [Bristol, University of the West of England] ▲
BSc (Hons): 3 years full-time or 4 years sandwich – BD71 A
Tariff: 200 IB: 30

Hartpury College [Bristol, University of the West of England] ▲
FdSc: 2 years full-time – D310 A
Tariff: 100 IB: 24

Sparsholt College, Hampshire [University of Portsmouth] S34
BSc (Hons): 4 years full-time – D310
Tariff: 120

Veterinary Nursing September entry (top-up)

Middlesex University M80
BSc (Hons): 1 year full-time or 3 years part-time – D312 E
HP

Veterinary Nursing (top-up)

Napier University N07
BSc/BSc (Hons): part-time – D311
HND, HP

Veterinary Pathogenesis

University of Bristol B78
BSc (Hons): 3 years full-time – DC35
A2: BBB BTEC: DDM SQA: BBBBB IB: 32

Veterinary Practice Management

Hartpury College [Bristol, University of the West of England] ▲
FdA: 2 years full-time – N220 A
Tariff: 100 IB: 24

Hartpury College [Bristol, University of the West of England] ▲
BA (Hons): 3 years full-time – DN32 A
Tariff: 200 IB: 30

Veterinary Science

University of Bristol B78
BVSc: 5 years full-time – D100
A2: AAB BTEC: DDD SQA: AAABB - AAAAB IB: 38
RCVS

University of Liverpool L41
BVSc: 5 years full-time – D100
A2: AAB BTEC: DDD ILC: AAAABB IB: 38
RCVS

Veterinary Science (with intercalated Honours year)

University of Liverpool L41
BSc (Hons): 6 years full-time BVSc: 6 years full-time – D101
A2: AAB BTEC: DDD ILC: AAAABB IB: 38
RCVS

Veterinary Sciences

Royal Veterinary College, University of London R84
BSc (Hons): 3 years full-time – D1B9
A2: BBB

Welfare of Animals (Collections)

Myerscough College [University of Central Lancashire] M99
FdSc: 2 years full-time – D329
Tariff: 80

Welfare of Animals (Management)

Myerscough College [University of Central Lancashire] M99
FdSc: 2 years full-time or 3 years part-time – D328
Tariff: 80

Welfare of Animals (Nursing)

Myerscough College [University of Central Lancashire] M99
FdSc: 2 years full-time or 3 years part-time – D311
Tariff: 80

Institution Address Listings

University of Aberdeen
Student Recruitment & Admissions
University Office, Regent Walk
Aberdeen
AB24 3FX

T: 01224 272090/272091
F: 01224 272576
E: sras@abdn.ac.uk
W: www.abdn.ac.uk
Institution code: A20

University of Abertay Dundee
Bell Street
Dundee
DD1 1HG

T: 01382 308000
F: 01382 308877
E: sro@abertay.ac.uk
W: www.abertay.ac.uk
Institution code: A30

University of Wales, Aberystwyth
Old College
King Street
Aberystwyth, Ceredigion
SY23 2AX

T: 01970 623111
F: 01970 627410
E: ug-admissions@aber.ac.uk
W: www.aber.ac.uk
Institution code: A40

Abingdon and Witney College
Northcourt Road
Abingdon, Oxfordshire
OX14 1NN

T: 01235 555585
F: 01235 553168
E: inquiry@abingdon-witney.ac.uk
W: www.abingdon-witney.ac.uk

Anglia Ruskin University
East Road
Cambridge
CB1 1PT

T: 01223 363271
F: 01223 352973
E: answers@anglia.ac.uk
W: www.anglia.ac.uk
Institution code: A60

Anglo-European College of Chiropractic
13 Parkwood Road
Bournemouth
BH5 2DF

T: 01202 436200
F: 01202 436312
W: www.aecc.ac.uk

Askham Bryan College
Askham Bryan
York
YO23 3FR

T: 01904 772211
F: 01904 772288
E: enquiries@askham-bryan.ac.uk
W: www.askham-bryan.ac.uk
Institution code: A70

Aston University
Aston Triangle
Birmingham
B4 7ET

T: 0121 204 3000
F: 0121 204 3696
E: prospectus@aston.ac.uk
W: www.aston.ac.uk
Institution code: A80

University of Wales, Bangor
Bangor, Gwynedd
LL57 2DG

T: 01248 351151
F: 01248 383268
E: admissions@bangor.ac.uk
W: www.bangor.ac.uk
Institution code: B06

Barnet College
Wood Street
Barnet, London
EN5 4AZ

T: 020 8440 6321
F: 020 8441 5236
E: info@barnet.ac.uk
W: www.barnet.ac.uk

Barnfield College, Luton
New Bedford Road
Luton
LU2 7BF

T: 01582 569700
F: 01582 492928
W: www.barnfield.ac.uk

University Centre Barnsley
Church Street
Barnsley
S70 2AN

T: 01226 606262
E: barnsley@hud.ac.uk
W: www.barnsley.hud.ac.uk
Institution code: H60

University of Bath
Claverton Down
Bath
BA2 7AY

T: 01225 388388
F: 01225 826366
E: admissions@bath.ac.uk
W: www.bath.ac.uk
Institution code: B16

Bath Spa University
Newton Park
Newton St Loe
Bath
BA2 9BN

T: 01225 875875
F: 01225 875444
E: enquiries@bathspa.ac.uk
W: www.bathspa.ac.uk
Institution code: B20

City of Bath College
Avon Street
Bath
BA1 1UP

T: 01225 312191
F: 01225 444213
E: enquiries@citybathcoll.ac.uk
W: www.citybathcoll.ac.uk
Institution code: B21

Bedford College
Cauldwell Street
Bedford
MK42 9AH

T: 01234 291000
F: 01234 342674
E: info@bedford.ac.uk
W: www.bedford.ac.uk
Institution code: B23

University of Bedfordshire
Park Square
Luton
LU1 3JU

T: 01234 400400
F: 01582 734400
E: admissions@beds.ac.uk
W: www.beds.ac.uk
Institution code: B22

Bell College
Almada Street
Hamilton, South Lanarkshire
ML3 0JB

T: 01698 283100
F: 01698 282131
E: inform@bell.ac.uk
W: www.bell.ac.uk
Institution code: B26

Berkshire College of Agriculture
Hall Place
Burchetts Green
Maidenhead
SL6 6QR

T: 01628 824444
F: 01628 824695
E: enquiries@bca.ac.uk
W: www.bca.ac.uk

Bexley College
Tower Road
Belvedere
Bexley, London
DA17 6JA

T: 01322 442331
F: 01322 448403
E: courses@bexley.ac.uk
W: www.bexley.ac.uk

Bicton College
East Budleigh
Budleigh Salterton, Devon
EX9 7BY

T: 01395 562300
F: 01395 567502
E: enquiries@bicton.ac.uk
W: www.bicton.ac.uk

rkbeck, University of London
et Street
don
1E 7HX
020 7631 6000/08456 010174
020 7631 6270
admissions@bbk.ac.uk
www.bbk.ac.uk

iversity of Birmingham
baston
ningham
2TT
0121 414 3344
0121 414 3971
admissions@bham.ac.uk
www.bham.ac.uk
titution code: B32

shop Auckland College
dhouse Lane
op Auckland, Durham
4 6JZ
1388 443000
1388 609294
ail.parkin@bacoll.ac.uk
www.bacoll.ac.uk

shop Burton College
op Burton
erley, East Riding of Yorkshire
7 8QG
1964 553000
1964 553101
nquiries@bishopburton.ac.uk
www.bishopburton.ac.uk
itution code: B37

ackburn College
en Street
burn
1LH
1254 55144
1254 263947
udentservices@blackburn.ac.uk
www.blackburn.ac.uk
itution code: E25

ackpool and the Fylde College
eld Road
am
pool
0HB
253 352352
1253 356127
sitors@blackpool.ac.uk
www.blackpool.ac.uk
itution code: B41

versity of Bolton
e Road
, Lancashire
5AB
204 900600
204 399074
quiries@bolton.ac.uk
ww.bolton.ac.uk
tution code: B44

Bournemouth University
Fern Barrow
Poole
BH12 5BB
T: 01202 524111
F: 01202 702736
E: prospectus@bournemouth.ac.uk
W: www.bournemouth.ac.uk
Institution code: B50

Bournemouth and Poole College of Further Education
North Road
Bournemouth
BH14 0LS
T: 01202 747600
F: 01202 205719
E: enquiries@thecollege.co.uk
W: www.thecollege.co.uk

University of Bradford
Richmond Road
Bradford
BD7 1DP
T: 01274 232323
F: 01274 236260
E: course-enquiries@bradford.ac.uk
W: www.brad.ac.uk
Institution code: B56

Bradford College
Great Horton Road
Bradford
BD7 1AY
T: 01274 433004
F: 01274 433173
E: admissions@bilk.ac.uk
W: www.bradfordcollege.ac.uk
Institution code: B60

Bridgwater College
Bath Road
Bridgwater, Somerset
TA6 4PZ
T: 01278 455464
F: 01278 444363
E: information@bridgwater.ac.uk
W: www.bridgwater.ac.uk
Institution code: B70

University of Brighton
Mithras House
Lewes Road
Brighton
BN2 4AT
T: 01273 600900
F: 01273 642825
E: admissions@brighton.ac.uk
W: www.brighton.ac.uk
Institution code: B72

Brighton and Sussex Medical School
Mithras House
Lewes Road
Brighton
BN2 4AT
T: 01273 600900
F: 01273 642825
E: medadmissions@bsms.ac.uk
W: www.bsms.ac.uk
Institution code: B74

University of Bristol
Senate House
Tyndall Avenue
Bristol
BS8 1TH
T: 0117 928 9000
F: 0117 925 1424
E: admissions@bristol.ac.uk
W: www.bris.ac.uk
Institution code: B78

Bristol, University of the West of England
Frenchay Campus
Coldharbour Lane
Bristol
BS16 1QY
T: 0117 965 6261
F: 0117 328 2810
E: admissions@uwe.ac.uk
W: www.uwe.ac.uk
Institution code: B80

City of Bristol College
College Green Centre
St George's Road
Bristol
BS1 5UA
T: 0117 904 5000
F: 0117 904 5050
E: enquiries@cityofbristol.ac.uk
W: www.cityofbristol.ac.uk
Institution code: B77

British College of Osteopathic Medicine
Lief House
120 Finchley Road
London
NW3 5HR
T: 020 7435 6464
F: 020 7431 3630
E: info@bcom.ac.uk
W: www.bcom.ac.uk
Institution code: B81

British School of Osteopathy
275 Borough High Street
London
SE1 1JE
T: 020 7407 0222
F: 020 7839 1098
E: admissions@bso.ac.uk
W: www.bso.ac.uk
Institution code: B87

Bromley College of Further and Higher Education
Rookery Lane
Bromley, London
BR2 8HE
T: 020 8295 7000
F: 020 8295 7099
E: info@bromley.ac.uk
W: www.bromley.ac.uk

Brooksby Melton College
Ashfordby Road
Melton Mowbray, Leicestershire
LE13 0HJ
T: 01664 855444
F: 01664 410556
W: www.brooksbymelton.ac.uk

Brunel University
Kingston Lane
Uxbridge, Middlesex
UB8 3PH
T: 01895 265599
F: 01895 269702
E: marketing@brunel.ac.uk
W: www.brunel.ac.uk
Institution code: B84

University of Buckingham
Hunter Street
Buckingham
MK18 1EG
T: 01280 814080
F: 01280 822245
E: info@buckingham.ac.uk
W: www.buckingham.ac.uk
Institution code: B90

Buckinghamshire Chilterns University College
Queen Alexandra Road
High Wycombe, Buckinghamshire
HP11 2JZ
T: 01494 522141
F: 01494 524392
E: admissions@bcuc.ac.uk
W: www.bcuc.ac.uk
Institution code: B94

Burnley College
Shorey Bank
Ormerod Road
Burnley, Lancashire
BB11 2RX
T: 01282 711200
F: 01282 415063
E: student.services@burnley.ac.uk
W: www.burnley.ac.uk

Calderdale College
Francis Street
Halifax, Calderdale
HX1 3UZ
T: 01422 357357
F: 01422 399320
E: info@calderdale.ac.uk
W: www.calderdale.ac.uk

University of Cambridge
Cambridge Admissions Office
Fitzwilliam House, 32 Trumpington Street
Cambridge
CB2 1QY
T: 01223 333308
F: 01223 366383
E: admissions@cam.ac.uk
W: www.cam.ac.uk
Institution code: C05

Canterbury Christ Church University
North Holmes Road
Canterbury, Kent
CT1 1QU
T: 01227 767700
F: 01227 470442
E: admissions@cant.ac.uk
W: www.cant.ac.uk
Institution code: C10

Canterbury College
New Dover Road
Canterbury, Kent
CT1 3AJ
T: 01227 811111
F: 01227 811101
E: admissions@cant-col.ac.uk
W: www.cant-col.ac.uk

Cardiff University
PO Box 921
Cardiff
CF10 3XQ
T: 029 2087 4404
F: 029 2087 4130
E: prospectus@cardiff.ac.uk
W: www.cardiff.ac.uk
Institution code: C15

University of Wales Institute, Cardiff
Student Recruitment & Admissions
Western Avenue
Cardiff
CF5 2SG
T: 029 2041 6070
F: 029 2041 6286
E: uwicinfo@uwic.ac.uk
W: www.uwic.ac.uk
Institution code: C20

Castle College Nottingham
Maid Marian Way
Nottingham
NG1 6AB
T: 08458 450500
F: 0115 912 8600
E: learn@castlecollege.ac.uk
W: www.castlecollege.ac.uk
Institution code: P40

University of Central Lancashire
Preston, Lancashire
PR1 2HE
T: 01772 201201
F: 01772 892946
E: cenquiries@uclan.ac.uk
W: www.uclan.ac.uk
Institution code: C30

University of Chester
Parkgate Road
Chester
CH1 4BJ
T: 01244 375444
F: 01244 392820
E: enquiries@chester.ac.uk
W: www.chester.ac.uk
Institution code: C55

Chesterfield College
Infirmary Road
Chesterfield, Derbyshire
S41 7NG
T: 01246 500500
F: 01246 500587
E: advice@chesterfield.ac.uk
W: www.chesterfield.ac.uk
Institution code: C56

University of Chichester
Bishop Otter Campus
College Lane
Chichester, West Sussex
PO19 6PE
T: 01243 816000
F: 01243 816080
E: admissions@chi.ac.uk
W: www.chiuni.ac.uk
Institution code: C58

Chichester College
Westgate Fields
Chichester, West Sussex
PO19 1SB
T: 01243 786321
F: 01243 539481
E: info@chichester.ac.uk
W: www.chichester.ac.uk
Institution code: C57

Cirencester College
Fosse Way Campus
Stroud Road
Cirencester, Gloucestershire
GL7 1XA
T: 01285 640994
F: 01285 644171
E: principal@cirencester.ac.uk
W: www.cirencester.ac.uk

City University
Northampton Square
London
EC1V 0HB
T: 020 7040 5060
F: 020 7040 5070
E: ugadmissions@city.ac.uk
W: www.city.ac.uk
Institution code: C60

City and Islington College
The Marlborough Building
383 Holloway Road
London
N7 0RN
T: 020 7700 9200
F: 020 7700 9222
E: courseinfo@candi.ac.uk
W: www.candi.ac.uk
Institution code: C65

Colchester Institute
Sheepen Road
Colchester, Essex
CO3 3LL
T: 01206 518000
F: 01206 763041
E: info@colch-inst.ac.uk
W: www.colch-inst.ac.uk
Institution code: C75

College of Agriculture, Food an[d] Rural Enterprise
22 Greenmount Road
Antrim
BT41 4PU
T: 028 9442 6601
F: 028 9442 6606
E: enquiries@dardni.gov.uk
W: www.cafre.ac.uk
Institution code: A45

ollege of Osteopaths
Furzehill Road
rehamwood, Hertfordshire
)6 2DG
020 8905 1937
020 8953 0320
: www.collegeofosteopaths.ac.uk

ornwall College
ad Office
gonissey Road
Austell, Cornwall
25 4DJ
01726 226526
01726 226666
enquiries@cornwall.ac.uk
: www.cornwall.ac.uk
stitution code: C78

oventry University
ry Street
entry
5FB
024 7688 7688
024 7688 8638
nfo.reg@coventry.ac.uk
www.coventry.ac.uk
titution code: C85

iversity of Cumbria
Martin's College
verham, Lancaster
3TD
01524 384384
www.cumbria.ac.uk
titution code: C99

Montfort University
Gateway
ester
9BH
116 255 1551
0116 255 0307
enquiry@dmu.ac.uk
www.dmu.ac.uk
titution code: D26

iversity of Derby
eston Road
y
2 1GB
1332 590500
1332 294861
dmissions@derby.ac.uk
www.derby.ac.uk
titution code: D39

iversity of Derby Buxton
vonshire Road
on, Derbyshire
6RY
1298 71100
1298 27261
nquiriesudcb@derby.ac.uk
www.derby.ac.uk/buxton
itution code: D39

Dewsbury College
Halifax Road
Dewsbury
WF13 2AS
T: 01924 465916/436221
F: 01924 457047
E: info@dewsbury.ac.uk
W: www.dewsbury.ac.uk
Institution code: D45

Duchy College
Stoke Climsland
Callington, Cornwall
PL17 8PB
T: 01579 372222
F: 01579 372200
E: admissions@duchy.cornwall.ac.uk
W: www.cornwall.ac.uk/duchy
Institution code: D55

University of Dundee
Perth Road
Dundee
DD1 4HN
T: 01382 383000
F: 01382 201604
E: srs@dundee.ac.uk
W: www.dundee.ac.uk
Institution code: D65

University of Durham
The University Office
Durham
DH1 3HP
T: 0191 334 2000
F: 0191 334 6250
E: admissions@durham.ac.uk
W: www.dur.ac.uk
Institution code: D86

University of East Anglia
The Registry
Norwich, Norfolk
NR4 7TJ
T: 01603 456161
F: 01603 458553
E: admissions@uea.ac.uk
W: www.uea.ac.uk
Institution code: E14

East Berkshire College
Station Road
Langley
Maidenhead
SL3 8BY
T: 01753 793000
F: 01753 793316
E: information@eastberks.ac.uk
W: www.eastberks.ac.uk

East Durham and Houghall Community College
Burnhope Way
Peterlee, Durham
SR8 1NU
T: 0191 518 2000
F: 0191 586 7125
E: enquiry@eastdurham.ac.uk
W: www.edhcc.ac.uk

University of East London
Docklands Campus
4-6 University Way
London
E16 2RD
T: 020 8223 3000
F: 020 8507 7799
E: admiss@uel.ac.uk
W: www.uel.ac.uk
Institution code: E28

Easton College
Easton
Norwich, Norfolk
NR9 5DX
T: 01603 731200
F: 01603 731200
W: www.easton-college.ac.uk

Edge Hill University
St Helens Road
Ormskirk, Lancashire
L39 4QP
T: 0800 195 5063
F: 01695 579997
E: enquiries@edgehill.ac.uk
W: www.edgehill.ac.uk
Institution code: E42

University of Edinburgh
Secretary's Office
Old College, South Bridge
Edinburgh
EH8 9YL
T: 0131 650 1000
F: 0131 650 2147
E: sra.enquiries@ed.ac.uk
W: www.ed.ac.uk
Institution code: E56

University of Essex
Wivenhoe Park
Colchester, Essex
CO4 3SQ
T: 01206 873333
F: 01206 873423
E: admit@essex.ac.uk
W: www.essex.ac.uk
Institution code: E70

European School of Osteopathy
Boxley House
The Street, Boxley
Maidstone, Kent
ME14 3DZ
T: 01622 671558
F: 01622 662165
E: kellyrose@eso.ac.uk
W: www.eso.ac.uk
Institution code: E80

Exeter College
Victoria House
33-36 Queen Street
Exeter, Devon
EX4 8QD
T: 01392 205222
F: 01392 210282
E: admissions@exe-coll.ac.uk
W: www.exe-coll.ac.uk
Institution code: E81

University of Exeter
Northcote House
The Queen's Drive
Exeter, Devon
EX4 4QJ
T: 01392 661000
F: 01392 263108
E: admissions@exeter.ac.uk
W: www.ex.ac.uk
Institution code: E84

Falmouth Marine School, Cornwall College
Killigrew Street
Falmouth, Cornwall
TR11 3QS
T: 01326 310310
F: 01326 310300
E: falenquiries@cornwall.ac.uk
W: www.cornwall.ac.uk/fal

Farnborough College of Technology
Boundary Road
Farnborough, Hampshire
GU14 6FB
T: 01252 407040
F: 01252 407041
E: info@farn-ct.ac.uk
W: www.farn-ct.ac.uk
Institution code: F66

Gateshead College
Durham Road
Gateshead, Tyne and Wear
NE9 5BN
T: 0191 490 0300
F: 0191 490 2313
W: www.gateshead.ac.uk

University of Glamorgan
Llantwit Road
Treforest
Pontypridd, Rhondda Cynon Taff
CF37 1DL
T: 0800 716925
F: 01443 480558
E: enquiries@glam.ac.uk
W: www.glam.ac.uk
Institution code: G14

University of Glasgow
Student Recruitment & Admissions
1 The Square
Glasgow
G12 8QQ
T: 0141 339 8855
F: 0141 330 4045
E: stras@gla.ac.uk
W: www.gla.ac.uk
Institution code: G28

Glasgow Caledonian University
City Campus
Cowcaddens Road
Glasgow
G4 0BA
T: 0141 331 3000
F: 0141 331 3005
E: helpline@gcal.ac.uk
W: www.gcal.ac.uk
Institution code: G42

University of Gloucestershire
PO Box 220
Cheltenham, Gloucestershire
GL50 2QF
T: 01242 532700
F: 01242 543334
E: admissions@glos.ac.uk
W: www.glos.ac.uk
Institution code: G50

Gloucestershire College of Arts and Technology
Brunswick Road
Gloucester
GL1 1HU
T: 01452 532000
F: 01452 563441
E: info@gloscat.ac.uk
W: www.gloscat.ac.uk
Institution code: G45

Goldsmiths, University of London
New Cross
London
SE14 6NW
T: 020 7919 7766
F: 020 7919 7509
E: admissions@gold.ac.uk
W: www.goldsmiths.ac.uk
Institution code: G56

University of Greenwich
Maritime Greenwich Campus
Park Row
London
SE10 9LS
T: 020 8331 8000/0800 005006
F: 020 8331 8145
E: courseinfo@gre.ac.uk
W: www.gre.ac.uk
Institution code: G70

Grimsby Institute of Further and Higher Education
Nuns Corner
Grimsby, North-East Lincolnshire
DN34 5BQ
T: 01472 311222
F: 01472 879924
E: infocent@grimsby.ac.uk
W: www.grimsby.ac.uk
Institution code: G80

Guildford College of Futher and Higher Education
Stoke Park
Guildford, Surrey
GU1 1EZ
T: 01483 448500
F: 01483 448600
E: info@guildford.ac.uk
W: www.guildford.ac.uk
Institution code: G90

Hadlow College
Hadlow
Tonbridge, Kent
TN11 0AL
T: 01732 850551
F: 01732 853207
E: enquiries@hadlow.ac.uk
W: www.hadlow.ac.uk

Harlow College
Velizy Avenue
Town Centre
Harlow, Essex
CM20 3LH
T: 01279 868000
F: 01279 868260/01279 868054
E: full-time@harlow-college.ac.uk
W: www.harlow-college.ac.uk

Harper Adams University College
Newport, Shropshire
TF10 8NB
T: 01952 820280
F: 01952 814783
E: admissions@harper-adams.ac.uk
W: www.harper-adams.ac.uk
Institution code: H12

Hartlepool College of Further Education
Stockton Street
Hartlepool
TS24 7NT
T: 01429 295111
F: 01429 292999
E: enquiries@hartlepoolfe.ac.uk
W: www.hartlepoolfe.ac.uk

Hartpury College
Hartpury House
Hartpury
Gloucester
GL19 3BE
T: 01452 702132
F: 01452 700629
E: enquire@hartpury.ac.uk
W: www.hartpury.ac.uk

Herefordshire College of Technology
Folly Lane
Hereford
HR1 1LS
T: 01432 352235
F: 01432 365357
E: enquiries@hct.ac.uk
W: www.hereford-tech.ac.uk

Heriot-Watt University
Riccarton
Edinburgh
EH14 4AS
T: 0131 449 5111
F: 0131 451 3630
E: admissions@hw.ac.uk
W: www.hw.ac.uk
Institution code: H24

University of Hertfordshire
College Lane
Hatfield, Hertfordshire
AL10 9AB
T: 01707 284000
F: 01707 284115
E: admissions@herts.ac.uk
W: www.herts.ac.uk
Institution code: H36

opwood Hall College
ochdale Campus
Mary's Gate
ochdale, Greater Manchester
L12 6RY
: 0161 643 7560
: 0161 643 2114
: enquiries@hopwood.ac.uk
/: www.hopwood.ac.uk
stitution code: H54

niversity of Huddersfield
ueensgate
uddersfield
D1 3DH
01484 422288
01484 516151
admissions@hud.ac.uk
: www.hud.ac.uk
stitution code: H60

ugh Baird College
lliol Road
otle, Merseyside
0 7EW
0151 353 4444
0151 934 4469
info@hughbaird.ac.uk
: www.hughbaird.ac.uk

niversity of Hull
missions Office
ttingham Road
gston-upon-Hull
6 7RX
01482 466100
01482 442290
admissions@hull.ac.uk
www.hull.ac.uk
stitution code: H72

ll College
een's Gardens
gston-upon-Hull
1 3DG
01482 329943
01482 598851
nfo@hull-college.ac.uk
www.hull-college.ac.uk
stitution code: H73

ll York Medical School
ersity of Hull
gston-upon-Hull
6 7RX
0870 124 5500
01482 464705/01904 321696
admissions@hyms.ac.uk
www.hyms.ac.uk
itution code: H75

perial College London
h Kensington Campus
don
' 2AZ
20 7589 5111
020 7594 8004
www.imperial.ac.uk
itution code: I50

International College of Oriental Medicine
Green Hedges House
Green Hedges Avenue
Crawley, West Sussex
RH19 1DZ
T: 01342 313406/7
F: 01342 318302
E: info@orientalmed.ac.uk
W: www.orientalmed.ac.uk

International Correspondence School
8 Elliot Place
Glasgow
G3 8EP
T: 0141 221 2926
F: 0141 248 4093
W: www.icslearn.co.uk

Isle of Man College
Homefield Road
Douglas, Isle of Man
IM2 6RB
T: 01624 648200
F: 01624 648201
E: enquiries@iomcollege.ac.im
W: www.iomcollege.ac.im

Keele University
Keele, Staffordshire
ST5 5BG
T: 01782 621111
F: 01782 632343
E: aaa30@keele.ac.uk
W: www.keele.ac.uk
Institution code: K12

Kendal College
Milnthorpe Road
Kendal, Cumbria
LA9 5AY
T: 01539 724313
F: 01539 733714
E: enquiries@kendal.ac.uk
W: www.kendal.ac.uk

University of Kent
Registry and Admissions
The Registry
Canterbury, Kent
CT2 7NZ
T: 01227 827272
F: 01227 827077
E: recruitment@kent.ac.uk
W: www.kent.ac.uk
Institution code: K24

King's College London, University of London
Strand
London
WC2R 2LS
T: 020 7836 5454
W: www.kcl.ac.uk
Institution code: K60

Kingston University
River House
53-57 High Street
Kingston upon Thames, London
KT1 1LQ
T: 020 8547 2000
F: 020 8547 7857
E: admissions-info@kingston.ac.uk
W: www.kingston.ac.uk
Institution code: K84

Kingston College
Kingston Hall Road
Kingston upon Thames, London
KT1 2AQ
T: 020 8546 2151
F: 020 8268 2900
E: info@kingston-college.ac.uk
W: www.kingston-college.ac.uk

Kingston Maurward College
Kingston Maurward
Dorchester, Dorset
DT2 8PY
T: 01305 215000
F: 01305 215001
E: administration@kmc.ac.uk
W: www.kmc.ac.uk

Lambeth College
Clapham Centre
45 Clapham Common South Side
London
SW4 9BL
T: 020 7501 5000
F: 020 7501 5325
E: courses@lambethcollege.ac.uk
W: www.lambethcollege.ac.uk

Lancaster University
Bailrigg
Lancaster
LA1 4YW
T: 01524 65201
F: 01524 846243
E: ugadmissions@lancaster.ac.uk
W: www.lancs.ac.uk
Institution code: L14

University of Leeds
Woodhouse Lane
Leeds
LS2 9JT
T: 0113 243 1751
F: 0113 244 3923
E: prospectus@leeds.ac.uk
W: www.leeds.ac.uk
Institution code: L23

Leeds Metropolitan University
Civic Quarter
Leeds
LS1 3HE
T: 0113 283 3113
F: 0113 283 3148
E: course-enquiries@leedsmet.ac.uk
W: www.leedsmet.ac.uk
Institution code: L27

Leeds Thomas Danby
Roundhay Road
Leeds
LS7 3BG
T: 0113 249 4912
F: 0113 240 1967
W: www.leedsthomasdanby.ac.uk

Leeds, Trinity & All Saints
Brownberrie Lane
Horsforth
Leeds
LS18 5HD
T: 0113 283 7123
F: 0113 283 7321
E: admissions@leedstrinity.ac.uk
W: www.tasc.ac.uk
Institution code: L24

University of Leicester
University Road
Leicester
LE1 7RH
T: 0116 222 2522
F: 0116 252 2400
E: admissions@le.ac.uk
W: www.le.ac.uk
Institution code: L34

Lews Castle College (UHI Millennium Institute)
Stornoway, Western Isles
HS2 0XR
T: 01851 770000
F: 01851 770001
E: aofficele@lews.uhi.ac.uk
W: www.lews.uhi.ac.uk
Institution code: H49

University of Lincoln
Brayford Pool
Lincoln
LN6 7TS
T: 01522 882000
F: 01522 882088
E: marketing@lincoln.ac.uk
W: www.lincoln.ac.uk
Institution code: L39

Lincoln College
Monks Road
Lincoln
LN2 5HQ
T: 01522 876000
F: 01522 876200
E: enquiries@lincolncollege.ac.uk
W: www.lincolncollege.ac.uk
Institution code: L42

University of Liverpool
The Foundation Building
765 Brownlow Hill
Liverpool, Merseyside
L69 7ZX
T: 0151 794 2000
F: 0151 794 2060
E: ugrecruitment@liv.ac.uk
W: www.liv.ac.uk
Institution code: L41

Liverpool Community College
Old Swan Centre
Broadgreen Road
Liverpool, Merseyside
L13 5SQ
T: 0151 252 3000
F: 0151 494 2796
W: www.liv-coll.ac.uk
Institution code: L43

Liverpool Hope University
Hope Park
Liverpool, Merseyside
L16 9JD
T: 0151 291 3000
F: 0151 291 3100
E: admission@hope.ac.uk
W: www.hope.ac.uk
Institution code: L46

Liverpool John Moores University
Roscoe Court
4 Rodney Street
Liverpool, Merseyside
L1 2TZ
T: 0151 231 5090
F: 0151 231 3462
E: recruitment@ljmu.ac.uk
W: www.ljmu.ac.uk
Institution code: L51

London Metropolitan University
Admissions Office
166-220 Holloway Road
London
N7 8DB
T: 020 7423 0000
F: 020 7753 3272
E: admissions@londonmet.ac.uk
W: www.londonmet.ac.uk
Institution code: L68

London South Bank University
103 Borough Road
London
SE1 0AA
T: 020 7928 8989
F: 020 7815 8273
E: enrol@lsbu.ac.uk
W: www.lsbu.ac.uk
Institution code: L75

Loughborough University
Loughborough, Leicestershire
LE11 3TU
T: 01509 263171
F: 01509 223905
E: admissions@lboro.ac.uk
W: www.lboro.ac.uk
Institution code: L79

Loughborough College
Radmoor Road
Loughborough, Leicestershire
LE11 3BT
T: 08451 662950/01509 215831
F: 08451 662951/01509 269723
E: info@loucoll.ac.uk
W: www.loucoll.ac.uk
Institution code: L77

University of Manchester
Oxford Road
Manchester
M13 9PL
T: 0161 275 2077
F: 0161 275 2106
E: ug.admissions@manchester.ac.uk
W: www.manchester.ac.uk
Institution code: M20

Manchester College of Arts and Technology
Openshaw Campus, Ashton Old Road
Openshaw, Greater Manchester
M11 2WH
T: 0161 953 5995
F: 0161 953 3909
E: enquiries@mancat.ac.uk
W: www.mancat.ac.uk
Institution code: M10

Manchester Metropolitan University
All Saints
Manchester
M15 6BH
T: 0161 247 2000
F: 0161 247 6390
E: enquiries@mmu.ac.uk
W: www.mmu.ac.uk
Institution code: M40

Matthew Boulton College of Further and Higher Education
Jennens Road
Birmingham
B4 7PS
T: 0121 446 4545
F: 0121 446 3105
E: ask@matthew-boulton.ac.uk
W: www.matthew-boulton.ac.uk
Institution code: M60

Merton College
Morden Park
London Road
Sutton, London
SM4 5QX
T: 020 8408 6400
F: 020 8408 6666
E: info@merton.ac.uk
W: www.merton.ac.uk

Mid-Kent College of Higher and Further Education
Horsted
Maidstone Road
Chatham, Medway
ME5 9UQ
T: 01634 830633
F: 01634 830224
E: course.enquiries@midkent.ac.uk
W: www.midkent.ac.uk

Middlesex University
Admissions Enquiries
North London Business Park, Oakleigh Road South
London
N11 1QS
T: 020 8411 5898
F: 020 8411 5649
E: admissions@mdx.ac.uk
W: www.mdx.ac.uk
Institution code: M80

ilton Keynes College
eadenhall
ilton Keynes
K6 5LP
: 01908 684444
: 01908 684399
: info@mkcollege.ac.uk
/: www.mkcollege.ac.uk

oulton College
est Street
oulton
rthampton
N3 7RR
01604 491131
: 01604 491127
: enquiries@moulton.ac.uk
/: www.moulton.ac.uk

yerscough College
yerscough Hall
sborrow
eston, Lancashire
3 0RY
01995 642222
01995 642333
mailbox@myerscough.ac.uk
: www.myerscough.ac.uk
stitution code: M99

apier University
9 Colinton Road
nburgh
14 1DJ
08452 606040
0131 455 3636
info@napier.ac.uk
: www.napier.ac.uk
stitution code: N07

ESCOT
gate Road
som, Surrey
17 3DS
020 8394 3038
020 8394 3030
info@nescot.ac.uk
: www.nescot.ac.uk
stitution code: N49

ew College Durham
mwellgate Moor Centre
ham
1 5ES
0191 375 4000
0191 375 4222
helpdesk@newdur.ac.uk
www.newdur.ac.uk
stitution code: N28

ew College, Swindon
College Drive
ndon
3 1AH
01793 611470
01793 436437
admissions@newcollege.ac.uk
www.newcollege.co.uk

Newcastle University
6 Kensington Terrace
Newcastle upon Tyne
NE1 7RU
T: 0191 222 5594
F: 0191 222 8685
E: enquiries@ncl.ac.uk
W: www.ncl.ac.uk
Institution code: N21

Newcastle College
Scotswood Road
Newcastle upon Tyne
NE4 7SA
T: 0191 200 4000
F: 0191 200 4517
E: enquiries@ncl-coll.co.uk
W: www.newcastlecollege.co.uk
Institution code: N23

Newman College of Higher Education
Genners Lane
Birmingham
B32 3NT
T: 0121 476 1181
F: 0121 476 1196
E: registry@newman.ac.uk
W: www.newman.ac.uk
Institution code: N36

University of Wales, Newport
PO Box 101
Newport
NP18 3YG
T: 01633 432432
F: 01633 432850
E: uic@newport.ac.uk
W: www.newport.ac.uk
Institution code: N37

North Devon College
Old Sticklepath Hill
Barnstaple, Devon
EX31 2BQ
T: 01271 345291
F: 01271 338121
E: postbox@ndevon.ac.uk
W: www.ndevon.ac.uk

College of North East London
High Road
London
N15 4RU
T: 020 8802 3111
F: 020 8442 3091
E: admissions@staff.conel.ac.uk
W: www.conel.ac.uk

North East Wales Institute of Higher Education
Plas Coch
Mold Road
Wrexham
LL11 2AW
T: 01978 290666
F: 01978 290008
E: sid@newi.ac.uk
W: www.newi.ac.uk
Institution code: N56

University of Northampton
Boughton Green Road
Northampton
NN2 7AL
T: 0800 358 2232
F: 01604 722083
E: study@northampton.ac.uk
W: www.northampton.ac.uk
Institution code: N38

Northumberland College
College Road
Ashington, Northumberland
NE63 9RG
T: 01670 841200
F: 01670 841201
E: thecollege@northland.ac.uk
W: www.northland.ac.uk
Institution code: N78

Northumbria University
Ellison Place
Newcastle upon Tyne
NE1 8ST
T: 0191 232 6002
F: 0191 227 4017
E: er.admissions@northumbria.ac.uk
W: www.northumbria.ac.uk
Institution code: N77

City College Norwich
Ipswich Road
Norwich, Norfolk
NR2 2LJ
T: 01603 773311
F: 01603 773301
E: information@ccn.ac.uk
W: www.ccn.ac.uk
Institution code: N82

University of Nottingham
University Park
Nottingham
NG7 2RD
T: 0115 951 5151
F: 0115 951 3666
E: undergraduate-enquiries@nottingham.ac.uk
W: www.nottingham.ac.uk
Institution code: N84

Nottingham Trent University
Burton Street
Nottingham
NG1 4BU
T: 0115 941 8418
E: marketing@ntu.ac.uk
W: www.ntu.ac.uk
Institution code: N91

University Centre Oldham
Oldham Business Centre
Cromwell Street
Oldham, Greater Manchester
OL1 1BB
T: 0800 085 0374
W: www.oldham.hud.ac.uk
Institution code: H60

Otley College
Otley
Ipswich, Suffolk
IP6 9EY
T: 01473 785543
F: 01473 785353
E: course.enquiries@otleycollege.ac.uk
W: www.otleycollege.ac.uk

University of Oxford
University Offices
Wellington Square
Oxford
OX1 2JD
T: 01865 279207
F: 01865 230708
E: undergraduate.ad@admin.ox.ac.uk
W: www.oxford.ac.uk
Institution code: O33

Oxford Brookes University
Gipsy Lane
Oxford
OX3 0BP
T: 01865 484848
F: 01865 483616
E: query@brookes.ac.uk
W: www.brookes.ac.uk
Institution code: O66

University of Paisley
Paisley Campus
High Street
Paisley, Renfrewshire
PA1 2BE
T: 0141 848 3000
F: 0141 887 0812
E: uni-direct@paisley.ac.uk
W: www.paisley.ac.uk
Institution code: P20

Park Lane College
Park Lane
Leeds
LS3 1AA
T: 0113 216 2000
F: 0113 216 2020
E: course.enquiry@parklanecoll.ac.uk
W: www.parklanecoll.ac.uk
Institution code: L21

Pembrokeshire College
Haverfordwest, Pembrokeshire
SA61 1SZ
T: 01437 765247
F: 01437 767279
E: info@pembrokeshire.ac.uk
W: www.pembrokeshire.ac.uk
Institution code: P35

Peninsula Medical School
Tamar Science Park
Plymouth
PL6 8BU
T: 01752 247444
F: 01752 517842
E: medadmissions@pms.ac.uk
W: www.pms.ac.uk
Institution code: P37

Penwith College
St Clare Street
Penzance, Cornwall
TR18 2SA
T: 01736 335000
F: 01736 335100
E: courses@penwith.ac.uk
W: www.penwith.ac.uk

Pershore Group of Colleges
Avonbank
Pershore, Worcestershire
WR10 3JP
T: 01386 552443
F: 01386 556528
W: www.pershore.ac.uk
Institution code: P50

Plumpton College
Ditchling Road
Lewes, East Sussex
BN7 8AE
T: 01273 890454
F: 01273 890071
E: enquiries@plumpton.ac.uk
W: www.plumpton.ac.uk

University of Plymouth
Drake Circus
Plymouth
PL4 8AA
T: 01752 600600
F: 01752 232141
E: admissions@plymouth.ac.uk
W: www.plymouth.ac.uk
Institution code: P60

City College Plymouth
Kings Road
Devonport
Plymouth
PL1 5QG
T: 01752 305300
F: 01752 305343
E: reception@cityplym.ac.uk
W: www.cityplym.ac.uk

University of Portsmouth
Winston Churchill Avenue
Portsmouth
PO1 2UP
T: 023 9284 8484
F: 023 9284 3082
E: admissions@port.ac.uk
W: www.port.ac.uk
Institution code: P80

Preston College
St Vincent's Road
Preston, Lancashire
PR2 9UR
T: 01772 225000
F: 01772 225002
E: marketing@preston.ac.uk
W: www.preston.ac.uk

Queen Margaret University, Edinburgh
Admissions Office
Clerwood Terrace
Edinburgh
EH12 8TS
T: 0131 317 3000
F: 0131 317 3248
E: admissions@qmu.ac.uk
W: www.qmu.ac.uk
Institution code: Q25

Queen Mary, University of London
Admissions Office
Queen's Building, Mile End Road
London
E1 4NS
T: 020 7882 5555
F: 020 7882 5500
E: admissions@qmul.ac.uk
W: www.qmul.ac.uk
Institution code: Q50

Queen's University Belfast
University Road
Belfast, Antrim
BT7 1NN
T: 028 9024 5133
F: 028 9024 7895
E: admissions@qub.ac.uk
W: www.qub.ac.uk
Institution code: Q75

University of Reading
PO Box 217
Reading
RG6 6AH
T: 0118 987 5123
F: 0118 378 8924
E: student.recruitment@reading.ac.uk
W: www.rdg.ac.uk
Institution code: R12

Reaseheath College
Reaseheath
Nantwich, Cheshire
CW5 6DF
T: 01270 625131
F: 01270 625665
E: reception@reaseheath.ac.uk
W: www.reaseheath.ac.uk

Richmond upon Thames College
Egerton Road
Twickenham, Middlesex
TW2 7SJ
T: 020 8607 8000
F: 020 8744 9738
E: courses@rutc.ac.uk.
W: www.rutc.ac.uk

Riverside College Halton
Kingsway
Widnes, Halton
WA8 7QQ
T: 0151 257 2020
F: 0151 420 2408
E: info@riverside.ac.uk
W: www.riverside.ac.uk
Institution Code: R30

obert Gordon University
erdeen
310 1FR
01224 262000
01224 263000
admissions@rgu.ac.uk
: www.rgu.ac.uk
stitution code: R36

odbaston College
nkridge
fford
19 5PH
01785 712209
01785 715701
rodenquiries@rodbaston.ac.uk
: www.rodbaston.ac.uk

oehampton University
smus House
ehampton Lane
ndon
15 5PU
020 8392 3232
020 8392 3470
enquiries@roehampton.ac.uk
www.roehampton.ac.uk
stitution code: R48

yal Agricultural College
ud Road
ncester, Gloucestershire
6JS
01285 652531
01285 650219
admissions@rac.ac.uk
www.rac.ac.uk
titution code: R54

yal Holloway, University of ndon
am, Surrey
20 0EX
01784 434455
01784 471381
dmissions@rhul.ac.uk
www.rhul.ac.uk
titution code: R72

yal Veterinary College, iversity of London
l College Street
don
0TU
20 7468 5000
20 7388 2342
egistry@rvc.ac.uk
www.rvc.ac.uk
titution code: R84

nshaw College
dale Road
on, Lancashire
5 3DQ
01772 622677
01772 642009
stask@runshaw.ac.uk
www.runshaw.ac.uk

University of St Andrews
St Katharine's West, The Scores
St Andrews, Fife
KY16 9AX
T: 01334 462150
F: 01334 463330
E: admissions@st-andrews.ac.uk
W: www.st-and.ac.uk
Institution code: S36

St George's, University of London
Cranmer Terrace
London
SW17 0RE
T: 020 8672 9944
F: 020 8725 0841
E: adm-med@sgul.ac.uk.
W: www.sgul.ac.uk
Institution code: S49

St Helens College
Brook Street
St Helens, Merseyside
WA10 1PZ
T: 01744 733766
F: 01744 623400
E: enquire@sthelens.ac.uk
W: www.sthelens.ac.uk
Institution code: S51

St Luke's Hospice (Education and Resource Centre)
Wilkes Education and Resource Centre
Little Common Lane, Off Abbey Lane
Sheffield
S11 9NE
T: 0114 236 9911
F: 0114 262 1242
E: j.roch@hospicesheffield.demon.co.uk
W: www.stlukeshospice.org.uk

College of St Mark & St John
Derriford Road
Plymouth
PL6 8BH
T: 01752 636890
F: 01752 636819
E: admissions@marjon.ac.uk
W: www.marjon.ac.uk
Institution code: M50

St Mary's University College, Twickenham
Waldegrave Road
Strawberry Hill
Middlesex
TW1 4SX
T: 020 8240 4000
F: 020 8240 4255
W: www.smuc.ac.uk
Institution code: S64

University of Salford
The Crescent
Salford, Greater Manchester
M5 4WT
T: 0161 295 5000
F: 0161 295 5999
E: course-enquiries@salford.ac.uk
W: www.salford.ac.uk
Institution code: S03

Salisbury College
Southampton Road
Salisbury, Wiltshire
SP1 2LW
T: 01722 344344
F: 01722 344345
E: enquiries@salisbury.ac.uk
W: www.salisbury.ac.uk
Institution code: S07

School of Pharmacy, University of London
29-39 Brunswick Square
London
WC1N 1AX
T: 020 7753 5800
F: 020 7753 5829
E: registry@pharmacy.ac.uk
W: www.pharmacy.ac.uk
Institution code: S12

Scottish Agricultural College
Recruitment and Admissions Office
Ayr
KA6 5HW
T: 01292 525359
F: 01292 525357
E: recruitment@sac.ac.uk
W: www.sac.ac.uk/learning
Institution code: S01

University of Sheffield
Western Bank
Sheffield
S10 2TN
T: 0114 222 2000
F: 0114 222 1415
E: ug.admissions@sheffield.ac.uk
W: www.sheffield.ac.uk
Institution code: S18

Sheffield College
PO Box 345
Sheffield
S2 2YY
T: 0114 260 2600
F: 0114 260 2601
W: www.sheffcol.ac.uk
Institution code: S22

Sheffield Hallam University
Howard Street
Sheffield
S1 1WB
T: 0114 225 5555
F: 0114 225 4023
E: admissions@shu.ac.uk
W: www.shu.ac.uk
Institution code: S21

Shipley College
Exhibition Road
Saltaire, Bradford
BD18 3JW
T: 01274 327222
F: 01274 327201
E: enquiries@shipley.ac.uk
W: www.shipley.ac.uk

Shrewsbury College of Arts and Technology

London Road
Shrewsbury, Shropshire
SY2 6PR
T: 01743 342342
F: 01743 342343
E: prospects@shrewsbury.ac.uk
W: www.shrewsbury.ac.uk
Institution code: S23

Shuttleworth College

Old Warden Park
Biggleswade, Bedfordshire
SG18 9EA
T: 01767 626222
F: 01767 626235
W: www.shuttleworth.ac.uk

Coleg Sir Gâr

Sandy Road
Llanelli, Carmarthenshire
SA15 4DN
T: 01554 748000
F: 01554 756088
E: admissions@colegsirgar.ac.uk
W: www.colegsirgar.ac.uk
Institution code: C22

Somerset College of Arts and Technology

Wellington Road
Taunton, Somerset
TA1 5AX
T: 01823 366331
F: 01823 366418
E: somerset@somerset.ac.uk
W: www.somerset.ac.uk
Institution code: S28

South Birmingham College

Cole Bank Road
Birmingham
B28 8ES
T: 0121 694 5000
F: 0121 694 5007
E: info@sbirmc.ac.uk
W: www.sbirmc.ac.uk
Institution code: S29

South Eastern Regional College

39 Castle Street
Lisburn, Antrim
BT27 4SU
T: 028 9267 7225
F: 028 9267 7291
W: www.serc.ac.uk

South West College

Circular Road
Dungannon, Tyrone
BT71 6BQ
T: 028 8772 2323
W: www.etcfhe.ac.uk

University of Southampton

Highfield
Southampton
SO17 1BJ
T: 023 8059 5000
F: 023 8059 3037
E: admissns@soton.ac.uk
W: www.soton.ac.uk
Institution code: S27

Southampton Solent University

East Park Terrace
Southampton
SO14 0YN
T: 023 8031 9000
F: 023 8022 2259
E: enquiries@solent.ac.uk
W: www.solent.ac.uk
Institution code: S30

Sparsholt College, Hampshire

Sparsholt
Winchester, Hampshire
SO21 2NF
T: 01962 776441
F: 01962 776587
E: enquiry@sparsholt.ac.uk
W: www.sparsholt.ac.uk
Institution code: S34

Staffordshire University

College Road
Stoke on Trent
ST4 2DE
T: 01782 294000
F: 01782 295704
E: admissions@staffs.ac.uk
W: www.staffs.ac.uk
Institution code: S72

Staffordshire University Regional Federation

Staffordshire University
College Road
Stoke on Trent
ST4 2DE
T: 01785 353517
F: 01782 292740
E: surf@staffs.ac.uk
W: www.surf.ac.uk
Institution code: S73

University of Stirling

Stirling
FK9 4LA
T: 01786 473171
F: 01786 466800
E: admissions@stir.ac.uk
W: www.stir.ac.uk
Institution code: S75

Stockton Riverside College

Harvard Avenue
Thornaby
Stockton
TS17 6FB
T: 01642 865400
F: 01642 865470
E: info@stockton.ac.uk
W: www.stockton.ac.uk

Stranmillis University College

Stranmillis Road
Belfast, Antrim
BT9 5DY
T: 028 9038 1271
F: 028 9066 4423
E: registry@stran.ac.uk
W: www.stran.ac.uk
Institution code: S79

Stratford upon Avon College

Alcester Road
Stratford upon Avon, Warwickshire
CV37 9QR
T: 01789 266245
F: 01789 267524
E: college@stratford.ac.uk
W: www.stratford.ac.uk
Institution code: S74

University of Strathclyde

16 Richmond Street
Glasgow
G1 1XQ
T: 0141 552 4400
F: 0141 552 0775
E: scls@mis.strath.ac.uk
W: www.strath.ac.uk
Institution code: S78

University Campus Suffolk

St Edmund House
Ipswich, Suffolk
IP4 1LZ
T: 01473 296451
F: 01473 343670
E: info@ucs.ac.uk
W: www.ucs.ac.uk
Institution code: S82

University of Sunderland

Edinburgh Building
Sunderland, Tyne and Wear
SR1 3SD
T: 0191 515 2000
F: 0191 515 3805
E: student-helpline@sunderland.ac.uk
W: www.sunderland.ac.uk
Institution code: S84

City of Sunderland College

Durham Road
Sunderland, Tyne and Wear
SR3 4AH
T: 0191 511 6060
F: 0191 564 0620
W: www.citysun.ac.uk
Institution code: C69

University of Surrey

Guildford, Surrey
GU2 7XH
T: 01483 300800
F: 01483 300803
E: admissions@surrey.ac.uk
W: www.surrey.ac.uk
Institution code: S85

University of Sussex

Falmer
Brighton
BN1 9RH
T: 01273 606755
F: 01273 678335
E: ug.admissions@sussex.ac.uk
W: www.sussex.ac.uk
Institution code: S90

ussex Downs College, Lewes ampus
ountfield Road
ewes, East Sussex
N7 2XH
: 01273 483188
: 01273 478561
: lewes@sussexdowns.ac.uk
: www.sussexdowns.ac.uk

utton Coldfield College
chfield Road
tton Coldfield, Birmingham
4 2NW
0121 355 5671
0121 355 0799
: infoc@sutcol.ac.uk
: www.sutcol.ac.uk
stitution code: S91

niversity of Wales, Swansea
gleton Park
ansea
2 8PP
01792 205678
01792 295874
admissions@swan.ac.uk
: www.swan.ac.uk
stitution code: S93

wansea College
och Road
ansea
2 9EB
0800 174084
01792 284074
admissions@swancoll.ac.uk
www.swancoll.ac.uk
stitution code: S94

wansea Institute of Higher ducation
unt Pleasant
ansea
6ED
01792 481000
01792 481085
enquiry@sihe.ac.uk
www.sihe.ac.uk
titution code: S96

windon College
ent Circus
ndon
1PT
01793 491591
01793 641794
admissions@swindon-college.ac.uk
www.swindon-college.ac.uk
titution code: S98

iversity of Teesside
dlesbrough
3BA
1642 218121
1642 342067
egistry@tees.ac.uk
www.tees.ac.uk
titution code: T20

Telford College of Arts and Technology
Haybridge Road
Wellington
Telford
TF1 2NP
T: 01952 642237
F: 01952 642263
E: studserv@tcat.ac.uk
W: www.tcat.ac.uk

Thames College of Professional Studies
35-41 Spring Road, Hall Green
Birmingham
B11 3EA
T: 0121 777 7050
F: 0121 777 8040
E: info@tcps.co.uk
W: www.tcps.co.uk

Thames Valley University
St Mary's Road
London
W5 5RF
T: 020 8579 5000
F: 020 8566 1353
E: learning.advice@tvu.ac.uk
W: www.tvu.ac.uk
Institution code: T40

Totton College
Water Lane
Totton
Southampton
SP40 3ZX
T: 023 8087 4874
F: 023 8087 4879
E: info@totton.ac.uk
W: www.totton.ac.uk
Institution code: T65

Trinity College Carmarthen
College Road
Carmarthen
SA31 3EP
T: 01267 676767
F: 01267 676766
E: registry@trinity-cm.ac.uk
W: www.trinity-cm.ac.uk
Institution code: T80

Truro College
College Road
Truro, Cornwall
TR1 3XX
T: 01872 267000
F: 01872 267100
E: enquiry@trurocollege.ac.uk
W: www.trurocollege.ac.uk
Institution code: T85

Tyne Metropolitan College
Embleton Avenue
Wallsend, Tyne and Wear
NE28 9NJ
T: 0191 229 5000
F: 0191 229 5301
E: enquiries@tynemet.ac.uk
W: www.tynemet.ac.uk
Institution code: T90

UCE Birmingham
Perry Barr
Birmingham
B42 2SU
T: 0121 331 5595
F: 0121 331 7994
E: prospectus@uce.ac.uk
W: www.uce.ac.uk
Institution code: C25

University of Ulster
Cromore Road
Coleraine, Londonderry
BT52 1SA
T: 028 7034 4141
F: 028 7032 4908
E: online@ulst.ac.uk
W: www.ulst.ac.uk
Institution code: U20

University College London, University of London
Gower Street
London
WC1E 6BT
T: 020 7679 2000
F: 020 7679 7920
W: www.ucl.ac.uk
Institution code: U80

Wakefield College
Margaret Street
Wakefield
WF1 2DH
T: 01924 789789
F: 01924 789191
E: courseinfo@wakcoll.ac.uk
W: www.wakcoll.ac.uk
Institution code: W08

Walsall College of Arts and Technology
St Paul's Street
Walsall
WS1 1XN
T: 01922 657000
F: 01922 657083
E: info@walsallcollege.ac.uk
W: www.walsallcollege.ac.uk
Institution code: W12

University of Warwick
Coventry
CV4 7AL
T: 024 7652 3523
F: 024 7646 1606
E: student.recruitment@warwick.ac.uk
W: www.warwick.ac.uk
Institution code: W20

Warwickshire College
Warwick New Road
Leamington Spa, Warwickshire
CV32 5JE
T: 01926 318000
F: 01926 318111
E: enquiries@warkscol.ac.uk
W: www.warkscol.ac.uk
Institution code: W25

West Kent College
Brook Street
Tonbridge, Kent
TN9 2PW
T: 01732 358101
F: 01732 771415
E: marketing@wkc.ac.uk
W: www.wkc.ac.uk

University of Westminster
Central Student Administration
115 New Cavendish Street
London
W1W 6UW
T: 020 7911 5000
F: 020 7911 5858
E: admissions@wmin.ac.uk
W: www.wmin.ac.uk
Institution code: W50

Weston College
Knightstone Road
Weston super Mare, North Somerset
BS23 2AL
T: 01934 411411
F: 01934 411410
E: enquiries@weston.ac.uk
W: www.weston.ac.uk
Institution code: W47

Wigan and Leigh College
PO Box 53
Wigan, Lancashire
WN1 1RS
T: 01942 761600
F: 01942 761533
E: admissions@wigan-leigh.ac.uk
W: www.wigan-leigh.ac.uk
Institution code: W67

Wiltshire College
Cocklebury Road
Chippenham, Wiltshire
SN15 3QD
T: 01249 464644
F: 01249 465271
E: info@wiltscoll.ac.uk
W: www.wiltscoll.ac.uk
Institution code: W74

University of Winchester
West Hill
Winchester, Hampshire
SO22 4NR
T: 01962 841515
F: 01962 842280
E: course.enquiries@winchester.ac.uk
W: www.winchester.ac.uk
Institution code: W76

Wirral Metropolitan College
Borough Road
Birkenhead, Merseyside
CH42 9QD
T: 0151 551 7777
F: 0151 551 7401
E: h.e.enquiries@wmc.ac.uk
W: www.wmc.ac.uk
Institution code: W73

University of Wolverhampton
Wulfruna Street
Wolverhampton
WV1 1SB
T: 01902 321000
F: 01902 322517
E: enquiries@wlv.ac.uk
W: www.wlv.ac.uk
Institution code: W75

City of Wolverhampton College
Paget Road
Wolverhampton
WV6 0DU
T: 01902 836000
F: 01902 423070
E: mail@wolvcoll.ac.uk
W: www.wolverhamptoncollege.ac.uk

University of Worcester
Henwick Grove
Worcester
WR2 6AJ
T: 01905 855000
F: 01905 855132
E: admissions@worc.ac.uk
W: www.worc.ac.uk
Institution code: W80

Worcester College of Technology
Deansway
Worcester
WR1 2JF
T: 01905 725555
F: 01905 28906
E: college@wortech.ac.uk
W: www.wortech.ac.uk
Institution code: W81

Writtle College
Writtle, Essex
CM1 3RR
T: 01245 424200
F: 01245 420456
E: info@writtle.ac.uk
W: www.writtle.ac.uk
Institution code: W85

Yeovil College
Mudford Road
Yeovil, Somerset
BA21 4DR
T: 01935 423921
F: 01935 429962
E: juc@yeovil-college.ac.uk
W: www.yeovil-college.ac.uk

University of York
Heslington
York
YO10 5DD
T: 01904 430004
F: 01904 433532
E: admission@york.ac.uk
W: www.york.ac.uk
Institution code: Y50

York College
Tadcaster Road
York
YO24 1UA
T: 01904 770200
F: 01904 770499
E: callcentre@yorkcollege.ac.uk
W: www.yorkcollege.ac.uk
Institution code: Y70

York St John University
Lord Mayor's Walk
York
YO31 7EX
T: 01904 624624
F: 01904 712512
E: admissions@yorksj.ac.uk
W: www.yorksj.ac.uk
Institution code: Y75

Index of Advertisers

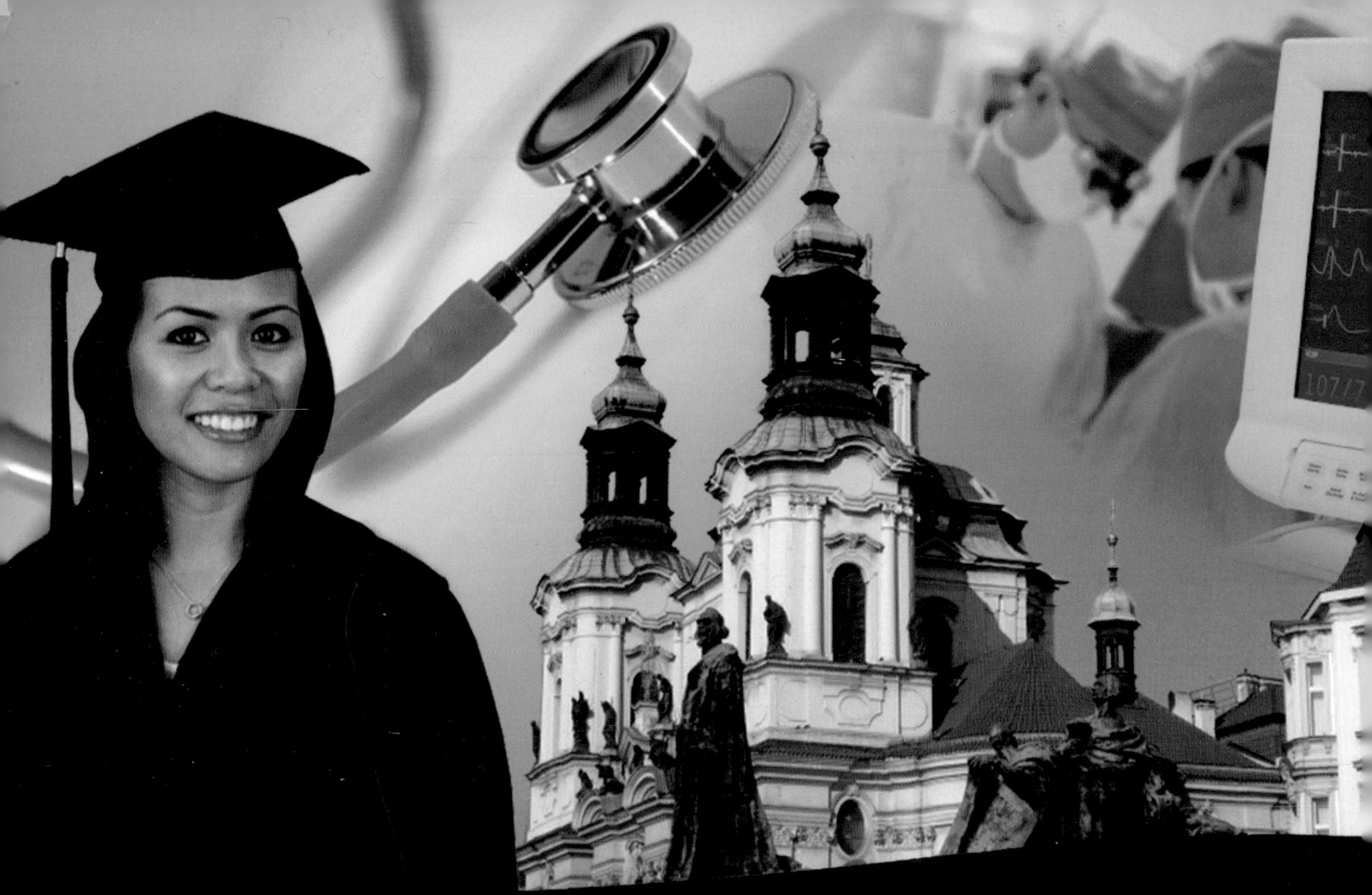

Medical/Dentistry Degrees

Courses are taught entirely in English at Charles University, the First Faculty in Prague.

For anyone determined to get into the medical or dental profession there is a established, fully GMC recognised route, to study for qualifications in one of world's oldest (est.1348) and finest universities (W.H.O world ranking).

Courses are taught entirely in English at Charles University, the First Faculty in Prague, the medical faculty in the heart of Prague. The Czech Medical Clearing System, C.M.U.C.A.S, has a representitive in Britain. Register directly now (with good A-Levels) for these courses recogr worldwide or for guaranteed reserved places after BAC (British Accreditation Council) accrec Foundation Year at The Abbey College in Malvern, Worcestershire, a British academic centre wit excellent reputation in this field.

REGISTER NOW FOR 2007/2008 ENTRY

UK C.M.U.C.A.S Office
253 Wells Road Malvern
Worcestershire WR14 4JF

Tel: 01684 892300 **Fax:** 01684 892757
Email: admin@cmucas.com
Website: www.cmucas.com